P9-CDX-558

Disrupted Dialogue

Disrupted Dialogue

Medical Ethics and the Collapse of Physician–Humanist Communication (1770–1980)

ROBERT M. VEATCH

Professor of Medical Ethics
Kennedy Institute of Ethics
Georgetown University
Washington, D.C.

OXFORD
UNIVERSITY PRESS
2005

OXFORD
UNIVERSITY PRESS

Oxford   New York
Auckland   Bangkok   Buenos Aires   Cape Town   Channai
Dar es Salaam   Delhi   Hong Kong   Istanbul   Karachi   Kolkata
Kuala Lumpur   Madrid   Melbourne   Mexico City   Mumbai
Nairobi   São Paulo   Shanghai   Taipei   Tokyo   Toronto

Copyright © 2005 by Oxford University Press, Inc.

Published by Oxford University Press, Inc.
198 Madison Avenue, New York, New York 10016
http://www.oup.com

Oxford is a registered trademark of Oxford University Press

Library of Congress Cataloging-in-Publication Data
Veatch, Robert M.
Disrupted dialogue : medical ethics and the collapse of physician-humanist
communication (1770–1980) / Robert M. Veatch.
p. ; cm.   Includes bibliographical references and index.
ISBN 0-19-516976-X
1. Medical ethics—England—History.   2. Medical ethics—Scotland—History.   3. Medical
ethics—United States—History.   4. Humanistic ethics—England—History.   5. Humanistic
ethics—Scotland—History.   6. Humanistic ethics—United States—History.   7. Physicians—
Professional ethics—England.   8. Physicians—Professional ethics—Scotland.   9. Physicians—
Professional ethics—United States.   I. Title.
[DNLM: 1. Ethics, Medical—history—England.   2. Ethics, Medical—history—Scotland.
3. Ethics, Medical—history—United States.   4. Humanism—England.   5. Humanism—Scotland.
6. Humanism—United States.   7. Physicians—England.   8. Physicians—Scotland.
9. Physicians—United States. W 50 V394da 2004]
R724.V414 2004
174.2'0941—dc22   2004050098

9 8 7 6 5 4 3 2 1

Printed in the United States of America
on acid-free paper

For Ann

Preface

I first conceived this book over a decade ago. The intense conversation of the past generation between humanists and physicians interested in ethics gave the appearance of something new. It was not the same old professionally articulated ethics of physician groups that had existed within medical professional associations for the past century. It was a true interdisciplinary conversation.

Exploring further back in the history of medical ethics, I discovered that, in another time and another place, physicians and humanists interested in ethics were also actively engaged with one another. As the research developed, I formulated and tested the hypothesis that the more isolated professional physician ethics in the English-speaking world of almost the past two centuries followed an earlier period of rich and close engagement among some of the leading humanists and physicians of the day. That period of engagement traces back to the 1770s and the Scottish Enlightenment, particularly in and around the University of Edinburgh. Soon after the end of the eighteenth century, however, something happened. The conversation stopped, and physicians became isolated, left to do their professional ethics on their own without the benefit of active engagement in the ethical debates in philosophy and religious ethics. Humanists retreated to do their ethics work without the benefit of those on the firing lines of clinical decision making.

That earlier, more engaged medical ethics had its foundation in the general religious and secular ethical controversies of the broader culture. Whether in the period of the ancient Hippocratic Oath, with its underlying Pythagorean and other Greek philosophical roots, or the common-sense empiricist tradition of the Scottish enlightenment, medical ethics at its best was an offshoot of important intellectual debates having nothing directly to do with medicine. My claim is that, beginning about 1800, the conversation that had fed medical ethics as a branch of important philosophical and religious debate ended, and physicians were left to work out their ethics on their own. Unfortunately, this occurred just when physicians ceased to receive a broad classical education that would prepare them to work at a sophisticated level on an ethic for their profession. Without the benefit of knowledge of the contemporary philosophical controversies of their day, physicians were reduced to reliance on simple slogans and to copying from their predecessors, who had written more sophisticated ethics for medical professionals. Those slogans and copies fit the philosophical conversations of an earlier era, but often were out of place in the philosophical climate decades later. The dialogue between humanists and physicians was interrupted until some 170 years had passed (that is, until about 1970), when it rather suddenly resumed in a major and dynamic way, giving rise to a new and more fitting ethic for a postmodern era of liberal political philosophy.

I will argue that during the late eighteenth century, the Age of Enlightenment, educated physicians were in rather close communication with humanists of the day. Professional physician ethics[1] was not developed as a separate entity in that period. Consequently, the Hippocratic Oath and the moral tradition surrounding it did not play a central role in the thought of late eighteenth century physicians. For some reason, however, physicians stopped talking to their colleagues in the humanities—at least about matters of medical ethics.

Is my impression correct and, if so, why did this happen? Before this volume is complete, we will need to explore the underlying culture and how it changed during these two centuries. We will examine the shifts in the scientific questions believed important for physicians to address, the changes in socioeconomic circumstances that influenced who chose to become physicians, and the social milieu that first forced physicians and humanists apart and then forced them back into the same conversation.

Let me suggest an initial typology—two ways of thinking about medical ethics. I will give them names for ease of reference. Think of these as ideal types. No one person is a pure case of either type. In no historical period was there a total manifestation of one or the other. These ways of thinking merely describe tendencies or patterns. In due course, I will try to show how cultural developments of the period account for these two patterns.

Some think of medical ethics as essentially the product of the profession of medicine. They tend to see the Hippocratic ethic as an all-purpose, timeless epitome of the proper ethic for the practice of medicine. I am going to call this the "Monro" approach to medical ethics and will explain why later. Others think of medical ethics as more closely associated with the broader underlying ethical milieu of a culture. For them, there are as many medical ethics as there are general ethics. This view derives the ethic for medicine from the general culture, not from the medical profession itself.

According to the latter view, every system of beliefs and values includes a general ethic from which an ethic for medicine can be derived. Talmudic ethics, for example, yields Talmudic medical ethics. Catholic moral theology yields Catholic medical ethics. Buddhist, Hindu, Confucian, and Marxist ethics yield their respective ethics for medicine. The ethic of liberal political philosophy is the most conspicuous and most important source of modern, secular medical ethics. Libertarianism, even Nazism, has implications for a medical ethic. This might imply ethical relativism—the notion that ethics are grounded merely in the beliefs and opinions of cultures. It need not require relativism, however. Those who hold these cultural views often believe that their view is the one universally correct position. Roman Catholic theologians, for example, believe that they are attempting to articulate the one correct, universal morality. Secular, liberal philosophers are not much different. They are trying to develop an ethical theory that they think is universal. Others have simply made an error. If these cultural views strive to be universal, they imply that there is really only one universally correct medical ethic, which is derived from the one universally correct system of ethical beliefs and values. For our purposes, it is not critical whether holders of this second view believe their religious or cultural tradition is the only correct one or whether they are more relativist. What is important is that they assume that an ethic for medicine is connected with and derives from a broader, more fundamental cultural or philosophical ethic.

Holders of this second view about the relation of medical ethics to the surrounding culture may see the Hippocratic ethic as one among competing systems of ethical thought derived from an underlying Greek mystery cult. Ludwig Edelstein (1967) tells us that it was probably Pythagorean in origin.[2]

Some who have refined this position, including Carrick (1985) and Temkin (1991), have said the Hippocratic ethic gained ascendency because it was compatible with early Christian ethical views. For example, the prohibition on abortion and condemnation of euthanasia were compatible with Christian views. However, Carol Mason Spicer and I have argued that the Hippocratic Oath is a manifestation of a peculiar ancient Greek mystery religion that was in many important ways at odds with the ethics of ancient Jewish and Christian culture (Veatch and Mason, 1987).

I shall call this second view, which sees medical ethics as derived from underlying cultural ethics, the "Gregory" view. Although the names I give these views, "Monro" and "Gregory," refer to individuals, I use them to refer to a much broader cultural phenomenon—whether the ethics of physicians is isolated from a broader cultural ethic (the Monro view) or an integrated part of that broader ethic (the

Gregory position). The project of this book is to distinguish these two views: the Gregory view is associated with the culture of the height of the Enlightenment and the Monro view with that of a more isolated group of medical scientists who are much less in communication with their humanist colleagues on matters of medical ethics.

The project undertaken in this volume is a complex one. It is a project in history—intellectual history, cultural history, political history, and the history of a number of nations, including Scotland and England within Britain, the United States, New Zealand, and Canada. This poses a problem. No one can be considered a specialist in philosophical and religious ethics, the history of ethics, the history of medicine, and cultural and national histories of all of these nations. Historians will justifiably complain that an ethicist who undertakes this project will be trespassing on the historian's turf. My training in the history of religions provides me with just enough exposure to admire the skills of formally trained historians, but not enough to claim such expertise myself. But this project is one that I am convinced needs to be done. If a professional medical historian were to undertake it, he or she would perhaps lack background in not only some of the national and cultural traditions explored but also the theories of philosophical or religious ethics. I undertake this as one committed to the value and importance of interdisciplinary research. I look forward to additions and revisions of what is said here from those who bring another mix of disciplinary skills to the subject.

I also need to add a note on method. I have never considered myself a proponent of the "great men" theories of history. That applies as well to the revolution in medical ethics. In the words of Joseph Ellis in his Pulitzer Prize–winning account of the "founding brothers" of the other American revolution, "all the heroic portraits of the great men were romantic distortions" (Ellis, 2000, p. 217). I am deeply committed to the view that an entire people shape a culture, not merely the handful who often command the pages of history books. Moreover, cultural developments are shaped not merely by the history of ideas, but also by the economic, sociological, and political developments of the time. But in writing this history I find myself following the same pattern that I would normally criticize, beginning by writing about a few men (and I mean males, almost exclusively) who illustrate the cultural patterns that I attribute to the generations whose stories are being told. Rather apologetically, I can offer two lines of defense.

First, as can be seen in Chapter 1, I use individuals as ideal types, individuals who symbolize their type in a broader culture, not pretending that they are unique but merely suggesting they are archetypes. Second, I intentionally seek out the best exemplars of their types. To make the claim that physicians writing ethics for over a century and a half in exile from the philosophical world were out of communication, I need to sustain it not merely with regard to the ordinary journeymen practitioners. They have always been and always will be something less than great philosopher healers. Rather, the claim needs to be defended with regard to the best and the brightest—those who have led the thinking of their era in medicine. By examining in depth the philosophical and ethical knowledge and interests, or lack thereof, of a few of the leaders, I hope to show that they represent the style and abilities of their group. It is this elite about whom we have extensive information. If they fail to manifest significant interest in the humanities, then their less distinguished colleagues are likely to as well.

After sketching the philosophical interests of these figures, I will turn to the underlying socioeconomic and political developments of the time—the shift in social class of physicians, the explosion of knowledge that would dramatically change the structure of medical education, and eventually the political revolution that would force physicians and humanists to resume their interaction. We will see that events as diverse as the invention of the ventilator and the Vietnam war played key roles. It was not that a few individual physicians developed by accident a fascination with the ethics of the humanists; it was that events of the broader culture pushed physicians very hard—first to turn away from ethics and then, nearly two centuries later, back towards it.

The book traces this pattern in Scotland in Part I before turning in Part II to England and in Part III to the United States and then, more briefly, New Zealand and Nova Scotia. In Part IV we move forward to the second half of the twentieth century to document a reconvergence. Throughout, the question will be, why did physicians and humanists quit talking to each other? Why was their dialogue disrupted, and what led them back together again over the past generation? We shall see that medical ethics does not evolve in isolation. It is part of a much more complex set of cultural factors. These cultural factors first disrupt the dialogue and then press the participants back into it.

Washington, DC   R.M.V.

Acknowledgments

The research for this volume took me and some very able research assistants to some of the great medical libraries of the English-speaking world, to the University of Edinburgh in Scotland, the Wellcome Institute in England, the University of Otago in New Zealand, and Dalhousie University in Nova Scotia, as well as many of the richest resources in the United States: the National Library of Medicine in Bethesda, the Library of Congress, Harvard's Countway Library, Philadelphia's resources at the College of Physicians, the Library Company, and the University of Pennsylvania. These supplemented the three wonderful resources at Georgetown University: the main campus Lauinger Library, the medical campus Dahlgren Library, and particularly the Kennedy Institute's own National Reference Center for Bioethics Literature. My travels were made possible by a sabbatical leave from the Kennedy Institute in 1996, which was supplemented by travel for research purposes within the United States and Canada since that time.

At the University of Edinburgh, I had the privilege of being appointed a fellow of the Institute for Advanced Studies in the Humanities. There I had the special joy of using the office whose previous occupant had been none other than Prince Phillip, who is the patron of the Scots at War Trust project of the Institute. Peter Jones, who at the time was the Center's director, was a delightful and gracious host, both at the Institute and in his home. Anthea Taylor, Assistant to the Director, arranged an apartment in the eighteenth century "New Town" row house of the university's president and provided countless bits of intellectual and logistic support. It was she who taught us that the Veitch ancestral home at Dawyck-on-the-Tweed was now a glorious part of the Edinburgh Royal Botanic Garden. In the university library's rare book collection, Dr. Michael Barfoot was not only a resourceful library professional, he also proved to be one of the world's experts on the history of Scottish medicine. I also had valuable help from Mr. A. T. Wilson, and, in the Registry Office, Mr. S. Stupart, Senior Administrative Officer, and Mrs. E. A. Carter, Administrative Secretary.

I did the research for the chapters on England while in residence at the Wellcome Institute for the History of Medicine in London, where the best library on the history of medicine in the English-speaking world is located. The librarians there helped me through a treasure of priceless original editions and obscure searches. I was resident in the Institute's Academic Unit (which has now become the Wellcome Trust Centre for the History of Medicine at University College London). I want to thank Sally Bragg, who was the administrator of the Academic Unit. The professional colleagues of the Academic Unit, particularly William Bynum, Vivian Nutten, Christopher Lawrence, and the late Roy Porter, were generous with their time and helpful in their comments on both the British and the New Zealand material.

I did much of the research for the developments in the United States from my office at the Kennedy Institute of Ethics, where we are blessed with the most wonderful staff of bioethics librarians in the world. The National Reference Center for Bioethics Literature, which is the library of the Kennedy Institute, is the library of record for American bioethics. That produces the remarkable fringe benefit for those working at the Institute of opening access to a group of a dozen or so of the most knowledgeable and dedicated library professionals. Their competence and dedication are reflected throughout this volume. I am also grateful to my professorial colleagues at the Institute for countless suggestions and for review of various parts of the draft manuscript. Several research assistants have worked with me on this project, including Brendan Howe, Nicholas Crosson, and Alexander Curtis. Nick was particularly helpful for the research in Philadelphia, especially at the College of Physicians. Julie Eddinger, Sally Schofield, and Linda Powell have been helpful in various ways in administrative and executive functions.

In Dunedin, New Zealand, I was received graciously at the Bioethics Research Centre. Alastair Campbell, who was then its director, was most generous, and Grant Gillett provided helpful comments on my work. I am also grateful to the staff of the medical library, particularly Donald Jameison, who was its head, and Mignon Pickwell, who was Senior Librarian and is presently librarian of the science library, for access to its fine resources on the history of New Zealand medicine and its Monro Collection. That is the library of the three generations of Monros who were chairs of anatomy at the University of Edinburgh during the period I was studying. I had wonderful help from Dr. Douglass Taylor, the retired Associate Dean of the Medical School, who was personally responsible for the Monro Collection and very knowledgeable about Scottish and New Zealand medical school history. I also got important help from Dr. Barbara Brookes, Senior Lecturer in the history of medicine, and from Suzanne Flemming in the office of the Dean of the Faculty of Medicine, who made the volumes of the minutes of the medical faculty meetings back to 1891 available to me.

On my all-too-brief visit to Nova Scotia, I was hosted graciously by Dr. Nuala Kenny, the former head of Pediatrics at Dalhousie and currently the chair of the Department of Bioethics. I also had stimulating conversations with several of the bioethicists in her program and with Dr. Jock Murray, the former dean of the medical school and resident historian on matters of medical ethics. Dilly MacFarlane, the Executive Director of the Dalhousie Medical Alumni Association was unusually generous and helpful, as were the personnel of the dean's office who assisted in providing documents. I am also grateful to the personnel of the Pictou County Genealogy and Heritage Society, administrators of the Hector Exhibit Centre and McCulloch House Museum, in Pictou, Nova Scotia.

In addition to these wonderful colleagues in Scotland, England, the United States, New Zealand, and Canada who helped me on specific pieces of this project, two long-term friends and colleagues deserve special mention as people who have led the way in scholarship, placing Gregory, Percival, and Rush back on the map of pioneers in professional medical ethics. Robert B. Baker, professor of philosophy at Union College, has stimulated scholarship on eighteenth and nineteenth century medical ethics in the English-speaking world, and Laurence McCullough, professor at Baylor College of Medicine, has produced the definitive study of John Gregory as well as the critical editions of Gregory's medical ethics. It is only with that background that I could go on to ask why the close communication between medicine and the humanities that existed at the end of the eighteenth century disappeared in the decades that followed.

In addition to all these wonderful colleagues at libraries and academic institutions throughout the world, I have had the great pleasure for over 20 years of working with Jeffrey House at Oxford University Press. He has shown unusual interest in this project, guiding it through several drafts and taking his skilled pen to the manuscript to show what a first-rate professional editor can do to a manuscript to improve on the author's sometimes excessive detail and unclear expressions. Without his commitment to this project, it never would have been completed.

All the material contained in this volume was prepared for this project and, with the exception of one chapter, has not been published previously. Chapter 8, which deals with the communication between physicians and religious ethicists in the United States, was the first research I did for this project. When invited to present a paper at the December 1990 Wellcome Institute symposium, "The Codification of Medical Morality," I agreed with the provision that I could present this one aspect of my research at that meeting and eventually incorporate it into the present manuscript. Chapter 8 constitutes a revised version of that paper.

It is apparent that, whatever one thinks of the thesis about the isolation of physician ethics, this has turned into a dream project for providing justifications for traveling to some of the most exciting, beautiful, and historical places in the English-speaking world and meeting a large group of wonderful and generous colleagues who have become friends. Finally, I am grateful to my wife, Ann, who has traveled with me to all of these places, tolerated the pursuit of some strange and time-consuming questions, and made it all worthwhile. When we first met, almost 50 years ago, she was an inspiration to me. She is still today.

Finally, a word needs to be said about the quotations from the historical material cited in this volume. The spelling and punctuation conventions of the eighteenth century are sometimes quite different from those of our time. I have generally retained all spellings and punctuation exactly as in the original in all direct quotations. This will often reveal commas occurring at places at which the twenty-first century reader is unaccustomed. Spellings and capitalization are different and sometimes inconsistent even within paragraphs. John Gregory, for instance, spells the word for truthful speech both as *candour* and *candor*. I have made one accommodation to the twenty-first century eye, systematically replacing the eighteenth century hard *s*, which is set with a type character *f* and appears to the twenty-first century reader much like an "f," with the standard letter "s."

Washington, DC   R.M.V.

Contents

I

SCOTLAND

1

MEDICAL ETHICS IN THE SCOTTISH ENLIGHTENMENT

Some who are interested in medical ethics in the twenty-first century might assume that, since the days of ancient Greece, the Hippocratic Oath and its ethic have always been at the center of Western medical ethics. That would be a mistake.

Aside from the brief and ambiguous flirtation with Hippocratic/Greek medical ethics in the Middle Ages, there is precious little surviving evidence of the Hippocratic influence in late medieval and early modern medical ethics in the Western world, at least in the English-speaking part of that world. By the seventeenth and eighteenth centuries surely the Hippocratic Oath was known, but I cannot find evidence that it played any significant role in the thought of the physicians, theologians, or philosophers of the time in the English-speaking world.[1] The ethics for medicine, like the ethics of any other aspect of life, was derived from the dominant religious and philosophical systems of the day. An ethic for medicine, as we shall see dramatically in Chapter 8, was crafted by theologians following the methods, organizational scheme, and content of the broader religious system. Among Catholic moralists, for example, comments on ethics, including ethics in a medical context, were organized according to the Ten Commandments or, occasionally, the classical virtues. The thought that theologians or talmudic scholars would abandon their underlying religious ethical system and turn to what they would have regarded as an obscure Greek medical cult for moral guidance is implausible. The same can be said for secular thought on medical ethics. For those in the culture of liberal political philosophy, the ideas that shaped their understanding of the nature of the world and laid the foundation of ethical claims, not an ancient, pagan cultic oath, would provide the basis for resolving a medical ethical problem.

The starting point for analyzing modern medical ethics in the English-speaking world is Scotland and, to a lesser extent England, in the eighteenth century. Part I examines the interactions between the physicians interested in medical ethics during the eighteenth-century Scottish Enlightenment and the theologians and philosophers who dominated the emergence of Enlightenment cultural thought. Part II covers similar ground in England.

BACKGROUND OF THE SCOTTISH ENLIGHTENMENT

The Enlightenment during the second half of the eighteenth century produced remarkable cultural changes that were stimulated by social and economic developments. Scholars trace this to the legal and educational system, the universities, and bold innovations in the church.[2] Building on the empiricism of Newton and Locke, the Calvinist religious reform of John Knox, and rapidly developing forces in economics and social science, the synergism of cultural developments in science, philosophy, medicine, the social sciences, literature, and art was, to use a term that captured the imagination of the period, electric.

Humankind, many believed, was finally getting close to catching a glimpse of God's blueprint, of the underlying structure of "natural laws" that humans had but to uncover to gain a full comprehension of the mechanics of the universe. These "laws," or universal truths, were not the domain of a single discipline but rather held true for all avenues of human endeavor. Liberal optimism was fueled by the belief that humanity was irreversibly set on an upwardly spiraling path of achievement. Georg Hegel's philosophy of history, particularly his dialectical method of thinking (thesis, antithesis, synthesis), was the first comprehensive theory to focus on these impersonal forces as a sort of preordained route of progress (Olson and Groom 1991, p. 27).

Medicine saw the founding of the Edinburgh medical faculty. Modern medical science could draw on leaders such as David Gregory in mathematics (1661–1708); James Hutton (1726–97) in geology; Joseph Black (1728–99) in chemistry; James Watt (1736–1819) in engineering; and, most critically for our purposes, the three Alexander Monros—Primus (1697–1767), Secundus (1733–1817), and Tertius (1773–1859)—William Cullen (1710–90), and John (1724–73) and James (1753–1821) Gregory in medicine. In philosophy the "common-sense" and "moral-sense" theories in epistemology and ethics emerged from such figures as Francis Hutcheson (1694–1746), Thomas Reid (1710–96), David Hume (1711–76), George Campbell (1719–96), James Beattie (1735–1803), and Dugald Stewart

(1753–1828). Hume's colleague and friend, Adam Smith (1723–90), along with William Robertson (1721–93), Adam Ferguson (1723–1816), and John Millar (1735–1801), provided leadership in economics and the social sciences. Allan Ramsay (1686–1758), James Thomson (1700–48), and Robert Ferguson (1750–74) contributed to literature, Robert Burns (1759–96) to poetry, and Tobias Smollett (1721–71) to the novel. Art and architecture saw such figures as Allan Ramsay, Jr. (1713–84), Henry Raeburn (1796–1823), David Allen (1744–96), Alexander and Patrick Nasmyth (1758–1840 and 1787–1831), and Gavin Hamilton (1730–97).[3] One might marvel that all of this creativity was going on at once, but something in the culture led to a cross-fertilization that permitted this innovation. The division of knowledge into distinct, technical disciplines had not yet occurred. These figures considered the universe of knowledge their domain.

The Age of Enlightenment held the seeds of its own downfall, however. The openness that had set the stage for innovation was ultimately replaced by increased positivism and scientific specialization as "experts" in various fields sought to define their boundaries of preeminence. The "philosophical century" (ca. 1750 to ca. 1850) was followed by the "scientific century." The impact of the Industrial Revolution was felt throughout society. Rather than trying to uncover God's or Nature's design, people then believed that the application of scientific method would allow humanity to carve out its own destiny. In particular it was hoped that humankind would finally be able to defeat its triple nemesis of famine, pestilence, and war. Certainly, the impact of the agrarian and industrial revolutions made considerable inroads against famine in the "civilized world." In the late nineteenth century, medicine was finally approaching the point where its practitioners were doing more good than harm to their patients. Knowledge increased at such a rate that the Enlightenment ideal of mastering the universe of knowledge would soon no longer be attainable. The grand intellectual with knowledge of both the sciences and the humanities was to be succeeded by more specialized, technical experts. Normative issues were pushed to the sidelines. This shift occurred for two reasons: first, the pace of development left little room for study in fields outside one's own area of specialization, and second, if humans were to be the masters of their own destiny, then utopian moralizing had to give way to hard-nosed realism.

CAMARADERIE BETWEEN MEDICINE
AND THE HUMANITIES

This book is concerned with the interplay between humanists and physicians and the later collapse of communication between them. It is from that remarkably close and fruitful interchange that modern medical ethics took it roots. The common-sense and moral-sense theories of Hutcheson, Hume, Smith, Reid, and Beattie stimulated the development of modern psychology and especially the close links between psychology and moral philosophy (Christie 1981). (The professorships in moral philosophy in eighteenth-century Scottish universities often carried the title "professor of mental and moral philosophy," a pattern that, as we shall see in Chapter 9, carries over to the development of university education in New Zealand in the nineteenth century.)

The Age of Enlightenment was an age in which physicians and humanists were talking to each other. To know the ethic of medicine, one conversed with the proponents of the ethical system of the day and then applied that system to medicine. For eighteenth century Britain that meant that one would consult Kant, Bentham, and especially the Scottish moralists such as Hutcheson (1728), Reid (1764), Hume (1739–40, 1751), and Adam Smith (1759).

The first and most important medical faculty of the Scottish Enlightenment was at the University of Edinburgh. Founded in 1726, this faculty was the source of a great deal of modern medical science (Lawrence 1985, 1988a, 1988b; Rosner 1991; Dow 1988). In the early eighteenth century, Scottish medicine was heavily under the influence of scholars at the University of Leyden. Every one of the initial faculty of medicine at Edinburgh studied under the great Hermann Boerhaave (1669–1738), professor of anatomy at Leyden.

Two members of the Edinburgh faculty are particularly critical in understanding the dialogue between physicians and humanists and how that dialogue became disrupted. The first was John Gregory (1724–73), professor of physic (medicine) at the University of Edinburgh from 1766 until his death in 1773. He published *Lectures on the Duties and Qualifications of a Physician* in 1772, which is based on his medical school lectures. Gregory was clearly in conversation with leading philosophical and theological figures of his day. A widely read intellectual, he produced for physicians a moral theory relying on *common sense* (a technical term in Scottish philosophy) with appeals to sympathy and the other buzzwords of the day (see Baker 1993, p. 94). The position of professor of medicine was occupied in succession by John Gregory (1766–73), William Cullen (1773–1790), and Gregory's son, James (1790–1821). Cullen and James Gregory, like John, had broad humanities interests that supplemented their teaching of medicine. Together they represent a rich ethical tradition in medicine that was in conversation with the humanities of the day. The project of this volume is to investigate why that culture dictated that elite physicians were very much a part of that conversation.

The other key member of the Edinburgh medical faculty was the first of three generations of Alexander Monros, who all held the chair as professor of anatomy. They are customarily referred to as Primus (from 1720 to 1759), Secundus (from 1759 to 1798), and Tertius (from 1798 to 1846). Together they dominated anatomy teaching at Edinburgh for 126 years. They shared a personal medical library that grew to approximately 600 volumes. That library ended up at The University of

Otago in Dunedin, New Zealand (Taylor 1979). It is clear from its contents that these scholars were educated in the classics. The existing library contains many works in Greek and Latin; however, all but six are what we would call works in medical science, for example, Monro Primus's *The Anatomy of the Human Bones*. Although Monro Primus was older than John Gregory, he represents the model for the beginning of isolation of physicians from the humanities. He is the precursor of the physician of the nineteenth century, when medicine emerged as a science with vast knowledge to be transmitted. He and his successors represent the beginning of the age of specialization.

Gregory and *Monro* are symbols of two very different cultural trends. They are alternative models (or ideal types) for linking medicine with the humanities at the end of the eighteenth century. The Gregories, especially John (the father), derived an ethic for medicine from the ethic of the Scottish Enlightenment. They were in conversation with the humanists of the day, humanists with serious interest in medicine. The Monros were serious medical scholars vaguely aware that medicine needs a humanistic or ethical dimension. They also assumed that this ethical orientation had something to do with Hippocrates, but they were not seriously involved in humanities. They were scientists of medicine.

In the pages that follow, I trace the thought of one group in medical ethics (including Gregory, Percival, and the Edinburgh-trained American physician/philosopher, Benjamin Rush) who were in conversation with the philosophical and religious ethics of their time. I will also show how that close relation collapses as medicine distances itself from the humanities. That humanities connection was gradually replaced with a gaze toward Hippocrates, a figure at best poorly understood, but romanticized as an ancient hero turned into a timeless ethicist. The task will be to understand the scientific, sociological, political, and economic forces that generated this shift.

John Gregory: The Beginnings of Anglo-American Professional Medical Ethics

While many people played important roles in developing the distinctive medical ethics of the period, John Gregory (1724–73), professor of the practice of medicine, first at Aberdeen (1754–64) and then at Edinburgh (1766–73), is certainly the culmination and most important of such figures.[4] He incorporated a series of lectures into the beginning of his course that were published from student notes (Gregory 1770). Students were known for taking detailed notes in shorthand and preparing them for distribution (Gregory 1770, p. iii). Unfortunately, Gregory had not approved the manuscript. When he saw what emerged, he prepared a revised text, which he published in 1772 as *Lectures on the Duties and Qualifications of a Physician*.[5]

Gregory's Background

John Gregory come from a remarkable Scottish family of mathematicians, clergy, philosophers, astronomers, and physicians in which several of these talents were often displayed in the same person. His great-great-grandfather, David Anderson, constructed the spire of St. Nicholas of Finyhaugh. The family is described as having "hereditary mathematical genius" (Clerke 1890, p. 98). Anderson's daughter, Janet, married Rev. John Gregory (d. 1653), who was a sufficiently prominent activist to be imprisoned by Covenanters. Their son, James (1638–1675), married the daughter of George Jameson, a rather well-known painter, and a remarkable family lineage was under way. With only modest effort, I was able to identify over the next five generations six physicians (all of whom were professors of medicine), four clergy, four mathematicians, a professor of modern language, a botanist, a metaphysician, two moral philosophers, a chemist, and an astronomer, plus assorted spouses. Had the women of that era been accepted in academic and intellectual careers, one wonders what more would have emerged from this family. The male members included the holder of the first exclusively mathematical professorship at Edinburgh, the inventor of the Gregorian telescope, the holder of the Savilian Professorship at Oxford, and the dean of Christ Church, Oxford. Two of these, James (1638–1675—John's grandfather) and David (1661–1708—related to John through his great-grandfather), were professors at Edinburgh and among the first to support Newtonianism (Wood 1993, p. 7). The professors of medicine included John Gregory's father, half-brother, a son, and two of his grandchildren. Although passing professorships from father to son was common during this period, the Gregories (and, as we shall see a bit later, the Monros and several other families of the medical faculties of Scotland's medical schools) were particularly skilled practitioners of the craft.

John Gregory's father, James (d. 1731), was Professor of Medicine at King's College, Aberdeen, a position he passed on to his older son, also named James (1707–55). John's maternal grandfather was principal of King's, making the family extremely influential in the college. John Gregory, the youngest son of the first James to teach medicine, was educated at Aberdeen—first in grammar school, then at King's College—and received the support of broad classical learning at home. In 1741, at age 17, he went to Edinburgh to study medicine and then studied in Leyden in 1745–46. In his absence at Aberdeen in 1746, a medical degree was conferred on him—a not uncommon practice of the time. Perhaps it was a device to lure him to the academic environment of his father and older brother. On June 3, 1746, he was given an appointment not as professor of medicine, a position already occupied by his older half-brother, but as regent, or what was sometimes called professor of philosophy.

The regency system, in which a teacher would take students through the whole course from the first to the fourth year, was still in place in Aberdeen at both King's and Marischal Colleges, the last two Scottish universities to use the system.[6] Over these years, Gregory would have taught mathematics, logic, metaphysics, and natural and moral philosophy (Wood 1993, p. 34).[7] These years were formative for Gregory in building a career irretrievably linking interests in medicine and philosophy.

The eighteenth century was a period of generalists. It was not at all uncommon for professors to move from one subject to the next. This was the norm not only within medicine (where, for example, at Edinburgh professors moved from chemistry to materia medica to the practice of medicine [Rosner 1991]) but across what a twenty-first-century academic would consider widely disparate fields. Adam Ferguson was professor of mathematics at Edinburgh and also professor of natural philosophy (what we would call natural science) before shifting to a professorship in moral philosophy (Espinasse, 1889). His successor in the moral philosophy chair, Dugald Stewart, had also previously held the chair in mathematics (Veitch 1858). Their predecessor, Sir John Pringle, was a distinguished physician who became president of the Royal Society after holding a professorship in moral philosophy (Payne 1896). Thus when John Gregory began his professorial career, it was common for professors teaching a group of students for several years in the regency system to develop a wide-ranging set of experiences that often led them to eventually assume more specialized professorships in more than one subject over the course of their careers.

We see here an Enlightenment pattern—an intelligentsia being broadly and classically educated without concern about the disciplinary boundaries separating the sciences from the humanities. These remarkable gentlemen—for they were, given the role expectations of the day, almost exclusively males—came from remarkable families that introduced classical literature, religious and philosophical studies, as well as mathematics and natural philosophy very early in life. Gregory's interests in and proficiency at natural science, medicine, metaphysics, and moral philosophy were impressive but not unique in this period.

In 1749, Gregory resigned his regency in Aberdeen to devote himself to his medical practice. With an older brother who had an established practice and reputation, John felt compelled in 1754 to move to London, where he immediately established ties with the cultural elite[8] and was elected fellow of the Royal Society. However, when his brother died, he was called back to Aberdeen to succeed him as the professor of medicine.

Gregory's Relation to Scottish Common-Sense Moral Philosophy

Gregory's philosophical thought was very much shaped during this period. Aberdeen was a center of common-sense philosophy, an approach reflected by Gregory throughout his writings.

MAIN TENETS AND FIGURES. Common-sense theory is a reaction to, and an attack on, philosophical paradox and skepticism. Thomas Reid describes these as "metaphysical lunacy" (Reid 1997, p. 68). Philosophers have variously understood common sense as the shared beliefs of rational beings that are based in intuition (intuitive, self-evident truths), "that constitution of human nature without which all the business of the world would immediately cease" (Stewart 1858, p. 307), and as that which is opposed to paradox. Proponents of this theory consider those skeptical or paradoxical theories that contradict or defy common sense to be nonsensical, absurd, and ridiculous. For instance, Thomas Reid argued that a belief in the existence of an external object is borne of the perception of the object itself and is not a separate, substituted "idea" within the mind. To posit that such "ideas" exist is, in his view, repugnant to common sense. Thus, the common-sense philosophers diverge from sceptics like Hume, whose conclusions, they argue, tend toward the absurd. Proponents of the Scottish school of common sense include Aberdeen professors Alexander Gerard, Thomas Reid (1997, p. 19), and James Beattie ("common Sense is the ultimate Judge of all reasoning" (cited in Wood 1993, p. 120), as well as Reid's student, Dugald Stewart.

GREGORY'S CLOSE CONNECTION TO SCOTTISH PHILOSOPHY. William Smellie, Gregory's contemporary and biographer, says of him, "In the company of literary men, his conversation flowed with ease; and on whatever subject, he delivered his sentiments without affectation or reserve" (1800, p. 117). Gregory's exposure to the figures of the philosophy of the Scottish Enlightenment was certainly intimate.

In addition to his Aberdeen exposure, he continued interaction with the great philosophical figures of the day when he was in Edinburgh.[9] Gregory's knowledge of contemporaneous key figures during his period of teaching of philosophy seems clear. He undoubtedly would have known the early work of Hume, whose initial effort, the *Treatise on Human Nature*, appeared in 1739, and of Francis Hutcheson, who is often credited with being the founder of the moral-sense tradition (Hutcheson 1728). Hutcheson, a precursor to Hume, taught moral philosophy at Glasgow from 1729 until his death in 1746. Gregory may have been familiar with Adam Smith, the Glasgow philosopher–economist famous for his *Wealth of Nations* (1776); Smith's most important work in moral philosophy, *The Theory of Moral Sentiments*, did not appear until 1759.

There is evidence that other philosophical figures probably played a more central role in Gregory's early philosophical life. A manuscript written in 1743 entitled "A proposall for a medicall society" shows that early in his career he had an intimate knowledge of Bacon's writings (Wood 1993, p. 31), an influence that remains apparent in his reading list during his years teaching at King's College and in the *Lectures on the Duties and Qualifications of a Physician* (1772). He left a book list prepared in 1748 that provides some idea of the books Gregory used or may have drawn upon for his teaching. In addition to figures in mathematics (including Newton, Cheyne, Bernoulli, Descartes, and Maclaurin) and natural philosophy (including Descartes, Galileo, and Boyle), the list named Descartes's *Opuscula Posthuma*, Montesquieu's *Considérations sur les causes de la grandeur et de la décadence des Romains* and *L'Esprit des lois*, and DeVries's *Metaphysica* (Wood 1993, pp. 31, 33–34). For our purposes it is perhaps most important that the list included Gerschom Carmichael's *Breviuscula Introductio ad Logicam*. Carmichael was Francis Hutcheson's predecessor in the professorship of moral philosophy and was considered by some to be the real founder of the common-sense school of Scottish moral philosophy (Wood 1993, p. 31). According to Paul Wood, whose recent study of the Aberdeen academic community in the eighteenth century provides the best available documentation of this community's teaching, Gregory's philosophy courses were in all likelihood rooted in the neoscholastic tradition, probably discussing Descartes and Locke, and likely relied on Gregory's knowledge of Bacon to attack the sterility of scholastic metaphysics and logic. This was a common pattern elsewhere in Scotland (Wood 1993, p. 34). Gregory's intellectual heritage is revealed in the explicit use he made of many of the key figures of British philosophy and especially the Scottish commonsense philosophers.

Gregory's *Lectures on the Duties and Obligations*, particularly the lectures on method, are grounded in the work of Bacon, Newton, and Boyle (Gregory 1772, p. 107; Smellie 1800, p. 21),[10] all precursors to British empiricism who were well known to Gregory from his Aberdeen days. *A Comparative View of the State and Faculties of Man with Those of the Animal World* was first presented as a series of six lectures to the Wise Club from October 1758 through August 1763 and was then published in 1765. This is Gregory's most straightforward philosophical work—a project of sophisticated analysis in faculty psychology and a clear reflection of Enlightenment Scottish empiricism. Part of this project is a defense of religion in an internecine feud with Hume and religious skeptics of the day, a subject creating a great emotional divide in eighteenth-century Britain (see Gregory 1765, discourse five, pp. 157–203; 1772, p. 66; and 1821). Gregory's attack on skepticism shows his belief that respectable philosophers were believers.[11]

Gregory is walking a tight rope here with regard to his critique of Hume. He was indebted to Hume for his concepts and method and did not want to be too critical of a colleague who was soon to become a personal friend. Descartes, another presence on Gregory's Aberdeen book list, was included in the *Lectures* (Gregory 1772, p. 153). But the most important sources were Gregory's contemporary colleagues, and it was Reid who was most visible (Gregory 1772, pp. 114, 153).[12] Although he was not immune from occasional criticism, Reid was an admirer of Bacon (Reid 1764, pp. 289–90) and Newton (Reid 1764, pp. 191, 232, 235, 316). This could be where Gregory got his interest in these figures.

I see no grounds for doubting Laurence McCullough's conclusion that Gregory based his concept of *sympathy* on Hume rather than on Smith (McCullough 1993, pp. 145–60).[13] Not only is the textual evidence cited by McCullough in favor of this conclusion, but the circumstantial evidence points in that direction as well. Gregory's knowledge of Hume may have been mediated though his more senior Aberdeen colleagues. Smith was 12 years younger than Hume and had not published during Gregory's formative period in the 1740s. Moreover, Hume was in Edinburgh soon after Gregory moved there and both were members of the Philosophical Society, where they were close associates.[14]

Gregory, however, was an intimate friend of other contemporaneous literati, including, most importantly, Thomas Reid (Bettany 1890, p. 102), as well as of faculty colleagues during Gregory's Aberdeen years. This group (with such now largely forgotten figures as George Turnbull [Reid's teacher], David Fordyce, Alexander Gerard, and James Beattie, as well as Reid), referred to as the "Aberdeen branch of the Scottish school of philosophy," is described as underappreciated (Wood 1993, xiv; on Turnbull, see especially pp. 46–7).[15]

In the critical years in Aberdeen during Gregory's philosophical formation— from 1746 when he began lecturing in philosophy to his departure in 1764— Thomas Reid was Gregory's intellectual mentor and companion. Although Reid did not begin as regent at King's College in Aberdeen until 1751, two years after Gregory stopped teaching the basic philosophy courses, Reid had been in Aberdeen as librarian at Marischal College for a time and then took a position as a cleric at New Machar (12 miles from Aberdeen) until he also became a regent. In 1758, Gregory and Reid founded a literary and debating society together, formally known as the Philosophical Society but often called the Wise Club (the club where Gregory's lectures were given beginning in 1758 that were to become the book *A Comparative View* [Gregory 1765]).

The relationship between Reid and Gregory was not just an intellectual one. They were also cousins, sharing a common great-grandfather—the Rev. John Gregory, the Gregory imprisoned by the Covenanters. Their relationship was even closer than the genealogy would suggest. When Gregory was seven his father died. According to some reports it was Reid (along with Gregory's maternal grandfather and half-brother) who raised young John (Gregory 1821, p. 147; Bettany 1890; cf. Smellie 1800, p. 2).[16] Reid was in Aberdeen during most of the time when John was educated in Aberdeen. During part of that time, Reid was librarian at Marischal College. He owed his appointment as professor at King's College to his connections with Gregory's father and half-brother (Wood 1993, p. 31).

James Beattie (1735–1803), another figure of the Scottish common-sense school, was also close with Gregory. It was he, however, who was the product of Gregory's influence, more than the other way around (Beattie 1790, 1793; Grosart 1885). Beattie went to Marischal College, which was to merge with King's College in 1860 to become the University of Aberdeen, as a student in 1749, just as Gregory was completing his brief career as philosophy professor at King's. After years away from Aberdeen, working first as a school master and parish clerk and then as a headmaster for two years at the grammar school of Aberdeen, Beattie was suddenly elevated to the chair of moral philosophy and logic at Marischal College. He began his lectures in 1760, near the end of Gregory's Aberdeen years. He was invited to become a member in the Wise Club, where he joined in the exchange with Reid, Campbell, Gregory, and the literati of Aberdeen. Beattie's affection for Gregory is revealed in his reference to Gregory's death in Beattie's most famous poem, "Minstrel," the second book of which appeared just after Gregory's death.[17] Three decades later, Gregory's son, James, wrote the Latin inscription for Beattie's tomb.

Gregory's involvement with this inner circle continued when he moved to Edinburgh in 1764 (Smellie, 1800, p. 117). Hume returned to Edinburgh in 1766, the year Gregory assumed his professorship, and resided there until his death, three years after Gregory's. At around this time, Smith, who had held the chair in moral philosophy in Glasgow from 1751 to 1764, accepted a traveling tutorship for Henry Scott, the third duke of Buccleuth. Smith was in Paris with the duke in 1764, then in London, and eventually retired to Kirkcaldy (some 20 miles from Edinburgh, but across the Firth of Forth). While residing at Kirkcaldy, he made several trips to London. He was in Edinburgh only for occasional visits during the period up until Gregory's death. Gregory's knowledge of Smith's ideas would have had to come through Smith's writings and reputation, along with these visits. At most, the two would have met on occasion.

Whereas McCullough has pursued the relative importance of Hume and Smith in shaping Gregory's concept of sympathy, the more fundamental question may be the importance of the Aberdonians, compared to that of the Glasgow and Edinburgh philosophers Hutcheson, Smith, and Hume. I find the evidence overwhelming that it is the Aberdonians, especially Reid, who had the most decisive influence on Gregory. For example, not only does the evidence from citations point almost exclusively to Reid (and to a lesser extent Beattie), so do the language and concepts. Gregory is not a moral-sense theorist in the tradition of Hutcheson and Hume; rather, he appeals epistemologically to the common sense and, to some extent, "good sense," phrases much more reminiscent of Reid and Beattie.

For the purposes of this book, however, we need not settle the exact philosophical pedigree of Gregory's thought. What matters is that the writers of medical ethics in the eighteenth century, work that became the foundation of Anglo-American professionally generated medical ethics, were serious participants in an interdisciplinary conversation that included leading philosophers of the day. It is clear that Gregory was a participant in that conversation. He was a philosopher (in both the eighteenth- and twenty-first-century meanings of the term) as well as a physician. Even if he was not the most significant philosopher of the period, he was a serious and respected colleague of a group of important philosophers.

GREGORY'S USE OF CURRENT MORAL LANGUAGE. It is apparent to anyone with even a modestly trained ear for language of the Scottish common-sense tradition that Gregory's vocabulary and concepts were a product of that movement. He uses phrases such as "enquiries into human nature." His ethics is based on *experience*. His key moral concept is *sympathy*. There are appeals to *common sense*, the concept for which the school takes its usual name, but he also frequently appeals to something he calls *good sense*, particularly in the early work, *A Comparative View*. He adopted a faculty psychology, a characteristic of the common-sense theorists.[18] This faculty psychology remained with him until the last days of his life when he wrote his advice to his daughters.

The virtues of Hume, Reid, and other contemporary philosophers were Gregory's virtues: *humanity*, *sensibility*, and *steadiness*. He made regular use of the notion of *improvement*. The focus of his ethics is on *sentiments*, a concept used often throughout Gregory's work, and *tastes*. Religion and ethics involve the *imagination* being warmed. Gregory commonly uses the term *imagination*, as it is used by the other writers of the tradition; it is often linked to taste and sentiments.[19]

The philosophical problems addressed were those of his time. Gregory took up the problem of the passions, particularly in his advice to his daughters (1821, pp. 155, 171, 179, 193), as well as whether reason could control the passions, an issue addressed by Hume.[20] He was more traditional than Hume in his claim that reason is sometimes seen in control (Gregory 1772, p. 17). His advice to his daughters is telling in this regard: "Do not marry a fool: he is the most untractable of all animals; he is led by his passions and caprices, and is incapable of hearing the voice of reason" (Gregory 1821, p. 191). Gregory often linked passion with *caprice*, as did Hume (Gregory 1821, p. 192). Still, in Gregory's early more philosophical work, he reached Hume's conclusion that passions, tempers, and instincts must be the immediately impelling principles of action, rather than reason (Gregory 1765, p. 14). His use of the concept of reason reflects the reason–passion controversy of the day, even if his formulation differs somewhat from Hume's.[21]

While Gregory's work is most conspicuous as a product of the common-sense empirical tradition of eighteenth century Scotland, he also reflects other characteristics of modern thought that sharply differentiate him from the more individualistic and paternalistic professional ethics of the nineteenth and twentieth centuries that are emotionally linked to the Hippocratic ethic. Gregory uses the language of *rights*, which is prevalent in the eighteenth century liberal tradition but absent from later professionally generated ethics (Gregory 1772, pp. 34, 218, 237). In general, he reflects the attitudes of eighteenth-century liberalism and brings them to medicine.[22] Whereas later professionally generated medical ethics follow Hippocratic individualism in which only one-on-one personal relations with an individual patient are the focus of ethics, Gregory's is much more the social ethic of *public utility* of Hume and other philosophers of his time (Gregory 1772, pp. 104, 105, 160).

In contrast with the Hippocratic tradition, Gregory was usually critical of professional authority. While the last decades of the eighteenth century saw regular practitioners fighting against what they considered to be quacks and the practice of medicine by those unschooled for the task, Gregory was remarkably blunt in defending lay authority in medical matters. He offered a marvelous analogy to the Protestant reformation's accepting the authority of the lay person in theology, referring to the religious battle that had recently been won in Scotland against papal authority.[23]

Even this scholar so thoroughly immersed in current Scottish philosophical culture was not totally immune, however, from the professional paternalism that would emerge unabated in the following decades when physician writers in medical ethics were increasingly isolated from the ethics of their broader culture. Gregory's handling of the subject of truth telling reveals an incipient tendency to bifurcate the duties of the medical professional from those of ordinary people. His advice to his daughters reflects the typical, blunt commitment to the morality of honesty in normal social discourse that would have been seen in any parent of his time: "Have a sacred regard to *truth*. Lying is a mean and despicable vice.—I have known some women of excellent parts, who were so much addicted to it, that they could not be trusted in the relation of any story" (Gregory 1821, p. 164). But in his advice to his medical students, Gregory abandoned veracity in favor of a proto-Hippocratism:

A physician is often at a loss in speaking to his patients of their real situation when it is dangerous. A deviation from truth is sometimes in this case both justifiable and necessary. It often happens that a person is extremely ill; but yet may recover, if he is not informed of his danger.

(Gregory 1772, p. 34)

The consequentialist reasoning seen in Hume and the other Scottish moralists also provided a consequence-based justification for physician paternalism.[24]

Lack of Interest in the Ethics of Hippocrates and Galen

Support for the claim that Gregory's incipient paternalism on truth telling came from the consequentialism of his contemporary philosophical environment rather than from a lapse into Hippocratism is based on his general lack of interest in the Hippocratic ethic. The ethics of Hippocrates is not mentioned at all by Gregory or any other figure who wrote on medical ethics during the eighteenth century. They simply had no interest in turning to a remote, cultic Greek source for their ethics when their thinking was so quintessentially the product of the vibrant culture in which they lived. They would no more have turned to the Hippocratic Oath than to the Ayurvedic medical ethical code from the ancient Hindu scriptures or the medical ethical texts from the Quran.

Gregory had a slight interest in the Hippocratic theory of medicine. He saw Hippocrates as advancing Greek medicine and occasionally referred to him as a competent physician (Gregory 1765, p. 47). He praised Hippocrates for moving beyond the "merely empirical" (Gregory 1772, pp. 130–31) and suggested that students canvass his opinions critically, urging them to show respect for Hippocrates's thought as well as that of Sydenham and Boerhaave (Gregory 1772, p. 43). He nonetheless referred to medicine from the time of Hippocrates to the present as being susceptible to facile credulity and reliance on authority rather than appealing directly to "Nature" (Gregory 1772, pp. 177, 182–83).[25] When he made reference to Greeks dividing medicine into dietetics, pharmacology, and surgery, however, he cited Celsus when he could have cited Hippocrates (Gregory 1772, pp. 43–45) and suggested that medicine had progressed considerably since Hippocrates's time (Gregory 1772, pp. 90–91).

In late eighteenth-century medical education, the cultured man was still expected to know Greek, and Gregory cited Hippocrates as a model for good Greek.[26] Apparently, at least partly as a device for testing in Greek, the medical student was expected to translate a Hippocratic aphorism as part of his graduation examination.[27] What is critical is that these cited references constitute every single mention Gregory made of Hippocrates during a long, prolific career. There is not a single reference to the Hippocratic Oath in any of Gregory's writings, at least those that I have been able to examine, including *A Comparative View* and *A Father's Legacy to his Daughters*, as well as the 1770 and 1772 versions of his lectures.

There are rare mentions by Gregory of other historical figures that would have been in a philosopher's vocabulary: Plato (Gregory 1772, pp. 133–34), Aristotle (Gregory 1772, pp. 134–136), and an occasional passing mention of Galen (Gregory 1772, p. 135). But the Hippocratic medical ethical tradition was not Gregory's orientation to any extent whatsoever; he was a philosopher of the eighteenth century.

In his view, the student had to be exposed to enough contemporary moral philosophy to be a man of culture. Thus he began his course in medicine with lectures on medical ethics and the philosophy of medicine that "are intended to have a relation to the proper subject of the profession, but not to be essentially connected with it" (Gregory 1770, pp. 1–2).[28] For Gregory, pursuit of "physick" was a profession of a learned gentleman. "To excel in it requires a greater compass of learning than is necessary in any other. . . . I think it will evidently appear, that no profession requires a greater variety of liberal accomplishments than that of physick" (Gregory 1772, p. 5). That included at least a basic knowledge in medical ethics, grounded not in an ancient Hippocratic cult but in the dominant philosophical movement of his culture, the common-sense school of the Scottish Enlightenment. In this school, students would join Gregory and his colleagues in the conversation that he lived between medicine and the humanities.

Other Scottish Enlightenment Figures with
Medicine and Humanities Links

Gregory was not the only figure of the Scottish Enlightenment with eclectic interests in humanities and medicine. The remarkable intellectual life of the cultural elite of Edinburgh, Glasgow, Aberdeen, and the estates of the countryside encouraged pursuit of classical languages, mathematics, and natural sciences, but also literature, the arts, theology, and philosophy. These members of the cultural elite continued an intellectual tradition of combining medicine with deep roots in theological and philosophical ancestry seen in John Locke (1632–1704) and biblical healing ritual.

Sir John Pringle

The 1772 version of Gregory's *Lectures* is dedicated to Sir John Pringle (1707–1782), who, until 1745, was the Professor of Moral Philosophy at the University of Edinburgh. He was also a physician, which suggests that Gregory was not unique in Enlightenment Scotland in combining interests in moral philosophy and medicine (see Ramsay 1888, p. 230). If Pringle and Gregory were unusual, it was only in the heights to which they took their transdisciplinary talents. Pringle took up the practice of medicine while continuing to hold his philosophy professorship, relying on a deputy to teach while serving as a military physician and eventually as physician to the king and as president of the Royal Society. He was intimate with Priestley, Franklin, and Boswell. He was considered a serious student of divinity, a significant contributor to our understanding of typhoid fever, and the founder of modern military medicine, but he apparently did not combine these interests by reflecting on medical ethics.

William Cullen

Gregory's fellow member of the medical faculty at Edinburgh, William Cullen (1710–1790), came close to combining medicine and philosophy to make a contribution in what we now call medical ethics (Bettany 1888). His interests lay more in what we would call philosophy of medicine. He had the misfortune to make commitments that have not proved durable—to a rather strange nosology and to an eighteenth-century version of ether theory. In this theory, the presence of a rarified substance called "ether" was used to explain various physical and chemical phenomena (see Christie 1981). Cullen became professor of medicine at Glasgow in 1751, moving to the chemistry chair at Edinburgh in 1755. He took over the lectures in materia medica in 1766 and was a candidate for the chair in the practice of physic that went to Gregory. Later that year he won the appointment of professor in the theory of physic, becoming a popular and successful lecturer. In 1768, he and Gregory agreed to alternate the practice and theory courses and did so until Gregory's death in 1773, when Cullen finally achieved the

Practice of Medicine chair. The practice of physic (or what we would call medicine) covered subjects now usually included in physiology, pharmacology, and pathology.

His work on nosology, or classification, of disease, "Synopsis Nosologiae Methodicae," reflected the work of a philosophically oriented theorist. Through J. R. R. Christie's analysis (1981), we can see the importance of the links between Cullen and his philosophical colleagues.

While a professor at Glasgow, Cullen was in conversation with Adam Smith; his interactions with Hume were also significant. The Philosophical and Select Societies provided an environment in Edinburgh in which the thought of Hume and Smith was disseminated. Cullen was among the members of both groups and offered papers on chemical theory and on improvement of the teaching and practice of chemistry (Christie 1981, pp. 90–91). Christie maintains that there is considerable evidence of the influence of Hume and Smith on Cullen. Moreover, both Cullen and Smith were sympathetic to Hume and pressed for his appointment to the chair of logic when Smith switched to that of moral philosophy. Hume expressed his gratitude to Cullen. According to Christie, "this occasion of Hume's attempt to enter academia lends credence to the view that Cullen should be seen as philosophically allied to Hume and Smith, particularly when one considers that Cullen's commitment was maintained in the face of by no means negligible clerical hostility" (Christie 1981, p. 91).[29]

In the end, however, even though he flourished during the height of the Enlightenment and had the knowledge, interests, and talent to contribute at the intersection of medicine and the humanities, Cullen, like Pringle before him, used his Enlightenment talents in ways that had no lasting impact on medical ethics.

James Gregory

Another figure who comes close to playing the role of ethicist–physician is James Gregory (1753–1821), son of John and successor to his father as professor of the medical faculty at the University of Edinburgh. Raised in the household of John Gregory and exposed to figures of the philosophical world, James Gregory showed philosophical interests early. He published a remarkably ambitious, if unimpressive, *Philosophical and Literary Essays* at age 39. In fact, it is misnamed, as it is actually one essay in two volumes that includes 331 pages of introduction, a text of 465 pages, followed by an appendix of 238 pages. I confess to not having read the entire text, but did read enough to see that it was a serious, if immature, effort at taking on the most critical issues of the day. His relation with Reid, who was perhaps the most important philosophical figure in his father's life, comes through dramatically. The volumes are dedicated to Reid while at the same time being aggressively critical of some of Reid's thought. The work has the quality of a graduate student's attempt to distance himself from his professor while remaining devotedly humble and simultaneously showing how dependent he is in his very choice of issues and philosophical phrasing. He attacks not only Reid but also Hume (Gregory 1792, p. clxx). He shows the reverence for Bacon and Newton seen in his father and other philosophers of the day but, with one exception, has few kind words to say about anyone since them. He accuses them of making unlucky, retrograde "discoveries" that contaminate the work of the masters.[30] James Gregory tried to position himself between Reid on the one hand and Hume, Priestley, and Leibniz on the other (see Gregory 1792, p. ccxii), but spent considerable ink establishing that he could attack his relative with equal heat.[31]

While James Gregory's philosophical interests were primarily in metaphysics rather than medical ethics, he did contribute to the latter by supervising a new edition of his father's *Lectures* (Gregory 1805). His energies were often wasted, however, with his argumentative style and penchant for extended academic squabbling with colleagues that not only generated their hostility but even inspired a lawsuit against him.[32]

Of all those with interests in both medicine and philosophy at this time, James Gregory probably came closest to having the broad knowledge, interest, and energy to continue the work of his father in medical ethics. He knew all the key figures. Reid was a household experience and a relative. James Gregory was intimate with other Scottish Enlightenment figures. (We have already seen that he wrote the Latin inscription for James Beattie's tombstone.) But that era was over. He was a generation too late. Medicine had begun the process of becoming an isolated scientific speciality. James Gregory was never taken seriously as a philosopher/medical ethicist. The conversation was over at least for the next 170 years. James Gregory did most of his publishing (aside from the fateful foray into writing a philosophical essay) in medical science, publishing papers on "De morbis coeli mutatione medendis" (1774) and "Conceptus medicinae theoreticae" (1780–82).

Dugald Stewart

The responsibility for ending the conversation between medicine and the humanities was by no means all that of the medical scientists. That can be seen in the life of one of the next generation of common-sense philosophers. Dugald Stewart (1753–1828) was Professor of Moral Philosophy at Edinburgh from 1785 to 1809. He took Reid's course at Glasgow in 1772 and was probably the best known propagator of the common-sense tradition in the next generation (Stewart 1858, pp. 303–308; Veitch 1858, pp. xcvii ff.; Stephen 1896, p. 437). Reid was known to travel to Edinburgh to visit both James Gregory and Stewart in 1796 (Stephen 1896, p. 438). In addition to being a serious student of and contributor to Scottish moral philosophy, Stewart was also closely connected with medical practice. His library, which is housed in the Special Collections of the University of Edinburgh Library, contains the existing copies of both John and James Gregory's works as well as a signed presentation copy of Thomas Percival's *Medical Ethics*. For some reason, however, Stewart never saw himself as a contributor to the field of medical ethics.

Moral philosophy was growing away from such practical, real-world areas. Stewart's published works were on moral philosophy, the human mind, and political economy, in addition to philosophical biographies of Thomas Reid, Adam Smith, and William Robertson. With very rare exceptions throughout the nineteenth century and the first two-thirds of the twentieth, no philosopher or theologian would again take up the issues of medical ethics. For these philosophers, the world of analytical philosophy was on the horizon. It would eventually become a badge of honor that moral philosophers worked on grand theoretical questions, sometimes called "metaethics," having to do with the meaning and justification of ethical terms. Other humanists, including the moral theologians, were almost as oblivious to the implications of ethics for an applied professional area such as medicine. They were attracted to the Great Revivals, the Oxford Movement, and other more pietistic spiritual quests. When they did turn to social problems of the world, it was to issues such as temperance, the anti-slavery movement, and eventually civil rights, the fight against the Vietnam war, and the women's movement. While we shall see in Chapter 10 that there were some precursors who made attempts to bridge medicine and the humanities, it would not be until about 1970— what can still be called the current generation of humanities—that applied and professional ethics would again be fashionable, for either physicians or humanists. The reasons are complex. They will be addressed in Chapter 11. But first, another piece of the story of the Scottish Enlightenment must be told, the beginnings of the emergence of medicine as an isolated science. It is to that story that we turn in Chapter 2.

2

THE BEGINNINGS OF MEDICINE AS AN ISOLATED SCIENCE

The medical elite of mid-eighteenth-century Scotland were a remarkable lot. They came from families that provided classical educations rich in Greek and Latin and study of classical rhetoric (which included the transmission of Greek and Roman moral insights) as well as natural and moral philosophy. But one of the unintended effects of the Enlightenment was to change the nature of the educated man.[1] The cadre of educated persons changed rather quickly from a group of generalists who regularly could converse, socialize with each other, and even gain employment in widely different fields to a group of more narrow, specialized experts. Of course, in any era it would be possible to find those of less profound education, and certainly more ordinary physicians, even more ordinary medical faculty members, could be cited as lacking broad cultural education and knowledge. But the story to be told here is the increasing isolation of even the elite of the medical world.

ISOLATION OF THE PHYSICIAN

The story of physician isolation begins even as Gregory and his colleagues were developing an ethic for physicians that was synchronized with the philosophical debates of the day.

Alexander Monro, Primus

The Monro family history[2] is as rich as the Gregories', starting with Primus's grandfather Sir Alexander Monro. He was an advocate (a lawyer) who fought in the battle of Worcester on the royalist side, opposing Cromwell and "alwaies with those who were in arms for the Royal Cause till there were no more such parties" (Erlam 1954, p. 80). Consequently, he was forced into hiding. His son (Primus's father) was John Monro, an Edinburgh surgeon who had visions of himself founding a medical faculty. He had great ambition for his son, Alexander, whom he pressed into the study of surgery. Alexander served an apprenticeship under his father, beginning sometime before he was 20 years of age. He then studied medicine in London, Paris, and eventually in Leyden, where he studied under Boerhaave. His father was so proud of his son's dissections that his father, without the son's knowledge, signed him up to give public lectures in front of the leading dignitaries of the College of Physicians.[3]

With his father's encouragement, he was named the first Professor of Anatomy at the University of Edinburgh in 1720 at the age of 23. He is recognized as a key figure in the founding of the medical faculty in 1726 and continued teaching for 39 years, at which time his son, Alexander, Secundus, was named to his chair. Primus's younger son, Donald, was also an Edinburgh medical graduate who practiced medicine in the army. The Edinburgh chair was gradually transferred to Alexander, Tertius, who was appointed conjoint professor in 1800, began teaching the whole course in 1808, and assumed the sole professorship in 1817. He held the position until 1846. Tertius's son, David, was also educated as a physician, but emigrated to New Zealand where he entered politics, served in the first general assembly in 1854, and was eventually knighted. In turn, David's son-in-law, Sir James Hector, was also a physician.

A family library started by Primus was passed through this line of physicians until Hector's wife (David's daughter) donated it to the parliamentary library in Wellington, New Zealand. Eventually, it was transferred to the Medical School Library at The University of Otago in Dunedin. (In Chapter 9, I trace the influence of the Edinburgh medical tradition on this medical school and the emergence of medical ethics there.)

The seven generations of Monros at first seem culturally and intellectually similar to the seven generations of Gregories—each representing an elite family of well-educated gentlemen, often with a penchant for medicine. But, as we shall see, something made a difference. Could that something be the fact that John Gregory's father was a physician, who steered his son toward a classical university education, whereas Alexander Monro's father was a surgeon, who pointed his son toward the apprenticeship that was normal for surgical training of the day?[4]

The Simple Analysis

A simple formulation of the difference between John Gregory and his more senior colleague suggests that, whereas Gregory's intellectual interests led him not
only to study ethics, metaphysics, logic, and pneumatology (the science of the
mind) but also to become a professor of philosophy and to publish in that area,
Monro's interests were much narrower. He was the quintessential modern medical scientist. Working as an apprentice to his father, he began to tend the sick at a
very early age. He attended the "Demonstration of the pharmaceutical Plants exhibited every Summer," took a course in chemistry, and attended "the dissection
of a human body which was shewed once in two or three Years by Mr. Robert
Elliot . . ." (Erlam 1954, pp. 80–81).

MEDICAL WRITINGS OF MONRO: ALL SCIENTIFIC. Monro published an enormous
number of books and articles, but they were almost without exception what we
would call technical medical science. His best known work was "Osteology, a
Treatise on the Anatomy of the Human Bones," which became a standard text.
He also published on such subjects as "Mechanism of the cartilages between the
true vertebrae," "Essay on the caries of bones," "Cure of a fractured tendo Achillis,"
"Cure of an ulcer of the cheek, with the superior salivary duct opened," all of which
appeared in the edition of his collected works published by his son, Alexander,
Secundus (Monro 1781).[5]

THE MONRO LIBRARY. One reaches a similar conclusion examining the library
of the Monros that passed through the three generations of anatomists at Edinburgh
and then on to New Zealand. Of an estimated 600 volumes, with six exceptions
all deal with technical aspects of medicine. They include manuscript copies of
the Monros' own writings and lecture notes, but many published volumes as well—
all titles that would be appropriate holdings for the modern medical scientist.
Among them are a copy of Monro's *Anatomy of Human Bones* and a manuscript
commentary on his *Osteology* (see Taylor 1979, for a carefully prepared catalogue).
Nothing resembles Gregory's *Lectures* or Thomas Percival's *Medical Ethics* or
shows the slightest evidence that any of the Monros were engaged with issues
related to the ethical practice of medicine or the more general ethical controversies of the day.

The Complex Account

John Gregory and Alexander Monro, Primus, represent two ideal types. The first
is of an engaged philosopher/physician whose rich exposure to philosophical
debates prepared him for doing medical ethics in a manner appropriate to his
environment, that is, the Scottish Enlightenment of Edinburgh in the middle

decades of the century. The other is the prototype of the modern medical scientist, deeply immersed in a rapidly evolving scientific literature in which a person could specialize for an entire lifetime not merely in medicine but in a particular branch of medicine, such as anatomy. The fact that the prototypical modern scientific specialist was about a generation older than the last of the Enlightenment generalists merely heightens the contrast.

MONRO AS A CLASSICALLY EDUCATED STUDENT. A closer examination of the lives of the Monros, however, reveals a slightly more complex picture. Alexander Monro, Primus, was in fact an important part of the literary culture of Edinburgh in the eighteenth century, a leading member of the literati. He was classically trained, studying Latin, Greek, and French as well as "philosophy, arithmatick, Mathematicks, and Book Keeping" in school (Erlam 1954, p. 80). It must be remembered, however, that philosophy included natural philosophy (i.e., natural science).

"ESSAY ON FEMALE CONDUCT". At least one publication of Monro, Primus, strays from the narrow domain of scientific and clinical anatomy and surgery. Following a pattern seen in many of the cultural elite of the time, late in life he composed for his daughter's use "An Essay on Female Conduct."[6] In it he treats "a Girls Education, her general Commerce in the World, a Woman's Conduct with Men, her Duty as a Wife, a Mistress of a Family and a Mother, to which is added a System of Religion consisting of the Laws of Nature, the Mosaical Institution and the Christian System, and that is followed by a short Dissertation on government" (Monro 1996; the summary in Monro's own words is from the published version by Erlam 1954, p. 94). Much of this essay, like the similar volume that John Gregory wrote for his daughters, reads today as quaint, paternalistic advice, but the sections on religion and government reveal the extent of Monro's knowledge of theology and philosophy (or lack thereof). Of particular importance is the section on religion, which includes considerable discussion of David Hume on religion. This makes clear that Monro at least understood Hume's reputation as a religious skeptic and provides a modest attempt at rebuttal. Its real theme, however, is support of the Christian religion. He refrains from entering more sectarian squabbles. What is important for our purposes is that Monro, at most, confronted Hume only on religious skepticism. There is no evidence that he engaged the philosopher on any issues of metaphysics or ethics the way that Gregory did.[7]

MONRO AS A MEMBER OF EDINBURGH SOCIETIES. The references to Hume's views on religion were not the only evidence of at least nominal interaction between Monro and Hume. Monro, Primus, was very active in Edinburgh's cultural societies, which were comparable in some ways to the Wise Club in Aberdeen started by Gregory and Reid. In about 1731, the professors of the different branches of medicine started a society for discussing unusual case histories and publishing them from time to time, known as the Society for the Improvement of Medical Knowledge (Erlam 1954, p. 87; Monro 1996, p. ix). Monro was the secretary and was responsible for several volumes of papers that emerged from the group. This society, however, was more narrowly medical. Moreover, it soon became inactive. It was reactivated and enlarged in 1737 as the Society for Improving Philosophy and Natural Knowledge, and now included "a "considerable Number of Noblemen and Gentlemen" (Erlam 1954, p. 88; Monro 1996, p. x). Once again, Monro served as secretary (and later, vice president). After another lapse, it was once again revived, apparently in 1752, and was then known simply as the Philosophical Society, but now the secretary was David Hume (Erlam 1954, p. 88; Monro 1996, p. x). Monro specifically says, however, that his papers were on medical subjects. Thus, although he might have heard more philosophical papers, there is no evidence that they influenced his scholarly work.

Soon after it was formed in 1754, Monro was invited to join still another group called the "Select Society," made up primarily of lawyers, but also including David Hume and Adam Smith. The purpose of this group was to acquire the habit of speaking easily in public. Monro eventually was elected its President. Here the focus was on questions of general utility. Monro claims to have been particularly good at questions where "physical Knowledge" was involved. This group evolved into The Edinburgh Society for The Encouragement of Arts, Science, Manufactures and Agriculture in Scotland; in about 1755 Monro was chosen as President. The Society was designed to promote arts and manufactures, with a focus on commercial and agricultural objectives. Monro was thus active in clubs of "nobles and gentlemen," some of whom permitted him to mingle with humanist thinkers; however, Monro specialized in medical, commercial, agricultural, and scientific questions, showing less interest in the philosophical issues even in those clubs where they were likely to arise. His association with Hume appears to have been more social than intellectual.[8]

This evidence leaves us with a complicated picture. Monro was an active participant in the cultural societies of the day and had ample opportunity to be exposed to its leading philosophical thinkers, but there is no evidence that Monro took great interest when the discussion turned from scientific and practical matters, such as animal husbandry and furthering of commerce, to metaphysical and moral subtleties. Whereas Gregory and Cullen were intellectually engaged in these gatherings and evidence of this shows in their work, the same cannot be said of Monro (see Christie 1981, p. 90).

EVIDENCE FROM THE MONRO LIBRARY: A FURTHER LOOK. An additional hint of Monro's lack of philosophical interest comes from the fact that the library that survives in Dunedin, while almost entirely consisting of books on medical science, contains six volumes that would catch the attention of the humanist.[9] If the

Monros are to be portrayed as archetypical medical scientists without interest in the humanities, these volumes need to be explained. That explanation exists, and it ends up furthering the impression that the Monros were not significantly engaged in contemporaneous philosophical conversation.

It is easy to account for the volume, *Commentary on the Hindu System of Medicine*, by Thomas Wise.[10] It is hardly the required reading for anatomists, but the copy is inscribed "Professor Monro sentiments of esteem and respect from the author, Edin, 13th Feby 1855." It is a presentation copy from the author, a fellow physician. Published in 1845 and presented 10 years later, the volume's recipient must have been Monro, Tertius, his father and grandfather being dead by then.

The second humanities volume in the collection, a secondary work entitled *An Account of Sir Isaac Newton's Philosophical Discoveries, in Four Books*, by Colin Maclaurin (1748),[11] is equally easy to account for. Maclaurin was a mathematician, first at Aberdeen, then Glasgow, and finally at Edinburgh. He is described as Primus's closest colleague in the university faculty (Monro 1781, p. xiv). The edition in the Monro library, however, was the fifth, published in 1801 and hence could not have been Primus's. It cannot be taken as evidence that Monro was intimately included in philosophical discourse in Edinburgh.

The next three volumes are intriguing. There is a Greek/Latin edition of Hippocratic writings containing 55 works.[12] It consists of all the critical works: the Laws, Aphorisms, Epidemics, and the Hippocratic Oath. In my rather extensive search of medical and philosophical writing of eighteenth-century Scotland, the Monro library is the only place I encountered any mention of the Hippocratic Oath. I have not been able to find a single mention of the Oath by either of the Gregories or the other Scottish common-sense moral theorists. It is thus clearly a mistake to assume that the Hippocratic Oath captured the essence of professionally articulated medical ethics in Greek culture, early Christianity, the Middle Ages, or the Scottish Enlightenment. They all had their own system of metaphysics and their own ethics—their own understanding of the source and justification of ethical requiredness, their own theory of moral authority, and their own notions of what made actions right and wrong.

Something important happened, however, when physicians became medical specialists focusing their education, starting at an early age, on the goal of mastering increasingly complex medical science. As they became isolated from the surrounding culture with its moral and religious concepts, they were left with nothing more than a vague notion that medicine was a profession with moral content. They sought in vain for a symbol for that content until Hippocrates was found to fill that role.

An Oath, not actually written by the historical Hippocrates but associated with his name, began to emerge as the symbol of the morality of the medical profession. Whereas John Gregory and the theological and philosophical leaders of the Scottish Enlightenment would have had no reason to turn to an obscure Greek mystery cult, and in fact would have been appalled at the idea, physicians like Monro, Primus, and his offspring, having no strong commitment to a careful understanding of current religious or secular ethical systems, saw no problem with a symbolic choice of the Hippocratic Oath for their ethic.

To be sure, Monro was just as strongly committed to a vaguely Christian perspective as Gregory, Reid, or Beattie, but it was a layperson's commitment in which no substantial difference was perceived between the tenets of that Oath and his chosen religion in the way that a more carefully sensitized scholar of a system would. For Monro there was no real tension between the Hippocratic symbol for the profession and his vague layman's commitment to Christianity. As we shall see momentarily, when the passionate commitment to the king and the Presbyterian Covenant fade, a secular world can import a hazily understood Hippocratic system without perceiving the tension. The Hippocratic writings were important to Monro not only in the way they were for Gregory—as documents from an ancient scientific literature that commands respect—but as a deontological literature for a secular age that no longer assigned the Presbyterian and Episcopal religious loyalties center stage. Thus the Oath gained a place for Monro not seen in Gregory.

The fourth work with humanities significance in the Monro collection is another Hippocratic work, a separate edition of the Epidemics.[13] Along with this was another volume from ancient medicine—Galen's works in five volumes.[14] These first five titles in the Monro library clearly show no signs that any of the Monros were serious about moral theory. To the contrary, they are a motley collection of samples from Hindu, Greek, Latin, and early modern writers, none of which were written by contemporary ethics authors.

The sixth volume potentially upsets the clean claim that the Monros are the prototype of the Hippocratic medical scientists isolated from contemporary humanities. The collection contains a copy of Reid's *An Inquiry into the Mind, on the Principles of Common Sense*.[15] While one volume does not a philosopher make, this is, from Gregory's point of view, probably the most important work of the eighteenth-century common-sense philosophers. If the Monros read it, the picture is more complicated.

But the evidence is to the contrary. The first edition of Reid's *Inquiry* appeared in 1764, just three year's before Primus's death. Certainly, Reid's *Inquiry* was not critical to Monro Primus's thought. He had basically finished his scholarly output by then. In fact, what appears in the Monro collection is the fifth edition, which did not appear until 1801 (Reid 1801). It had seen previous editions in 1765, 1769, and 1785, in addition to the first publication. We can assume that this was acquired sometime after 1801, probably by Monro, Secundus. Still, it muddies a clean typology, even if only Secundus was a reader of Reid. The evidence is still to the contrary, however. Nothing appears in Monro, Secundus, that suggests Reid's influence. More important, when I went to the rare book room in Dunedin,

New Zealand, to see the copy, I found that many of the pages had not even been cut open. Clearly, none of the Monros studied this volume carefully.

An examination of the existing library of the Monros leads us to the following inescapable conclusion: the Monros were well educated in the classics and possessed many works in Greek and Latin, but were otherwise prototypical modern medical scientists. Their attention was on medical science. When they turned to the humanities, it was to Hippocratic and Galenic medicine, and then largely for historical and symbolic purposes. No evidence was found of any working knowledge of eighteenth-century Scottish philosophy.

Gregory and Monro are the two models at the end of the eighteenth century for linking medicine with the humanities. Gregory, though years younger, is the Enlightenment generalist teaching the entire curriculum to arts students and publishing serious efforts in philosophy before becoming a professor of medicine. His medical ethics is little more than his common sense philosophy worked out for the medical role. The Monros, by contrast, are well educated in the classics, but their real interest is in the science of medicine and the ever-increasing scientific literature.

The Faculty of 1826

If Alexander Monro, Primus, is the archetype of the modern medical scientist who has dropped out of the conversation with the humanists and has no real interest in the ethics of his profession, the effects of that archetype can be seen in the following decades, not only in the thought of the Monros, Secundus and Tertius, but now penetrating virtually the entire medical faculty. In 1826 a remarkable set of hearings took place under the control of a Scottish Royal Commission established by the king to review the universities of Scotland. The commission had hearings at each university lasting sometimes for months. It eventually published verbatim transcripts of the entire proceedings (Commission for Visiting the Universities and Colleges in Scotland, 1837). In the case of Edinburgh, the hearings included the testimony of every professor. Sometimes a professor's testimony lasted more than a day. Some were recalled for additional testimony.[16] The result is a 900-page volume of small-print, 1200-word pages with every imaginable detail of the off-the-cuff remarks of faculty about their interpersonal squabbles as well as a record of attitudes about educational philosophy. The medical faculty testimony gives a good record of the priorities and pressures under which the faculty operated. It shows a complete lack of interest in ethics or the humanities of the profession and a rigorous commitment to increasing the quality of the science in the curriculum while at the same time responding to what they perceived to be strong competitive pressures from lesser schools. This led to efforts to shorten the curriculum, such as by reducing or eliminating the requirements for Greek and Latin.

William Pulteney Alison

A representative example of the views of the medical faculty of 1826 is that of William Pulteney Alison, Esq., M.D., Dean of the Faculty of Medicine and Professor of the Theory of Physic, essentially the same position held by Gregory 50 years earlier (Commission 1837, pp. 190–218, 248–250).[17] The most compulsively pursued questions include whether an arts degree should be a prerequisite for the medical degree or whether the practice of admitting students directly from the grammar (high) school preparation should be continued and whether classical languages, especially Greek, should be required of all students (Commission 1837, p. 191). The faculty, especially the seven regular faculty members, appear to have rehearsed their answers, all insisting that it would be wrong to require preparation in the arts, philosophy, and languages beyond what the students bring with them from school training (where "school" refers to grammar and other pre-university education).[18] The following passage reveals the current mood, in which Dr. Alison feels compelled to provide an apology for streamlining medical education by focusing on practical matters rather than on more elaborate arts and literature:

It has been said by some that the medical profession ought to have a more aristocratic form than it has at present in this country, and that this might be given by the degree in the University being made to require a greater outlay of time and expense than it does just now, and by the graduate in the University acquiring in return a higher rank in society. But we conceive the idea that that could be done by University education, is attributing more to education in the University than experience entitles us to suppose it can do. . . . For example, if it were found that our graduate, after a more expensive education than they have now, and after the acquisition of a good deal more literature and science, were continually passed in practice by men whose education had been cheaper, and who did not pretend to any attainments, but those which were merely professional, the consequence would be, that our degree would become unpopular; we should lose, and the public would not gain by the change.

(Commission 1837, pp. 193–4)

The pressure was perceived as coming from the physicians with lesser rather than more training in the arts and literature.[19] Alison pointed out that many of the students were "strangers," that is, from foreign lands and that "very few of these gentlemen have had a University education;—they come here as medical students, and for medical instruction only" (Commission 1837, p. 198). In other words, they came as apprentices with little opportunity for study of philosophy or the arts. A choice had to be made between having background in the arts and in the branches of their medical preparation, that is, in the relevant sciences. The report shows that, when asked, Alison states that the rest of the faculty have read the statement and are in agreement (Commission 1837, p. 199). An exchange between a commissioner and Dr. Alison summarizes the faculty's minimalist stance.[20] The humanities are simply no longer on the agenda of the medical faculty, as indicated by the following exchange:

"Is there any other distribution of the Philosophical courses that you would propose different from that which exists?"

"No, I have not thought of that subject."

(Commission 1837, p. 208)

Instead of philosophy classes (whether natural or moral philosophy), Alison suggested more classes in anatomy (Commission 1837, p. 209). Given the earlier suggestion that Aberdeen retained a strong commitment to the regenting system and a more integrated philosophy curriculum, it is noteworthy that only Aberdeen among the Scottish universities in 1826 was still insisting on an arts degree for its medical students (Commission 1837, p. 210). Alison was not even sure that Aberdeen really insisted on the arts background and recommended that, if it wanted to be a great medical school, it would drop any such requirement (Commission 1837, p. 210).

Other Faculty Testimony

MEDICAL FACULTY. The other faculty that testified before the commission were in remarkable agreement with Alison. Robert Graham, Professor of Medicine and Botany, and Thomas Charles Hope, Professor of Chemistry and Chemical Pharmacy (Commission 1837, pp. 259, 270) added their second, as did Alexander Monro, the grandson who has by now had succeeded to the Anatomy Chair (Commission 1837, pp. 272, 277). The requirement for an arts background was a luxury that the nineteenth century could not afford. Rather than worrying about increasing the admission and graduation requirements for their medical students, they needed to worry about the increasingly stiff competition from lesser schools. More and more time was needed for the core courses of the medical faculty. As knowledge proliferated in medicine, languages and philosophy, along with other "ornaments" in education, had to be set aside. No member of the regular medical faculty dissented from this view. The closest thing to the old view was expressed by Dr. Andrew Duncan, Senior, the professor of medical theory whose duties were increasingly taken over by the young dean. He held out for giving exams in Latin and for the obligatory commentary on a Hippocratic aphorism, something that, as we have seen, Gregory supported not so much out of commitment to Hippocratic deontology but rather as an exercise in classical language skill.

The only other resistance came from the Regius Professors who were not technically members of the medical faculty and who obviously were not as much a part of the consensus. There was clearly tension between the regular faculty and the Regius Professors, who resented their second-class status and decried the fact that they were excluded from the lucrative splitting of student fees. For example, James Russell, Regius Professor of Clinical Surgery, argued for the requirement of literature, complaining that at the time, "there is nothing at all exacted" by way of an admission requirement (Commission 1837, p. 288). Robert Christison, the Regius Professor of Medical Jurisprudence, expressed doubt that the time could be afforded for such a course (Commission 1837, p. 290). He commented that the current training methods, in which many students started out as apprentices and spent several years with a family practitioner, was in his mind the best qualification (Commission 1837, p. 290). He was in line with the regular faculty in worrying about a drop in enrollment if additional requirements were added. Dr. George Ballingall, the Clinical Professor of Military Surgery, supported the requirement for Greek and Latin (Commission p. 300). In general, however, even the regius professors were not strong advocates for the arts and humanities.

PHILOSOPHERS. This acquiescence to the isolation of medicine from the humanities was accepted not only by the core medical faculty but by the humanists as well. While the previous professor of moral philosophy, Duncan Stewart, was at least engaged in applied medical ethics to the extent of acquiring the key books and retaining personal friendships with his physician colleagues, his successor, John Wilson, was oriented toward the divinity students, who were required to take his course (Commission 1837, p. 114).[21] Medicine was no longer on the radar screen.

In addition to Wilson, another faculty member showed significant sophistication in moral philosophy: Macvey Napier, the Professor of Conveyancing (Commission 1837, pp. 227–33). While a member of the law faculty, he was interested primarily in the various branches of philosophy (in the narrower sense in which twenty-first century philosophers use the term). He made elaborate proposals for a restructuring of the philosophy curriculum into three distinct professorships: Physiology of the Mind and Moral Philosophy, Political Philosophy, and Logic and Rhetoric, but never ventured to comment on their implication for any of the professions, whether medicine, divinity, or his own faculty of law. Clearly, the move to isolate moral philosophy and the other philosophical disciplines from application in the professions was supported as much by the philosophers as it was by the members of the faculties for the professional schools. It is safe to say that by 1826, if not two or three decades earlier, the isolation of medicine had been firmly established.[22] There was no longer anyone on the faculty at Edinburgh (or anyplace else in Scotland) with John Gregory's vision that knowledge in general is the province of the cultured person.

EMERGENCE OF HIPPOCRATIC-TYPE OATHS AT GRADUATION

In addition to examining the individuals who synthesized medicine and the humanities in the eighteenth century and let them drift apart in the nineteenth, there is another way of getting a picture of medical ethics in the medical school setting. It is sometimes assumed that throughout Western history, at least at graduation from medical school, students have been asked to take the Hippocratic Oath. While they may not study it, have their professors exegete it, or learn its historical context, it is sometimes assumed that they at least recite it on this one ceremonial occasion. Such ceremonies should not be taken lightly because, even if students do not comprehend the content of any oath they recite, some individual or some group must think about its content. Such oaths or codifications cannot survive long if their content is radically at odds with the beliefs of the faculty or student body. I have therefore attempted to study the evolution of medical ethics during the period of its isolation from the humanities by examining how the oaths, or pledges, or "declarations," as they are sometimes called, have evolved. On the basis of what has been said thus far, one would predict that, at least until well into the eighteenth century, any oaths taken during medical gradation would have been related to the theological, philosophical, and ethical context of contemporaneous Scotland rather than to some Hippocratic-type oath. History never conforms perfectly to theoretical frameworks, but, in this case, it comes close.

The Aberdeen Oath

The first evidence in the secondary literature I encountered on the subject of medical school oaths in Scotland appeared in the *British Medical Journal* in October 1994 ("The Hippocratic Oath," 1994; see also Nutten 1995). Here the editor printed several letters responding to a proposal for revisions in the Hippocratic Oath, and included a summary of the current oaths used at all 27 British schools of medicine. He reported that 13 schools used no oath at all, 3 used the Hippocratic Oath or a modern version of it, 11 used the Declaration of Geneva (which is often described as a modern version of the Hippocratic Oath), and 6 used what he called the "sponsio academica." Among the latter group were Aberdeen, Edinburgh, and Glasgow—the three Scottish medical schools in the report. Included in the series of letters was one from T. H. Pennington and C. I. Pennington of the University of Aberdeen, confirming that Aberdeen has used the sponsio academica since 1888. T. H. Pennington was a "sometime medical dean and promoter of graduates at Aberdeen" (Pennington and Pennington 1994, p. 952). That letter tells an important story. After describing the current Aberdeen oath as "something in principle . . . not too far removed from [the Hippocratic Oath]," the letter states that "it was introduced in 1888 by the medical faculty in response to the discontinuation of the graduation oath hitherto taken by students in all faculties. The university had done this because the centuries-old oath contained religious sentiments to which a qualified candidate for the medical degree had been unable to subscribe on grounds of conscience, thereby preventing him from obtaining his degree."

I have been unable to verify the full history of the Aberdeen Oath, but this account certainly fits the prediction made above. The year 1888 seems late for the abandonment of the more religiously based oath in favor of one with a more Hippocratic character, but this shift at least fits the pattern I have been tracing. The sponsio quoted is, in fact, very close to the Declaration of Geneva—so close, that any one placing them side by side would have to conclude that the sponsio influenced the authors of the Declaration of Geneva.

The Edinburgh Oath

Locating the text of oaths, particularly the older versions, is not an easy task. The story at Edinburgh is especially long and complicated. I was able to examine the volumes of what at Edinburgh is called the "Laureation book," an official register that contains the original signature of every graduate appended to a declaration, or what is called the "sponsio academica." The sponsios date from the first university graduate in 1587.[23] That first graduate, Robert Rollock, was asked to sign a short confession of faith, or covenant, that is written on the first page of the book. The text was first subscribed to by King James I and his household in 1581 and soon after by "all persons of rank" (Dalzel 1862, p. 100). It eventually was made the first part of the National Covenant of 1638. Thus the original purpose was clearly one involving loyalty to the King and the Scottish religion. Beginning in 1604—more than a century before the beginning of the medical school—the professors as well as the graduates were required to sign the oath and the graduates were also required to sign a pledge to remain affectionate and dutiful to the University of Edinburgh. Changes were made during the seventeenth century, including a new, shorter oath with a renunciation of popery that the university began using in 1635 (Dalzel 1862, p. 100). Beginning in 1639, the formal religious covenant portion was omitted, while religious language continued in the sponsio document itself. In 1687 the promise included a commitment to perseverance in the Christian religion. It is clear that the function of the sixteenth- and seventeenth-century oaths was the articulation of patriotic, religious, and academic loyalty. This was the case before there was ever a medical graduate of the university.

Although the medical faculty was not created until 1726, the university granted several medical degrees prior to that time, the first to David Cockburn in 1705. As the first medical graduate he was asked to sign a sponsio that varied from that of other students, but the document varied only modestly from that being used at the time. It commited Dr. Cockburn to "maintain the Christian religion in truth and purity purged of all Popish errors."[24] The same document was signed by the second medical-degree recipient in 1710 and by 16 others before the establishment of the medical faculty, as well as by two between 1726, when the medical school was established, and 1731.[25]

In 1731 a new, shorter form was adopted that still contained the Reformation Christian pledge.[26] In no way is any of the language of this form reminiscent of the Hippocratic Oath; it is much more similar to the sponsio used by other students at the time. In a published list of medical graduates from 1846, the next version of the sponsio is dated 1803. This newer version is significantly different in that it contains no reference to the Christian religion or to popish errors (though it still includes the pledge before God) ("Nomina Eorum . . ." 1846, p. vi). The opening line now reads, "Whereas the distinction of a degree in Medicine is now to be conferred upon me, I solemnly promise before God, the Searcher of hearts, that I will to my latest breath abide steadfast in all due loyalty to the University of Edinburgh." Although this still cannot be described as Hippocratic wording, a confidentiality sentence is included that is virtually verbatim from the Hippocratic Oath. That language is peculiar and could not have found its way into the Edinburgh sponsio without some awareness of the Hippocratic text as a referent. The closing line also is very similar to the close of the Hippocratic Oath and is alien to Christian theology. (The medieval "Hippocratic Oath Insofar as a Christian May Swear It" dropped this Hippocratic closing, presumably because it was too Pelagian, that is, it had the appearance of permitting humans to earn their way to heaven rather than relying on God's grace). The full text of the medical oath carrying the 1803 date reads as follows:

Whereas the distinction of a degree in Medicine is now to be conferred upon me, I solemnly promise before God, the Searcher of hearts, that I will to my latest breath abide steadfast in all due loyalty to the University of Edinburgh. Further, that I will practise the art of Medicine with care, with purity of conduct and with uprightness, and, so far as in me lies, will faithfully attend to everything conducive to the welfare of the sick. Lastly, that, whatever things seen or heard in the course of medical practice which ought not to be spoken of, I will not, save for right reason, divulge. This I promise, as I hope for the gracious blessing of Heaven.[27]

A second version was available to be used by Quakers, which omitted the language of promising before God. A small number of Quakers in the nineteenth century signed this version of the Oath, as recorded in the Laureation book.

While this is not the Hippocratic Oath or even a loose, modernized translation, it certainly eliminates the explicitly religious and anti-Roman perspective. Except for the reference to God, which we can presume was still the Judeo-Christian God, and the loyalty pledge to the university, this oath could reasonably be called Hippocratic in character.

This seems to support the conclusion that, throughout the eighteenth century, the medical graduate at the University of Edinburgh took a pledge that was Protestant Christian and had its roots in loyalty oaths to religion, king, and university rather than having any Hippocratic connections. As the Enlightenment integration collapsed at the turn of the century and medical ethics became isolated, a new Hippocratic symbolism found its way into the medical graduation ceremony.

Unfortunately, there is a slight problem with this chronology. Although the 1846 published register of medical graduates contained the new version, which we have labeled Hippocratic, with an 1803 date, in fact, the new version was adopted with the graduating class of 1762. The original hand-written Laureation book clearly made the transition after the 1761 class, with the last graduate's signature dated

16 September, 1761. There is then a page with a portion of the 1761 sponsio written as if prepared for the 1762 class's signatures. That ends abruptly, and the remainder of the page is blank. On the next page, the new version appears verbatim as in the text dated 1803 in the published volume. That text, with no substantive change, appears into the present Laureation book. When I read the book in 1996, the last group of signatures was dated 1995.[28]

What this means is that, if we are correct in describing the latest version of the declaration as Hippocratic in character, the Hippocratizing of the university's medical sponsio occurred in 1762, rather than when the published version would have us believe—that is, 1803. From the point of view of this chapter, this means that the process of separating medical ethics from the broader culture—from the Protestant Christian and secular Enlightenment moral philosophy of the mid-eighteenth century—began at Edinburgh earlier than we might have expected. We see the Hippocratic influence, modest as it was, as early as 1762. Given that Monro, Primus, was finishing his tenure by that time and he represents the prototypical secular, medical scientist who would be willing to use the Hippocratic Oath symbolically to fill this function, this date is not too early, even though Gregory was still making the Enlightenment generalist's presence felt in the curriculum for another decade. Certainly, by the turn of the century, this process of increasing isolation was finished. Essentially no trace remained within the medical faculty of Enlightenment men who were comfortable crossing disciplinary boundaries to work simultaneously in what we would now call the disciplines of philosophy, theology, classics, the natural sciences, and medicine. Only when that isolation of medicine occurred did medical ethics completely lose its connections with the culture in which it rested and fill that void by grasping at the Hippocratic symbol.

WHY THE ISOLATION?

Why the isolation after the beginning of the nineteenth century? It is a question we can begin to address at this point for Scotland. In Part II we will ask the same question for England, and in Part III, for the United States, New Zealand, and Canada. What happened at the end of the eighteenth century that stopped the dialogue between the medical community and the humanists?

Young Age of Entry into College or Medical School

One striking feature of the Scottish medical education system of the nineteenth century is the young age of entry into medical school. The full story is more complicated, however. Whereas nineteenth-century Scottish physicians were entering college or medical school at a very young age, the pattern was not necessarily different in the eighteenth century. Thus our account will have to consider the age of entry into medicine in the eighteenth century and what the differences were sociologically as well as in age.

In Scotland in the nineteenth century (and, as we shall see, in England and in New Zealand), students could move directly into medical school from secondary school, giving them no real exposure as young adults to the great literature, history, philosophy, or theological thought of the day. A great deal of evidence about the young age and poor preparation of early nineteenth-century university and medical school students is found in the report of the Commission for Visiting the Universities and Colleges in Scotland (1837).

Age of Entering College

The transcript includes considerable evidence of the young age and the poor preparation of students. Consider first the general problem of university students and then more specifically those in medical studies. In responding to a query from a commission member, the Principal of the university, The Very Rev. Dr. George Husband Baird, D.D., addressed the age of students at the college (not the medical school): "The greater portion of them, on first entering to the college, which they do at an average from the age of 12 to 15, are nearly of the same age" (Commission 1837, p. 80).

Even younger ages were apparently possible, though unlikely. Since admission to classes was under the control of the individual professor, who issued the student a "ticket" for a fee, the principal was unable to rule out even a 10-year-old attending a class. He noted, "I cannot conceive that any Professor would give a ticket to a boy of 10 or 12 years of age to go to Moral or Natural Philosophy . . . , but I know no regulation of the University, or any statute of the Town-council, prohibiting it" (Commission 1837, p. 84).

He went on to report that the typical age for students in the "Humanity Class" was 13 to 15, though "many of them enter[ed] much sooner" (Commission 1837, p. 85). Greek professor George Dunbar confirmed this to be the average age (Commission 1837, p. 89). The principal acknowledged that some students came at a somewhat older age, but they were still very young and apparently poorly prepared.[29]

Medical Students

This pattern was found among medical students as well. The minimum age at Edinburgh for the degree of Doctor of Medicine was normally 21[30] (Commission 1837, p. 195). Apparently, a minimum age had to be adopted because some students were claiming to have finished their studies before that age.

But some eighteenth-century medical students also went directly to medical school and graduated at an early age. Born in 1724, Gregory entered the University of Edinburgh in 1742 to study medicine. By then he had graduated from King's College and served as an apprentice to his physician brother (McCullough 1998, pp. 31–32; Haakonssen 1997, p. 46). We shall see, however, that the key figures in medical ethics in England and the United States in the eighteenth century began their medi-cal education much later. Nevertheless, the age alone of entering students cannot explain the differences between a Gregory and the nineteenth-century figures.

Changing Social Class and More Practical Interests of Medical Students

If young age alone is not the explanation for the difference between the last de-cades of the eighteenth century and the first years of the nineteenth, then some-thing else is critical: the shift in social class and more practical interests of the students of the nineteenth century.

Social Class Shift

One critical factor can be gleaned from a closer look at Gregory's family environ-ment. Gregory's blood line ran very blue. In Chapter 1 we traced the long line of distinguished, academic Gregories from which he descended. His ancestors were distinguished in mathematics, mechanics, and astronomy. They included clergymen as well. Relatives included Rob Roy and Thomas Reid. His father was a physician and professor of medicine at King's College, as was his half-brother. His father's second wife, John's mother, was the daughter of a King's College Principal. Greg-ory took the classical course of study at Aberdeen Grammar School and enrolled at King's College under the supervision of his grandfather, who not only played a role in raising him after his own father died but also was the principal of the school. According to A. F. Tytler, Gregory's eighteenth-century biographer, "he was a good classical scholar, and entered warmly into the beauties of the ancient authors; thence deriving a faculty of acutely discriminating the excellencies and defects of literary composition, and forming for himself that pure, simply-elegant, and perspicuous style, which is the characteristic of his writing" (Tytler 1788, p. 27, quoted in McCullough 1998, p. 31). Thus, even though he entered King's Col-lege at a young age, his education was as much the responsibility of his re-markable family. His study under his father, half-brother, cousin, and maternal grandfather as well as his study at college made him, by age 16, richly prepared in the classics, mathematics, ethics, and natural philosophy.

   By contrast, in the nineteenth century, the students, as assessed by their faculty, had much weaker social and intellectual connections. There was a noticeable shift in social class from the aristocratic families, who could prepare even young stu-dents in the home and in the elite preparatory schools, to a much more modest fa-milial and academic environment. The 1826 Commission, questioning William Pulteney Alison, Dean of the faculty of Medicine and Professor of the Theory of Physic, was told that students of the 1820s were not like those of old. The students of former times were more aristocratic, a well-prepared elite. Students of Alison's day, by contrast, entered the school more easily and with less preparation.[31]

Part of the reason for this lower standard in literary and philosophical education was, undoubtedly, a lack of commitment of the faculty. When it was Alexander
Monro, Tertius's turn to be interviewed, he spent almost all his time explaining
his teaching of anatomy and defending the claim that the professor of surgery could
do the job of teaching anatomy. Like almost all the other faculty, he was pressed
on the importance of literary education for medical students and failed to see its
importance (Commission 1837, p. 277).

As Haakonssen (1997, pp. 134–35) has described, Gregory saw the medical
profession as being connected with the gentry and aristocracy. He saw British
physicians as "gentlemen of the best families, distinguished for their spirit and
genius . . . well born and genteely educated" (Gregory 1772, p. 7) This applies to
what Christopher Lawrence has called the "old order" (see also Lawrence 1985,
pp. 153–76, especially p. 170), but "the forty years 1790–1830 saw the draining
of power and patronage from the old order of physicians, lawyers, landed gentry
and literati" (Lawrence 1988b, p. 278).

Poorer Preparation of Students

Correlated with the change in social class of the medical student was a decline in
the quality of students' preparation. The problem was a more general one in the
nineteenth-century university. During the 1826 commission hearings, a questioner
asked George Dunbar, the professor of Greek, about making a Master of Arts a
requirement for students entering the Divinity Hall, which, he pointed out, had
been a requirement "in the middle of the last century." Dunbar strongly endorsed
restoring the requirement (Commission 1837, p. 95).

In response to a query about attendance at classes, the Edinburgh principal re-
plied, "In the higher classes I do not know that it is possible to take means to ascertain whether each student is daily in attendance; and I have no reason to believe
that means are so taken to ascertain it" (Commission 1837, p. 83). Regarding the
medical students, he revealed the minimalist standards: "It is necessary for every
medical student to enrol his name in the album of the University every month, for
it was found, some years ago, that occasionally individuals came down from
England, and took out class tickets, and pleaded this as a ground of graduation;
and now, by making them enrol their names once a-month [sic], we are such that
at least six times in the course of the winter they are in town" (Commission 1837,
p. 83).[32] Nor can we assume that the medical student was expected to have advance preparation in the college (Commission 1837, p. 84).

John Leslie, Esq., professor of natural philosophy at Edinburgh, also emphasized to the 1826 commission that the quality of preparation of medical students
had declined:

Till beyond the beginning of the last century our young men, after they had finished their
course of Philosophy at home, generally went to France or Holland for the study of Law

or Medicine. The title of A.M. was an indispensable requisite to the obtaining the degree of Doctor in Physic and at Glasgow and some other Universities, it is the practice, even at present, to bestow that title *pro forma*, before the Medical Degree is conferred. I am persuaded, however, that it would be inexpedient and impracticable now to exact from the candidate in Physic an attendance upon all the regular classes in Literature and philosophy. It will be more judicious, at least for some time hence, to rest satisfied with a moderate share of classical knowledge. . . . To require higher attainments would only repel strangers from our gates. They would either abandon the hope of obtaining a degree, and remit their exertions, or they would seek that boon in other quarters.

(Commission 1837, p. 154)

To Leslie the real controversy was the relative emphasis on general science classes and those in medicine. Leslie was an advocate for more general science (Commission 1837, p. 155). Leslie's proposal was for more "philosophical" classes, but by "philosophical" he meant what we would call "natural sciences," not moral philosophy. Leslie was acutely aware of the decline in preparation of medical students in comparison with former times. He testified, "my object is to raise the character of the medical profession, which at a former period, was the most distinguished by its various and extensive learning" (Commission 1837, pp. 155–56).

Compounding the problems of early age of entry into the medical curriculum and poor preparation was the fact that there were no examinations prior to entering classes (Commission 1837, p. 81). A course in moral philosophy was offered, but, according to John Wilson, Esq., Professor of Moral Philosophy, only those in the Divinity Hall had to take it (Commission 1837, p. 114). When Edinburgh professor of Greek, George Dunbar, was asked whether students in the medical school had attended the more basic "junior" classes prior to medical school, his answer was, "I do not think that of those who are going forward to the study of Medicine, more than four or five have attended the junior classes" (Commission 1837, p. 99). The faculty of arts wanted to extend the requirement that medical students take literary and philosophical classes. A proposal to that effect was put before the Senatus Academicus, but it was not sanctioned as being necessary to form a part of the education of medical students (Commission 1837, p. 100).

Professor Dr. Andrew Duncan, Junior, the professor of Materia Medica and son of a professor of the Theory of Physic, was put on the spot on this issue. The questioner attempted to get him to admit that medical students were not as well prepared in "liberal study" as they were in earlier years. Duncan did not want to admit it, but could not support his claim to the liberal education of current students in anything other than modern languages (Commission 1837, pp. 235).

The Problem of "Strangers"

The questioner then opened the door for Duncan to defend the lesser preparation of current medical students. In his response, Duncan hit on a theme that occurs repeatedly in the commission hearings: "strangers," that is, foreign medical students, were populating the school and their preparation was inferior, watering down the entire class. The question and Duncan's response are revealing:

"What particular objection occurs to you to requiring evidence of having attended Philosophical classes in the Universities previously to taking the degree of Medicine?"

"The objection which occurs to me, and which is in my own mind quite conclusive against it, is, that a very large proportion of our graduates come from England and Ireland, where, during the period of their life before they begin their professional study, they have no means of attending those branches in a University, although they may acquire a moderate knowledge of them in schools, both public and private, and from their own private exertions. If we were to require evidence of their having attended them in Universities in addition to the four years of professional study, the degree here could not be obtained without a residence of not less than six or eight years, the effect of which would be that these gentlemen would take no degree at all."

. (Commission 1837, p. 236)

In the 13-year period before the Commission hearings, only 422 of the 1354 graduates had been Scots. As the dean put it:

When we contemplate the imposition on all graduates of a preliminary course of academical education, not only in the classes but likewise in Mathematics, Natural Philosophy, Natural History, Moral Philosophy, and Logic, . . . we must remember that a great proportion of the strangers have not the means of acquiring information in all these. . . . To require a full course of study on all these subjects previously, of all our candidates, would be to place the medical degree in many cases beyond their reach, and compel them to practise upon inferior degrees only.

(Commission 1837, p. 197)

Competition with Inferior Medical Schools

The Edinburgh faculty felt that the public was satisfied, indeed more satisfied, with physicians who had a more modest, practical education. When the Commission turned to Dean William Pulteney Alison, he spoke of education that was "cheaper" and "merely professional" in ways that were not particularly negative. At least in the eye of the public, these seemed to be virtues. The school at Edinburgh was faced with meeting this public demand or losing its students.[33]

A Faculty Content with a More Pragmatic and Technical Curriculum to Meet the Competition

The dean was a clear supporter of the more practical, technical education of medical students to meet the competition and supply what the public demanded. When asked if he would support a requirement that students take the degree of Master of Arts before going to medical school, Alison opposed it, saying, "I think I would require a knowledge of French, Latin, and Mathematics. I do not say that I would go farther than that." (Commission 1837, p. 203).

In page after page of the commision's report, commission members pressed their concern about the lack of philosophical and literary preparation of medical students. It was clearly a sore point for them. Yet one faculty member after another rejected proposals to add "philosophical classes" (Commission 1837, pp. 239, 253). The same tolerance of thin preparation in philosophical and scientific subjects existed at the other Scottish medical schools. Only The University of Aberdeen required a Master of Arts. St. Andrews and Glasgow did not (Commission 1837, p. 210).

Scientific Data Overload

The third possible explanation of the isolation of physicians is the emergence of medicine as a science with an enormous literature to be mastered. By the end of the eighteenth century, medicine was generating a rapidly expanding scientific knowledge base, which must have left students feeling that it was all they could do to keep up with the narrower, more technical subject matter. Those familiar with the medical school admissions process recognized the pressure on the young aspirants to become proficient in the sciences. One strayed into the humanities at great peril.

In Scotland of the eighteenth century, Enlightenment scholars took the world's knowledge as their domain. As a regent at Aberdeen, Gregory taught the entire range of knowledge before turning his attention more narrowly to medicine. Gregory published in philosophy and clinical medicine as well as in medical ethics. To a lesser degree, these eclectic interests were also seen in Gregory's predecessor, the philosopher–physician Sir John Pringle, his contemporary; William Cullen; and his son, James, as well as in the late eighteenth-century to early nineteenth-century philosopher Dugald Stewart.

By contrast, another group of Scottish physicians had much narrower interests. This pattern can be traced back to the first Alexander Monro, Gregory's older faculty colleague. He also wrote for his daughter, as Gregory did, but most of his writing was narrowly medical, scientific, and technical. Medicine was on the verge of becoming a highly specialized field in which whole careers would have to be spent mastering tiny areas in which a great deal of knowledge had been and was continuing to be generated. These features of the early nineteenth century—the young age of medical students, the change in social class of physicians, and the explosion of scientific knowledge—make the Enlightenment goal of mastering all of human knowledge an impossibility. This meant that Scottish medical students were getting a substantially different education than their predecessors a few decades earlier. Determining that these same forces occur in England and the colonies will require further work. That is the task of the next chapters.

II

ENGLAND

3

EIGHTEENTH-CENTURY ENGLAND'S INTEGRATION OF MEDICINE AND THE HUMANITIES

> Last night I received a copy of your work on medical Jurisprudence, and this morning I have given to the perusal of it all the time I could. . . . I have found opportunities for conversation and friendship with a class of men, whom after a long and attentive survey of character, I have found to be *the most enlightened* professional persons in the circle of human arts and sciences
>
>   Letter from the Rev. Samuel Parr, LL.D. to Dr. Percival. Hattan,
>   Sept. 24, 1794 regarding Thomas Percival's *Medical Jurisprudence*
>   (E. Percival 1807, pp. cxci, cxciii)

In the second half of the eighteenth century, while Scotland was teeming with life in the humanities and medicine and its leading physicians were pursuing vigorous discussions with its leading philosophers and theologians, England was also emerging into the era of modern medicine. It also had a history of philosophers and theologians who practiced medicine and the sciences. This was, after all, the land of Bacon and Newton. It was the home of the physician/philosopher, John Locke. As was observed by A. W. Hill, a student of John Wesley's linking of theology and medicine, the "study of physic formed part of a gentleman's education alongside classical and philosophical studies" (Hill 1958, p. 29). Just as Gregory was awarded a medical degree with the benefit of completing formal study at the institution that awarded the degree, sometimes clergy were given similar university recognition in medicine. For example, in 1719 a medical doctorate was awarded gratis by

Aberdeen's King's College to the Reverend Alexander Anderson, Minister of Duffus, as "being a gentleman of approved skill in physic" (Hill 1958, p. 29). Sometimes medical credentials were even awarded by the church. Joseph Cam and John Spink, two graduates of Marischal College, Aberdeen, already possessed licenses to "practise physick" that had been awarded by the Archbishop of Canterbury (Hill 1958, p. 30). It is not known when, if ever, William Cullen, the philosophically inclined colleague of John Gregory encountered in the previous chapter, ever received formal sanction to practice medicine (Hill 1958, p. 30). This chapter will explore the thought of several participants in the English version of this interaction, men who jointly were responsible for the shaping of Anglo-American medical ethics.

A good early example of a clergyman who also practiced medicine was James Clegg (1679–1755). He was a Presbyterian minister, serving a church at Chapel-en-le-Firth, and a practicing physician. At age 50 he began a diary that he kept for the next 25 years (Clegg 1981). It incorporated earlier written notes and provides a view of a life that intermixed parish work with visits to the sick. From the early 1720s Clegg practiced medicine, even though he was not formally credentialed. He was threatened, not by physicians, but by ecclesiastical authorities, for practicing without a license. This troubled him, so he applied for a university credential, first unsuccessfully to Edinburgh and then with more success to Aberdeen University. In October 1729 he recorded the following:

Being this month created Doctor of Physick by a Diploma Medicum from the University of Aberdeen in North Brittain upon the Testimonials and Recommendations of Dr. Nettleton of Halifax, Dr. Dixon of Bolton and Dr. Latham of Finderne I think it is now proper to keep a more exact account of my patients, their diseases, ye remedies prescribed.

(Clegg 1981, p. 50)

Clegg maintained active medical and clerical practices until his death in 1755.

JOHN WESLEY

In recounting the story of physician–humanist interaction, one figure is particularly intriguing. John Wesley (1703–1791), founder of the religious denomination of Methodism, might not be the most obvious character to explore in this regard. Some think of him as a horseback-riding evangelist to England's lower classes, whose heart was "strangely warmed" after a mid-Atlantic crisis that brought him in contact with Moravian Brethren who reoriented his views of religion.

Wesley as Humanist Intellectual

Wesley fits that description, but he was a much more complex figure.[1] He was also an Oxford don—a fellow of Lincoln College. In addition to many volumes of sermons, letters, hymns, and theology, he did a remarkable amount of scholarship.

Admittedly in the looser style of the eighteenth century, borrowing copiously from other authors, he wrote grammars for five languages (English, French, Latin, Greek, and Hebrew). He also published *The Complete English Dictionary, The Concise Ecclesiastical History* (in four volumes), *The Concise History of England from the Earliest Times to the Death of George II*, and *A Survey of the Wisdom of God in the Creation, or a Compendium of Natural Philosophy* (in five volumes) (Shepherd 1966, pp. 83–96). The edition of his collected works that was published while he was alive extended to 32 volumes (Wesley 1771–74).[2] In addition, he was responsible for producing a 50-volume *Christian Library* (Wesley 1749–55) that contained his abridgements of what he considered to be the essential English-language literature of the history of the world. The library included classical works of the early church fathers as well as many Puritan and other seventeenth- and eighteenth-century works.[3] He was also something of a Locke scholar (Brantley 1984).

Wesley as a Serious Student of Medicine

While many know of Wesley's contribution to Protestant religious denomination-alism, fewer are aware of his influence in science and medicine. Yet for good reason, he has been called the most influential figure in *medicine* of eighteenth-century England. He was widely read in medicine as well as philosophy and theology. He ran what we might call storefront health clinics for his parishioners and others who could never afford the costly care of the formally educated and credentialed physician. He was the author of the best-selling *Primitive Physick* (1747), a book of simple medical remedies, which went through at least 23 editions before his death to a total of at least 35, appearing regularly well into the nineteenth century.[4] Its reception in the new world is marked by the appearance of an American edition annexed to a book by an American physician providing advice to families who could not consult regularly with physicians (Wilkins, 1795). The book is still in print (Wesley, 1999).

Wesley was also a social reformer. His Arminianism led him to a more aggressive social activism.[5] As might be expected from his focus on evangelizing the lower classes, he was committed to improving the welfare of the poor. He crusaded for the elimination of poverty and preached often on the subject (MacArthur 1936; Marquardt 1992, pp. 27–48). His views on the evils of slavery evolved so that by the last decades of his life he was a fervent spokesperson in the antislavery movement (Marquardt 1992, pp. 70–75). He was also active in the reform of prisons (Marquardt 1992, pp. 77–86).

Wesley's Feuds with Orthodox Medical Practitioners

The Oxford don, Locke scholar, Arminian theological revolutionary, failed missionary, evangelist to coal miners, social reformer, writer of hymns, and reluctant founder of a denomination was also a serious student of medicine. In fact, his passionate commitment to the poor was directly related to his aggressive pursuit of medicine. In his medicine as well as in his theology he was firmly committed to the Protestant doctrine of the priesthood of all believers. His hostility toward orthodox, establishment physicians was palpable. The small number of practitioners meant that the ordinary lower-class citizen had no possibility of obtaining their services. Moreover, Wesley was convinced that physicians intentionally practiced "polypharmacy," the combining of many drugs when one would work at least as well, to increase the physician's prestige and fee. He appealed to the Enlightenment principle of common sense to support this view:

The common method of compounding and de-compounding medicines, can never be reconciled to Common Sense, Experience shews, that one thing will cure most disorders, at least as well as twenty put together. Then why do you add the other nineteen? Only to swell the Apothecary's bill: nay, possibly, on purpose to prolong the distemper, that the Doctor and he may divide the spoil.

(Wesley 1785, p. xi)

Wesley firmly believed that elite physicians, like their Hippocratic ancestors, were intentionally obscure, the more to increase their god-like images as well as their profits.[6]

To this the Protestant reformer, who believed the text should be rendered plain and simple and placed in the hands of the layman, rebelled. He claimed that he first tried to get his parishioners treated in hospitals, but, as he made clear in a letter to the Reverend Vincent Perronet, Vicar of Shoreham, "upon the trial [of the hospital] we found there was indeed less expense, but no more good than before" (cited in Hill 1958, p. 11). He goes on to explain to the vicar that this led him to pursue medical knowledge himself:

At length I thought of a kind of desperate expedient. "I will prepare and give them physic myself." For six or seven and twenty years I made Anatomy and Physic the diversion of my leisure hours: though I never properly studied them, unless for a few months when I was going to America, where I imagined I might be of some service to those who had no regular physician among them. I applied to it again. I took into my assistance an apothecary and an experienced surgeon: resolving at the same time not to go out of my depth, but to leave all difficult and complicated cases to such physicians as the patients should choose.

(Quoted in Hill 1958, p. 11)

When one compares this quarter century of study with the sometimes irregular education of those who passed as full-fledged practitioners, the claim of Wesley to be a physician to the poor is not as preposterous as it might appear to the twenty-first–century reader. He opened dispensaries in London, Bristol, and Newcastle, and wrote some of the most important and widely read medical literature of his day.

Primitive Physick

These medical interests led to publishing the first edition of *Primitive Physick* in 1747. It could be thought of as the "Dr. Spock" for adults of Wesley's time. It consists of a provocative preface and an alphabetically presented "collection of receipts." The exact number changed over the years. For example, my 21st edition contains 288 sections arranged from "Abortion, (to prevent)" to five paragraphs on "Wounds." The latter, in addition to a general discussion of wounds, includes "Inward Wounds," Putrid Wounds, "Wounded Tendons," and "To open a Wound that is closed too soon." Each section contains a list of "home remedy" treatments, normally presented from the simplest to the most complex (Wesley 1785, pp. 114–15).

In keeping with Wesley's suspicion of complex and harsh new remedies from elite physicians, he preferred simple, easily available treatments. For example,

22. *To prevent Swelling from a Bruise.*
Immediately apply a Cloth, five or six times doubled, dipt in *cold Water*, and new dipt when it grow's warm : Tried.

(Wesley 1785, p. 24)

He would always indicate the treatments he had tried personally, but he was exceedingly hostile to some of the standard, more harsh therapies of the day. He aggressively attacked more orthodox physician practices such as blood-letting and the use of mercury compounds. In his journal for April 5, 1756, he wrote,

Inquiring for one whom I saw three or four days ago in the height of a violent pleurisy, I found he was perfectly recovered, and returned into the country. A brimstone-plaster in a few minutes took away both the pain and the fever. O why will physicians play with the lives of their patients!

(Wesley 1958, Vol. 2, p. 360)

Though not rigidly critical, he was also skeptical of the widespread use of mercury, which, in his 1755 postscript, he considered "extremely dangerous."[7]

Wesley's general philosophy of medicine was that new, complex, "Herculean" remedies were not only dangerous but could be part of a conspiracy of apothecary and physician to obfuscate treatment and increase income. Even if regular practitioners were acceptable for serious cases, they were not accessible to the ordinary masses and probably were not good for them even if these physicians could be obtained. Fresh air, clean water, and clean living were, for Wesley, the best of God's gifts to humans.

Hawes

As one might expect, this attitude left Wesley with no more friends among the elite physicians than he had among the Anglican clergy. He showed proper reverence for the great physicians of an earlier generation, referring to "the great and good Dr. *Sydenham*" (Wesley 1785, p. ix) and "the great *Boerhave*" (Wesley 1785, p. xi) as well as "the learned and ingenious Dr. *Cheyne*" (Wesley 1785, p. ix). In fact, it is from George Cheyne (1674–1743) that Wesley took his "few plain, easy rules" for health, which emphasized good air, cleanliness, moderation in diet, consumption of plenty of water, sleep, and exercise.[8] We have also noted the implied endorsement of American physician, Henry Wilkins (1795), who included the full text of the 24th edition of *Primitive Physic* in his own advice to those without physicians. Wesley's preferred appeal, however, was to the Protestant and Enlightenment standard of "Experience, Common Sense, and the common Interest of Mankind" (Wesley 1785, p. x).

His attitude particularly incensed the London physician William Hawes (1736–1808). Hawes came to the defense of the gentleman of the medical faculty. Hawes is remembered in a memoir as a humane man who took up the cause of hundreds of silk workers when their livelihood was threatened by cotton. He was devoted to the development of the humane society and was a well-known promoter of precautions to make sure people were not interred prematurely when they were not yet dead, but merely in a state of "suspended animation" (Hawes 1802). With Wesley, however, he was less humane. The title of his 1776 diatribe reveals his attitude well: *An Examination of The Rev. Mr. John Wesley*'s Primitive Physic: *Shewing That great Number of the Prescriptions therein contained, are founded on Ignorance of the Medical Art, and of the Power and Operation of medicines; and that it is a Publication calculated to do essential Injury to the Health of those Persons who may place Confidence in it. Interspersed with Medical Remarks and Practical Observation.* Hawes critiqued Wesley's recommendations on fever, in the process revealing that Hippocrates (and Galen) were emerging as the physician's standard of authority. He sarcastically noted,

What were *Hippocrates* and *Galen*, compared to John Wesley! [he then quotes Wesley] *Stamp . . . a handful of leaves of woodbine; put fair water into it, and use it cold, as a clyster. It* COMMONLY *CURES IN AN HOUR.* A more expeditious remedy need scarcely be wished for; much is it to be regretted, that its efficacy is not somewhat better authenticated!

(Hawes 1776, p. 45)

That Hawes's dialogue with Wesley included an understanding of Wesley's theology as well as his medicine is revealed in Hawes's hostile comments. He not only impugned Wesley's motives for publishing, suggesting that his interests were financial, but accused him of being "far enough from perfection," a dig at Wesley's unique doctrine of "Christian perfection." Wesley held that, through grace, it was possible for humans in this world to become "perfect" in their conduct (see "A Plain Account of Christian Perfection" in Wesley 1958, Vol. 11, pp. 366–446).[9] The conversation between theologian and orthodox practitioner remained a serious, sustained one.

Electricity

Wesley's innovation in medicine was influenced by the excitement over developments in the understanding of electricity. In Wesley's journal from February 17, 1753, he referred to letters from Benjamin Franklin that explained Franklin's understanding of the phenomenon (Wesley 1958, Vol. 2, p. 280). Wesley saw himself as one who could synthesize existing knowledge on subjects such as electricity, presenting it in a collected form to the broader public as well as to his own parishioners. In the last week of October 1759, he recorded in his journal that he spent Wednesday and Thursday "revising and perfecting a 'Treatise on Electricity'" (Wesley 1958, Vol. 2, p. 517). The result was the book *The Desideratum: or, Electricity Made Plain and Useful. By a Lover of Mankind, and Common Sense* (Wesley 1771). In the preface he claimed to "have endeavoured to comprize the sum of what has been hitherto published, on this curious and important subject by Mr. *Franklin*, Dr. *Hoadly*, Mr. *Wilson*, *Watson*, *Lovett*, *Freke*, *Martin*, *Watkins*, and in the *Monthly Magazines* (Wesley 1771, p. iii).[10]

While acknowledging his lack of expertise, Wesley revealed that he was actively engaged in the current scientific conversation, showing his commitment to the contemporary ether theory propounded by Newton, Cullen, and others. Indeed, Richard Lovett's volume had been published in 1756, only three years before Wesley took up the subject. In Wesley's essay he also showed his enthusiastic commitment to electricity as a desirable (hence, his title) all-purpose remedy.[11] At the same time, he continued on his criticism of the "gentleman of the faculty" for their resistance to these scientific innovations:

> Be this as it may, Mr. *Lovett* is of opinion, "the electrical method of treating disorders, cannot be expected to arrive at any considerable degree of perfection, till administered and applied by the gentlemen of the faculty." Nay then, *quanta de spe decidi!* All my hopes are at an end. For when will it be administered and applied by them? Truly *ad Græcas Calendas*. Not till the gentlemen of the faculty have more regard to the interest of their neighbours than their own, at least, not till there are no apothecaries in the land: Or till physicians are independent of them.
>
> (Wesley 1771, p. vi).[12]

That Wesley's study of electricity and the scientific literature was sustained over a considerable period of time is seen by another journal entry some eight years after completing the *Desideratum* volume. Clearly, his enthusiasm for electricity's medicinal uses had not decreased, nor had his sense that he could judge the accuracy of the work of distinguished writers. On January 4, 1768, he makes the following comment:

> At my Leisure hours this week, I read Dr. Priestley's ingenious book on Electricity. He seems to have accurately collected and well digested all that is known on that curious subject. But how little is that all! Indeed the use of it we know; at least, in some good

degree. We know it is a thousand medicines in one: In particular, that it is the most effica-
cious medicine, in nervous disorders of every kind, which has ever yet been discovered.

(Wesley 1958, Vol. 3, p. 311)[13]

All of this may sound bizarre, like a theologian out of his depths, until one real-
izes what Wesley's three major uses for electricity in his clinical practice were:
first, for nervous disorders and "lunacy," including what we would call depression (Wesley 1785, pp. 77, 81); second, for heart problems, including what we
would consider abnormal heart rhythms (Wesley 1785, p. 83); and third, in spite
of his earlier qualifications regarding "palsies," for paralyzed muscles. It is striking that at the beginning of the twenty-first century, electrical shock is current, if
controversial, therapy for depression, is standard treatment for cardiac arrhythmias,
and is experimental treatment for muscle paralysis. In Wesley's era, bleeding and
mercury were standard treatments from more fashionable physicians serving the
elite.

Our conclusion is not that Wesley was a professional medical practitioner like
Gregory or Monro or Hawes. Quite obviously he brought to his practice of medicine a radical reformist, Protestant clerical perspective that was hostile to the establishment medical practitioners. Our conclusion must instead be that Wesley
was in a sustained conversation with these practitioners, often a heated one, but a
conversation nonetheless. He was reading the latest theories, was in correspondence with the likes of Franklin, and knew when his theological commitments
forced him to part company with the beliefs and practices of the mainstream.
Moreover, the mainstream—Hawes and Franklin, for example—knew enough of
his thought to know when they disagreed.

Wesley's Contact with Gregory, Monro, and Hamilton

One last episode deserves mention before we turn to others in the eighteenth-
century English conversation. It turns out that Wesley's contact with medicine, at
least on one occasion, brought him into direct communication with several in the
Scottish scene we encountered in Chapter 1. In the spring of 1772, Wesley was
preaching in Scotland. On May 5 he recorded in his journal that, during his travels, he read Beattie's "Inquiry after Truth," which Wesley described as "ingenious"
(Wesley 1958, Vol. 3, p. 462). He couldn't resist recording his opinion of Hume,
whom he called a "minute philosopher," and "the most insolent despiser of truth
and virtue that ever appeared in the world" (Wesley 1958, Vol. 3, p. 462).

He traveled on to Leith, near Edinburgh, where he was scheduled to preach.
On May 18 he was seen by "Dr. Hamilton," who "brought with him Dr. Monro
and Dr. Gregory." Wesley, a world-class circuit rider, had been injured some three
or four years previously when his horse stumbled, throwing him on the pommel
of his saddle (Hill 1958, p. 43). The Hamilton referred to was not either of the
Hamiltons who were professors of medicine at Edinburgh (and the targets of James

Gregory's hostility), but rather a practitioner (who lived from 1740 to 1827) who was a friend of Wesley's and a member of the Methodist Society at Dunbar. His two colleagues, however, were physicians we have previously encountered: James Gregory (son of John) and Alexander Monro, Secundus. According to Wesley, they assured him of his diagnosis and that there was "but one method of cure" (Wesley 1958, Vol. 3, p. 463). Unfortunately, that cure was not recorded by Wesley. However, his continuing skepticism about physicians was. He added in his journal, "perhaps but one natural one; but I think God has more than one method of healing either the soul or the body" (Wesley 1958, Vol. 3, p. 463).

Wesley's radical Protestant belief that each person should know his or her condition and be responsible for the use of simple therapies, and his long-term skepticism about the authority of the physician surface once again. He shows the intimate connection between one's ethical and religious beliefs and the foundations for the practice of medicine. Moreover, he was in close communication about these matters with the scientists and medical people of his day. No matter how they disagreed, as often they did, they were in the same conversation. He did not, however, move to a formal and explicit discussion of health professional ethics.

GISBORNE

More directly in this conversation was an Anglican clergyman named Thomas Gisborne (1758–1846).[14] Descended from a distinguished family that included mayors of Derby, not far from Clegg's home, Gisborne was a student at St. John's College, Cambridge. In 1783 he received a perpetual curacy at Barton-under-Needlewood near an estate he had inherited from his father.

Gisborne was a college friend and neighbor of the anti-slavery leader, William Wilberforce (1759–1833), who was also a correspondent of John Wesley's (see Wesley 1958, Vol. 13, p. 153). Gisborne wrote against slavery (Gisborne 1792), but was also known for his more theoretical interest in philosophical ethics. His *Principles of Moral Philosophy* was an attack on the utilitarian reasoning of William Paley and a defense of a more rigorous moral stance, a view that would eventually be reflected in his medical ethics as well (Gisborne 1789).

For our purposes, Gisborne's most important work is his 1794 volume, *An Enquiry into the Duties of Men in the Higher and Middle Classes of Society in Great Britain Resulting from their Respective Stations, Professions and Employments*. It contains 15 chapters, one each devoted to the special "duties of station" attached to such roles as that of the sovereign, peers (of the house of lords), members of the House of Commons, military officers, lawyers, clergy, persons engaged in trades and business, and "private gentlemen." A crucial chapter, "On the Duties of Physicians," played an important role in shaping Anglo-American professional medical ethics (Gisborne 1794, pp. 383–426). The book went through six editions by 1811. The key chapter on physicians appeared separately as late as 1847.

Gisborne provides vivid evidence of the communication among the intelligentsia and how their thought passed back and forth among theologians and philosophers on the one hand and members of the other learned professions, including physicians, on the other. An introductory footnote acknowledges the interchange:

In some part of this chapter I am indebted for several hints to Dr. Gregory's Preliminary Lecture on the Duties and Offices of a Physician: and for others to the first part of a treatise entitled "Medical Jurisprudence, or a "Code of Ethics and Institutes adapted to the Professions of Physic and Surgery," by my excellent friend Dr. Percival of Manchester; which, as far as it was then composed, was communicated to me by him in the kindest manner.

(Gisborne 1794, p. 383).[15]

The first section of Gisborne's chapter constitutes advice to the medical student. He is not only knowledgeable about the late eighteenth-century medical education curriculum but bold in presuming to give the student advice on which courses were most important. Theory and practice of physic and anatomy are on the one hand "foremost in point of importance, but the student should have acquaintance with the principle of surgery" (Gisborne 1794, pp. 387–88). On the other hand, "the peculiar object of the Student is not to distinguish himself as a chemist, as a botanist, or as a natural philosopher" (p. 388). Also, "a portion of his leisure will be usefully and laudably devoted to a deeper study of the various works of God, of the laws to which they are subject, and of the properties which they possess" (p. 388). He presumes a knowledge of Greek and Latin and a "certain degree of legal knowledge." He urges reading "works of general information and of taste" (p. 390). But no studies, whether professional or otherwise, ought to encroach on "higher duties," i.e., public worship and "private perusal and investigation of the Scriptures" (p. 390). In short, he presupposes a classical education of the eighteenth-century English gentleman.

The next section is devoted to the peculiar situation of the physician when he begins practicing. Gisborne warns of the dangers of assuming that one knows more than one actually does, of parading one's knowledge and imposing on the unwary "solemn, pompous, and consequential deportment" (p. 395). Sounding like Wesley, he warns of using "technical terms and learned trifling" to cause oneself to be more highly esteemed.

It is in the third section, devoted to the general duties of practice, that Gisborne's dialogue with his physician colleagues, Gregory and Percival, become most apparent. Gisborne's list of the virtues of the physician reflects the moral psychology of the period. He endorses "sympathy with the sufferer" and a list of virtues—steadiness, authority, kindness, compassion, tenderness, and benevolence—which overlaps the list endorsed by Percival (Gisborne 1794, p. 397). He is particularly attuned to the tendencies of physicians to withhold troublesome information and provide exaggerated optimism. Gisborne comes down four-square in favor of avoiding lies: "[The physician] is at liberty to say little; but let that little be true" (p. 401).

Gisborne's use of his texts is revealing. Even though he claims to have had access to Gregory, at least the 1770 version of his lectures the discussion of deceiving patients does not make reference to Gregory. Since Gregory's endorsement of benevolent deception appears essentially unchanged in both the 1770 (p. 32) and 1772 (p. 33) versions, it leads one to wonder why Gisborne spares Gregory here.

Instead he provides gentle, but clear criticism of Percival, whose ambivalence about deceiving the patient places him in between Gregory and Gisborne on this issue. Citing Percival's *Medical Jurisprudence*, the early version of what, as we shall soon see, will become the most critical founding document of Anglo-American physician ethics, Gisborne endorses Percival's view that a surgeon "assure the patient that every thing goes on well, *if that declaration can be made with truth*" (Gisborne 1794, p. 401, italics in original). He goes on to say, however, that this view can be extended to the situations at the hand of the physician and even of "nature." But, says, Gisborne, "truth and conscience forbid the Physician to cheer him by giving promises, and raising expectations, which are known or intended to be delusive" (p. 401). He accepts Percival's view that there is a duty to reveal the diagnosis to the relatives, but adds, "on many occasions it may be the duty of the Physician spontaneously to reveal it to the patient himself" p. 402). This is clearly pushing Percival to go beyond his more timid stance, a position that fits Gisborne's deontological critique of Paley's consequentialism.

Later in the third section Gisborne takes up the crucial problem for intraprofessional relations of the day, the relations among physicians, surgeons, and apothecaries. Here Gisborne is promoting a harmony among the practitioners that is in accord with Percival's views. Gisborne quotes Gregory (1770, p. 45), who points out that physicians, who have the best education and the "best parts," must depend on apothecaries for their success and that the apothecary is often repaid with "pain and indignation" (Gisborne 1794, p. 413, quoting Gregory 1770, p. 45).[16]

Later, in Part IV, in which Gisborne turns to the ways a physician should spend his leisure time in study, he returns once again to quoting Gregory's *Observations*. In addressing the charge that physicians have shown infidelity and contempt of religion (p. 421), Gisborne claims that this charge has been "strenuously repelled by Dr. Gregory," perhaps reflecting his knowledge that Gregory, along with Reid and Beattie, was an active defender of religion against the likes of Hume. In a potent footnote, Gisborne shows his dislike of Hume, referring to his views as a prejudice that is "truly surprising." He cannot resist adding, "I had almost said childish" (p. 423, note q).

THOMAS PERCIVAL

While the previous discussion should make clear that Gisborne, the philosopher/ cleric, was reading the scholarly physicians of the Enlightenment, it needs to be stated that the reverse is true regarding the physicians in England, just as in Scotland. To see this dialogue at its best we should turn to Thomas Percival.

A Man of the Enlightenment

Thomas Percival (1740–1804), who lived most of his adult life in Manchester, was a distinguished physician with remarkable accomplishments in cultural and philosophical undertakings.[17] He played a role in the English conversation between physicians and humanists that is, in many ways, analogous to that played by John Gregory in Scotland. More than any other figure in Anglo-American history, he is responsible for shaping physicians' professional medical ethics. His literary and philosophical interests are reflected in the title page of his posthumous *Works*, collected by his son, Edward, in 1807, which describes him as "Late Pres. of the Lit. and Phil. Soc. at Manchester; Member of the Royal Societies of Paris and of Lyons, of the Medical Societies of London, and of Aix en Provence, of the America. Acad. of arts, &c. and of the America. Phil. Soc. at Philadelphia" (E. Percival 1807, title page).

Edward prefaces the *Works* with a 262-page introduction to Thomas's life. It provides the best account of the development of his father's life. Thomas Percival was born in 1740 at Warrington in Lancashire, where his grandfather had practiced physic. It is a town about halfway between Liverpool and Manchester. Both of his parents died when he was three, leaving him in the care of an older sister. His father's older brother, also named Thomas, was a physician as well, having been a student of Boerhaave at Leyden. According to the biographical information provided by Edward Percival, the physician uncle had "combined with his medical pursuits the study of various other branches of knowledge. Following the steps of his great master, he directed his attention to Natural History, Chemistry, Ethics, and theology" (E. Percival 1807, p. iii). The uncle, however, died when young Thomas was 10, leaving him with a valuable library, "accession to his patrimonial fortune," a resolve to study medicine, and apparently an interest in combining medicine with ethics.

The young man developed an early proficiency in Greek and Latin at a private seminary near Warrington (E. Percival 1807, p. vi). Then, in 1757, he was the first student enrolled at the Warrington academy, which was established to provide education for dissenters who could not subscribe to the thirty-nine articles and were thus barred from English universities. There he pursued classical studies. Edward continues, revealing Percival's early interest in ethics: "The study of ethics, however, which formed an important branch of academical discipline, attracted his early curiosity. Guided by an able master, he explored the various and fascinating regions of moral science; and imbibed a partiality for these pursuits." (E. Percival 1807, p. viii).

Percival's Early Education

The "able master" to which Edward Percival referred was the Rev. John Seddon, who was a dissenting clergyman who became the *Rector Academiae*, or head of the institution at Warrington (E. Percival 1807, p. viii). In fact, it was soon after Percival's association with the Rev. Seddon that the family quit the Church of England to associate themselves with the Protestant dissenters.

The Warrington Academy catered to the needs of the dissenters.[18] It and the congregation in Warrington shared Presbyterian and Scottish intellectual influences. John Seddon's sermons and his theological and philosophical views reflected the positions of the clergy of Scotland with whom he had trained (Haakonssen 1997, pp. 96–97 and notes 3 and 4). He was a graduate of Glasgow University and was a disciple of Francis Hutcheson (McLachlan 1943, p. 11). The school exhibited a theological and philosophical pluralism, welcoming a diverse group of students from throughout Britain as well as the American colonies and the West Indies. The students studied Scottish thinkers such as Adam Smith and Adam Ferguson as well as the ethics of commerce and other vocations. But there was also a decided commitment to a liberal education with a sense that teachers were not preparing mere "professionals," that is, those merely proficient in a particular set of skills (Haakonssen 1997, p. 98). The third- and fourth-year students spent a great deal of time studying moral philosophy and theology (McLachlan 1943, pp. 39–40).

According to Haakonssen (p. 99), "most of the Warrington tutors, including all of Percival's teachers, received part of their training at Scottish universities, which at the time boasted some of Britain's foremost philosophers." McLachlan (p. 21) observes that "few nonconformist academies . . . owed nothing to the Scottish universities, and Warrington owed more than most." Four tutors had studied at Glasgow, two at Edinburgh, and one at Aberdeen. The Warrington curriculum was substantially influenced by George Turnbull, Francis Hutcheson, William Leechman, and Adam Smith.

All three tutors at Warrington while Percival was in residence (1757–1761) were graduates of Scottish universities.[19] John Taylor (1694–1761) was a graduate of Glasgow University. He taught divinity, Hebrew, and moral philosophy. Taylor's moral philosophy was more critical of Hutcheson than was Seddon's.[20] Taylor was a critic of moral-sense theory whereas Seddon defended it. Thus Percival was thrust into the midst of one of the great controversies of moral philosophy through two of his first teachers of the day. It is no wonder that he eventually emerged as a person capable of arbitrating between competing factions, whether they were philosophical or medical professional realms. I would suggest that far more important than the side that Percival took in this introduction to moral philosophical dispute is the fact that he was pressed into the debate. This was much less likely to occur among his nineteenth- and early twentieth-century medical ethics counterparts.

Haakonssen (p. 103) suggests that Percival ended up being more shaped by Taylor than by Seddon, but that the real influence of Scottish philosophy was not so much where Percival landed on the highly abstract theoretical issue of moral-sense theory, but rather the importance of the specification of practical moral duties or rules of virtuous conduct. As long as one did not completely reject the idea of the moral sense, this ethics of duty was not challenged. That clearly Percival did not do. Haakonssen concludes, "it is the knowledge of these duties that both the followers and antagonists of Hutcheson's system could agree upon and this was the primary lesson taught in the classes of both Seddon and Taylor" (Haakonssen 1997, p. 104).

The other tutor at Warrington who was a major influence on Percival was John Aiken, Sr. (1713–80). After study at Northampton Academy, he was educated at King's College, Aberdeen—Gregory's intellectual home. In fact, Aiken was a lifelong friend of Thomas Reid (McLachlan 1943, p. 49–50). Aiken taught languages, belles lettres, logic, and history, and incorporated his interest in the Greek classics in his courses so much as to make them almost a course in natural religion and ethics (McLachlan 1943, pp. 41, 50, 115; Haakonssen 1997, p. 104).

Scientist, philosopher, theologian, and fellow Royal Society member, Joseph Priestley (1733–1804), was another of the Warrington professors who was a long-term friend of Thomas Percival (E Percival 1807, p. xxvi). Priestley came to Warrington in September of 1761, just after Percival had completed his studies (McLachlan 1943, p. 115). At Warrington he taught languages and belles lettres, and developed his interest in what we would call the sciences (McLachlan 1943, pp. 57–60, 115). Although Percival had already left Warrington by this time, he did meet with Priestly while home on vacations. He probably was interested in Priestley's electrical experiments. It was through Rev. Seddon that Priestley was introduced to a distinguished group of London scientists as well as to Benjamin Franklin. These contacts would lead to Priestley's fame. Priestley wrote his *History and the Present State of Electricity* while at Warrington in 1767, just months before John Wesley recorded in his journal on January 4, 1768, that he had read this work. This remarkable early education nurtured Percival's lifelong love of philosophy and ethics, provided the basis for friendships with some of England's most distinguished thinkers, and oriented him toward the intellectual fervor to the north.

Percival's Medical Education

Since Percival could not enter Oxford, he began, at the age of 21, the study of medical science at the University of Edinburgh, placing him by 1761 in the midst of one of the great intellectual environments of all times. And he apparently availed himself of the opportunities this presented. According to his son Edward, his medical studies "did not preclude him from using with care the opportunities he possessed of forming an extensive acquaintance with the literary characters and person of distinction in Edinburgh. He had the good fortune, in particular, to enjoy frequent and friendly intercourse with the rival candidates for historic fame, Mr. Hume, and Dr. Robertson" (E. Percival 1807, p. xiii).

Percival was a frequent houseguest of William Robertson, the principal of the university, putting him in the same company that John Gregory would associate with so intimately just a few years later. Gregory, though 16 years Percival's senior, did not arrive in Edinburgh until just after Percival's departure. Nevertheless, as we shall see below, it is clear that Percival knew Gregory's work well. (By contrast, even though Percival would have been at Edinburgh when Alexander Monro, Primus, was teaching there, I have been unable to find any mention of Monro in Percival's writings.)

Percival maintained a lasting friendship with Robertson, arranging for Robertson to participate in a project to abolish the slave trade that had been suggested by the French finance minister. Percival also suggested to Robertson that the university confer an honorary doctorate to his friend Joseph Priestley.

In addition to Percival's contact with Hume in Edinburgh was his renewed acquaintance with him in France. As Percival later recounted in *A Father's Instructions*;

With Mr. Hume I was personally acquainted at Edinburgh; and was afterwards introduced to his particular notice by a letter from Dr. Robertson, the historian, addressed to him during his residence at Paris in 1765, when secretary to the British embassy. It was impossible to know him, without admiring his talents and various learning, and loving him for the suavity of his manners.

(T. Percival 1807, p. 335)

Through Hume, Percival met many of Paris's leading philosophers, including Voltaire and Diderot. He also met Mme Necker, the wife of the French finance minister, which explains how Percival was in a position to connect Robertson to the finance minister's slave trade project.

Percival remained at Edinburgh for three sessions, interspersing time in London where he cultivated many friendships with individuals of eminence (E. Percival 1807, p. xv). One of these was Lord Willoughby de Parham, described as "a nobleman of considerable learning and various accomplishments" (E. Percival 1807, p. xv) and vice president of the Royal Society of London. Willoughby became Percival's patron, which, in 1765, led to Percival becoming the youngest person ever elected to the Royal Society.

That year he left Edinburgh, because there were "local circumstances of difference" between the faculty and students (E. Percival 1807, p. xvi). Many of the students, including Percival, moved to Leyden, where he received his degree on July 6.[21] He then returned to Warrington, intending to practice in London, but in 1767 he moved to Manchester, where he resided for the remainder of his life.

Percival's Early Essays: Medical and Philosophical

His leisure time was occupied with preparing essays, some of which were presented at the Royal Society. They were later published in various periodicals and then gathered and published in three volumes over the next five years under the titles *Essays, Medical and Experimental* (Percival 1772, 1773a) and *Philosophical, Medical, and Experimental Essays* (Percival 1776b). (Still more versions of the collected essays appeared a decade later under the title *Essays Medical, Philosophical, and Experimental* [Percival 1788–89]). Many of these essays did not deal with clinical, medical topics. They covered matters of public health[22] as well as a wide range of philosophical and social issues such as the antislavery movement.[23] He wrote on matters of population "in conjunction with his friend Dr. Price [Richard Price, the philosopher who was Percival's friend and fellow member of the Royal Society], a copious and well-known writer on subjects of this nature" (E. Percival 1807, p. xxix). The interest in public health matters was not accidental. Both William Robertson and Edinburgh professor of physic William Cullen encouraged their students to pursue statistical activities, as did Sir John Pringle, the president of the London Royal Society from 1772 to 1778. Thomas Reid was also a participant in this activity, having contributed an account of the population of Glasgow to the *Statistical Accounts of Scotland* (Haakonssen 1997, p. 113 and note 75, p. 179). Percival prepared an enumeration of Manchester in 1773, an effort he saw as being of interest to physician, statesman, and philosopher alike. For the moral philosopher he hoped to show a correlation among disease, intemperance, and the life of luxury. He and fellow physicians involved in the hospital movement were deeply committed, for religious and political reasons, to provide services to the poor. They were convinced that only by improving their living conditions would contagious disease be overcome, a view quite compatible with Wesley's.

During this period Percival also corresponded with Benjamin Franklin, the Archbishop of York, and many other illustrious figures. He soon rose to become the principal official of the Manchester Infirmary and is described as a zealous supporter of many benevolent institutions in Manchester (E. Percival 1807, p. xxxvii).

In the second volume of his *Essays* he includes an account of the medical use of coffee, of which he was a firm advocate. In that essay he recounts that he was "subject to periodical attacks of fevere head-ache, which no caution could prevent, and no remedy could effectually alleviate" (E. Percival 1807, p. xxxvi). By 1775, for reasons of health, he was forced to retire and take a country residence near Manchester called Hart-Hill.

His essays include evidence that Percival was engaged in the philosophical issues of his day. For example, in "A Socratic Dialogue on Truth," Percival cites not only Hutcheson but also Beccaria, the Italian philosopher who was a favorite of Immanuel Kant (T. Percival 1807, Vol. 2, pp. 12–13).

Percival's Humanities Writing Addressed to His Children

That summer he turned his attention to a collection of narratives. In the manner of Gregory and many others of the period, they were designed to be presented to his children. The first volume was soon published as *A Father's Instructions to His Children* (Percival, 1776a). It appeared in many editions between 1776 and Percival's death. The edition in the 1807 *Works*[24] carries the dedication:

"To T.B.P.–A.P.–F.P.–J.P. &c.
  My dear children, . . ."

It is a charming compendium of moral guidance and religious instruction, but sometimes drifts well beyond the normal conversation between a father and his children. It includes a long chapter, "The Evidences of Christianity," an extended discussion of David Hume's views on religion, and a chapter on the virtues of truthfulness (to which we shall turn shortly).

Percival's attitude about Hume was ambiguous. While he clearly admired Hume's intellectual rigor and character, he, like Gregory, found fault with Hume's views on religion. He devotes a long chapter in *A Father's Instructions* to discussing Hume's position (T. Percival 1807, pp. 327–350). He recommends that his children peruse the discourses of a Dr. Erlington (T. Percival 1807, p. 335), saying, "the author's animadversions on Mr. Hume at first shocked my feelings: but though I still regret their severity, I am compelled to acquiesce in their truth and justice." He goes on to devote a significant discussion to Hume's empiricist critique of religious miracles (T. Percival 1807, pp. 336–346),[25] concluding, "thus fallacious is Mr. Hume's attempt to give dignity, solemnity, and strength of attestation to the alleged miracles of Vespasian" (T. Percival 1807, p. 343). He ends by criticizing Paley as well.[26]

This is a remarkable commentary for a physician to make, showing his knowledge not only of Hume's views on miracles but also his moral theory and its relation to Paley's thought. He also displays his familiarity with Hume's *History of England* and its alleged biases. Percival is placing himself not entirely outside the sphere of Hume or Paley, but conveying that he is aware of the criticism of their views. He is deeply immersed in the philosophical debate of the day, carving out a nuanced intermediate position, one of a dissenting utilitarian who is nevertheless distancing himself from Hume and Paley. We shall see in a moment how he similarly attempted to create space between himself and one of Paley's adversaries, the anti-utilitarian Gisborne.

This is the kind of intellectual agility that befits one who is actively in the midst of the intellectual controversies of his day. He is self-consciously committed to the value of that conversation. Percival's son quotes his father's endorsement of a broad and classical education:

It is a fact, I believe, not to be controverted, that the most distinguished physicians, philosophers, and metaphysicians, in ancient as well as in modern times, have been persons of general erudition. The names of Hippocrates, Aristotle, Cicero, Pliny, Bacon, Boyle, Newton, Hoffman, Haller, and Priestley, authenticate the remark, and encourage our imitation.

(E. Percival 1807, pp. li–lii)

One wonders how many physicians of the nineteenth or twentieth centuries knew enough about these figures to make such a statement.

In the following years Percival wrote *A Socratic Discourse on Truth and Faithfulness* (Percival 1781), which, three years later, was included in a 332-page volume, *Moral and Literary Dissertations* (Percival 1784), that he intended to be another installment in his advice to his children. In the discourse on truth and faithfulness he reveals his anti-utilitarian tendencies, at least when he is considering his desire to see his children manifest the virtue of veracity.[27]

We shall see below that, in spite of this defense of truthfulness with regard to his children, his views on physician truthfulness pull him back in the direction of Paley (and Gregory). The project of advising his children continued with a third and final volume entitled *The Discourse on the Divine Permission of Evil*, which was not completed until nearly the end of his life (T. Percival 1807, p. cciv). His moral, philosophical, and religious pursuit, both as a scholar and as a father, was clearly central to his life project.

Percival's Role in Philosophical Societies

Percival's interest in and commitment to philosophical, moral, and other humanities scholarship is evident not only in his extensive writings but also in his long-term involvement in that special characteristic of the Enlightenment, the philosophical society. In addition to his membership in the Royal Society of London, together with other leading inhabitants of Manchester, he established that city's Literary and Philosophical Society. It originally met at Percival's house (E. Percival 1807, p. lxvii). Percival was its joint president, together with the lawyer James Massey. After Massey's death, Percival became its sole president, a position to which he was unanimously re-elected yearly for the rest of his life (E. Percival 1807, p. lxx).[28]

In 1787 Percival was elected to the American Philosophical Society "in consequence of the recommendation of his friend Dr. Franklin, the illustrious President of that body" (E. Percival 1807, p. lxxxii). About the same time he became a member of the Royal Society of Edinburgh and the Medical Society of London. He was a regular correspondent with the elite of the Anglo-American intellectual world, including James Beattie, Franklin, Priestley, and Paley.[29]

Percival's *Medical Ethics*

Occasion of the Writing

In February 1793, Percival's second son, James, died of a "malignant fever" while studying medicine at Edinburgh. Another son, Thomas, who was a clergyman, had left for St. Petersburg to be chaplain to British merchants. The younger Thomas became seriously ill, suffering attacks of rheumatic fever, from which he died in 1798. The third son, Edward (the writer of the memoir[30]), suggested that this produced a "dejection of the mind," which led Percival to an "investigation of the interesting but difficult question respecting the purpose of moral and physical evil" (E. Percival 1807, p. clxxxi). Whether for these reasons or not, the following days would lead to Percival's most important contribution to professional physician ethics.

His *Medical Ethics; or, a Code of Institutes and Precepts, adapted to the Professional Conduct of Physicians and Surgeons* (1803)[31] was first privately published in 1794 under the title *Medical Jurisprudence.*[32] Percival claims on the opening page that he wrote the first chapter in the spring of 1792 "at the request of the physicians and surgeons of the Manchester Infirmary" (p. 1). He says he was then induced "by an earnest desire to promote the honour and advancement of his profession" to enlarge upon it and "frame a general system of MEDICAL ETHICS; that the official conduct, and mutual intercourse of the faculty, might be regulated by precise and acknowledged principles of urbanity and rectitude" (p. 1).

The 1794 edition was circulated to friends. According to Percival, many of them warmly encouraged him and honored him with suggestions for improvement. He provides a list of some of the names, but adds that there were "many other respectable friends, to whom copies of the Medical Ethics were transmitted, subsequently to the first circulation of the scheme" (Percival 1794, Note II, p. 140). The names he does provide make clear that his communicants were both interdisciplinary and distinguished. The physicians included John Aiken (the son of his Warrington teacher and friend at Edinburgh), S. A. Bardsley, James Currie, Erasmus Darwin, William Falconer (another friend at Edinburgh), John Ferriar, John Haygarth (whom his son described as "the most intimate of his professional friends" [E. Percival 1807, p. xiii]), Edward Holme, Robert Percival of Dublin, Richard Warren, and William Withering. Ferriar, Currie, Haygarth, and Falconer are all acknowledged in the 1803 edition for their suggestions of specific changes (Percival 1803, pp. 22, 151, 152, 186, 206; see also McLachlan 1943, p. 75). He refers to Aiken as "an excellent writer" and quotes him at length to support his own recommendation that justice and humanity are demonstrated when a physician or surgeon exercises discretionary power to refuse to consign to the hospital those who cannot be cured quickly (Percival 1803, p. 17).[33] Lawyers included Thomas Butterworth Bayley (his longtime friend and classmate at Edinburgh), Foster Bower, John Cross, Samuel Heyward, George Lloyd, Sir G. O. Paul, and

Charles White. From the clergy he identifies Thomas Gisborne, Archdeacon Paley, and Right Rev. Richard Watson, Bishop of Landaff. Two final friends, not otherwise identified, were Thomas Henry and "Mr. Simmons" (Percival 1803, pp. 139–140, see also p. 152). Thus he confirms that Thomas Gisborne was a recipient of the 1794 version, as was Paley.[34]

Conversation with the Scottish Philosophers

Since Percival's teachers were educated in Scotland and his medical education began in Edinburgh, it is not surprising that *Medical Ethics* contains many influences of the Scottish Enlightenment. In the critical discussion of truthfulness to patients (which we shall take up below), Percival relies, to some extent, on Hutcheson, providing two separate long quotations from his *System of Moral Philosophy* (Percival 1803, pp. 162–64). He relies on his friend, William Robertson, the Principal of the University of Edinburgh, for various historical points (pp. 174, 216, 219). In a significant note on "Caution or Temerity in Practice," Percival proposes that the best character is one not swayed by temper "but alternately employs enterprise and caution." The words are a part of a quotation from Hume's *Essays*, quoted without a hint of disapproval. Percival was able to separate his criticism of Hume's views on religion from his approval of his notions of good character. This quotation is followed immediately by a reference to Adam Smith's *Theory of Moral Sentiments* (Percival 1803, pp. 152–53). In another note Percival pokes fun at Rousseau, saying he combines "morbid sensibility and depraved imagination" (p. 211). This is followed by a reference to a more moderate Scottish character we encountered in Chapter 1: "The reader is referred to the Elements of the Philosophy of the Human Mind, Sect. V by Professor Dugald Stewart, for some admirable remarks on the evils which result from an ill-regulated imagination" (p. 212 note).

The most important of the Edinburgh elite for Percival, however, was John Gregory.[35] In his preface he refers to "the excellent lectures of Dr. Gregory" (Percival 1803 p. 6), saying that he hopes that his work and Gregory's "rather illustrate than interfere with each other" (p. 6). In a rich, 20-page note, Percival takes up the charge that physicians are guilty of skepticism and infidelity. He wanders through references to Sir Thomas Brown, Locke, David Hartley, Samuel Parr, a long section on Gisborne, and then turns to "the late Dr., Gregory, of Edinburgh." Percival says that "though his excellent lectures are, doubtless, in the hands of most physicians, yet I am tempted to make a transcript from them, because I wish the present important subject to be viewed in the several lights, in which it has been presented to the mind by different writers, of acknowledged probity, information, and judgment" (Percival 1803, p. 189). He proceeds to quote from Gregory for two pages, rehearsing Gregory's defense of his profession against the charges, after which Percival adds, "the judicious and animated considerations which are here delivered, could proceed only from a mind actuated by the principles of virtue and religion. And I trust, the great majority of physicians have their feelings in unison with those of the amiable writer I have quoted" (p. 191).

Percival and English Philosophy and Theology

As an Englishman, however, Percival's conversations in philosophy and theology were not limited to Scotsmen. He made liberal use of historical figures: Bacon, Locke, and Thomas Brown, for example.[36] Lord Shaftesbury appears in a long note on dueling (Percival 1803, p. 221). The really significant English humanities influences on Percival's *Medical Ethics*, however, appear to have been Paley and Gisborne, to whom we will turn below. This is in addition to the influence of Priestley and Price, who, although not explicitly mentioned in *Medical Ethics*, are nevertheless significant both as personal friends and in their shaping of Percival's philosophical thought. Along with these Scottish and English figures, Franklin and Montesquieu make appearances.[37]

Percival Writing in the Tradition of Literature on the Duties of Office

Percival wrote in a genre that was strongly represented in his time. He introduces *Medical Ethics* by stating his desire to "promote the honour and advancement of his profession" (1803, p. 1). The "duties-of-office" literature was prominent during this period. It traces back to Bacon, whom Percival quotes at length when he sets out his project (p. 3). This literature is, of course, manifest in Gisborne's *Enquiry into the Duties of Men* (1794) and in John Gregory's *Lectures on the Duties and Qualifications of a Physician* (1772) and the earlier unauthorized edition.

PERCIVAL'S TEMPERED CONSEQUENTIALISM. Percival is best understood as a "qualified consequentialist." The consequentialist influences of Scotland—of Hutcheson, Smith, Hume, and Gregory—as well as those of Paley in England so shape the intellectual climate of Percival's environment that, in spite of necessary qualifications, the single most appropriate designation is "consequentialist."[38] Nevertheless, Percival went out of his way to seek contrary opinion. He sent copies of *Medical Jurisprudence* to Gisborne and Paley and wrestled with the wisdom of conflicting opinion. The result was a moderated and nuanced consequentialism. Just as he admitted having been tempted by Hume's view of religion until he read Butler, so he was tempted by the latitudinarianism of physicians like Gregory when considerations of humaneness conflict with more robust nonutilitarian moral prohibitions. But in this case, anti-utilitarians, especially Gisborne and Price, forced him into a complex and qualified position that reflects the conclusions of one sampling the moral opinion and theory of his surroundings.[39] In fact, McCullough (1998, p. 274) considers Price to be Percival's main philosophical source. There is no doubt of Price's influence, but the conflicting sources are present as well.

PERCIVAL AS CONTRACTARIAN. Percival's formulation of ethics was explicitly built on the concept of a tacit social compact (Percival 1803, p. 45), a notion that can be traced back to both Bacon and Blackstone (Haakonssen 1997, p. 123). For Percival, as for Bacon, the compact was among members of the profession, but it generated professional duties to the members of the society at large. This was a notion that, by the latter part of the twentieth century, would become very controversial. Critics of professionally generated physician ethics have asked how a professional group, by agreement among its members, can generate duties to those outside the group, particularly if it is questionable whether those outside the group will accept the behavior to which professionals mutually pledge themselves. For example, benevolent paternalism has long been taken as a duty of physician–professionals, yet by the end of the twentieth century, physician paternalism was militantly opposed by some laypeople. The idea that a closed professional group could legitimate its actions by mutual pledging among its members, even when the outsiders whose lives are affected may not approve of this legitimation, is now morally controversial, but in Bacon's or Percival's time, this was not an issue.

For example, in the section of *Medical Ethics* where Percival invokes the social compact, he goes on to advise that, if there is a controversy among members of the profession, the relevant group (the physicians or surgeons or a combination thereof) should arbitrate, but that "neither the subject matter of such references, not the adjudication, should be communicated to the public; as they may be personally injurious to the individuals concerned, and can hardly fail to hurt the general credit of the faculty" (Percival 1803, p. 46). Since what is being adjudicated directly affects the lay population, today this social compact would be grossly offensive. The public is not only excluded from participating in the discussion of the norms for proper conduct of physicians and surgeons; it is actually prohibited from knowing there is even a dispute.

To Percival's credit, he qualifies his contractarianism in an important and little-noticed way. After enjoining medical professionals to submit to the laws generated by compact among professionals, he adds that these laws should apply "so far as they are consistent with morality, and the general good of mankind" (Percival 1803, p. 46). Thus, even though the norms for professional conduct are produced by agreement among professionals in a closed session, he is aware that the professional norms must conform to a more fundamental moral standard outside the professional compact. For social contractarians, those more fundamental norms for morality themselves can be thought of in contractarian terms. That, in fact, is the foundation of ethics I have proposed elsewhere (Veatch 1981).

The immediate source of Percival's contractarianism insofar as it extends outside the profession is not Locke or Hobbes or Rousseau, but rather Blackstone. In his *Commentaries on the Laws of England*, William Blackstone claims that public office holders contract with those who employ or entrust them (Blackstone, Vol. 3, p. 163 as cited in Haakonssen 1997, p. 124). Note, however, the striking asymmetry. Whereas Blackstone's contract is between the office holder and those affected by the office holder's actions, Percival's professional contract is among professional group members, not between the profession and the public affected by the professional's actions.

Regardless of this controversial and novel application of contract theory to provide an account of professional duties, what is important here is that Percival, like Gregory, knew enough about Blackstone and Bacon to recognize a currently fashionable jurisprudential concept and adapt it to professional medical ethics. It is not as if he had invented these notions out of whole cloth.[40]

Percival and Truth: Mediating the Ethical Controversy

The best example of Percival's sophisticated ambivalence in negotiating various ethical theories is his set of positions on the morality of truth telling. At first his views seem paradoxical. As we have seen, he had earlier advised his children that lying is wrong. He had also offered "A Socratic Discourse on Truth and Faithfulness" to the Manchester Literary and Philosophical Society (Percival 1781). However, 22 years later in *Medical Ethics*, he provided a remarkable and important 12-page endnote that essentially authorizes benevolent, consequence-driven deception by physicians who confront patients who would be distressed by bad news (Percival 1803, Note VII, pp. 156–168).

Percival's nuanced views on truth telling are explicitly drawn from Cicero, Horace, "The Fathers of the Christian Church" ("Origin, Clement, Tertullian, Lactantius, Chrysostom, and various others"), Augustine, Grotius, Puffendorff, Hutcheson, Samuel Johnson, Grove, Balguy, Cambray, Butler, Paley, and Gisborne. (But Kant is not in the list, nor is Bentham.) Pecival's dialogue with Gisborne, which we encountered in the discussion of his *Duties of Men*, is instructive. Percival seems to find himself trapped between two competing claims. He respects Augustine, Gisborne, and his Christian rigorist heritage, but Cicero, Hutcheson, Gregory, and Paley are an even more powerful pull. In the end, he cautiously and reluctantly yields, at least in extreme cases, to the combined pressures of his consequentialist and physician mentors to adopt what he calls the "latitudinarian" view, but with the sense that he feels the weight of the appeals of the other side. What is perhaps more important than this guarded consequentialist conclusion is the breadth of philosophical knowledge Percival displays. No physician until the last decades of the twentieth century would again be able to display such encyclopedic knowledge of the philosophical and theological literature.

Percival and Social Consequentialism

This qualified consequentialism has led some analysts of the history of medical ethics to see Percival as being essentially in the Hippocratic tradition. The Hippocratic Oath is, beyond doubt, a consequentialist ethic for physicians. It has physicians pledge to benefit the patient according to their ability and judgment. That seemingly benign core principle of Hippocratism does, in fact, appear to be consistent with Percival's support of lying to patients.

An affinity undoubtedly exists between both Percival's and Gregory's medical ethics and Hippocratism, but I am now convinced that it is a mistake to place them in the Hippocratist camp. First, as we shall see, Percival had even less active interest in the Hippocratic literature than Gregory did. More substantively, there are some significant differences between the eighteenth-century physician of the Enlightenment and the ancient, pagan, Greek. One of the important differences is the extent to which their consequentialism takes into account benefits to persons beyond the patient.

The Hippocratist had no social ethic. His view of the practice of medicine was one of service to the individual patient. The practitioner had no duty to take as patients persons whom the physician did not want to serve. In fact, the Hippocratic author advised physicians that it was bad for the physician's reputation to take as patients those whom the physician believed were inevitably terminal.

By contrast, Percival's ethic was vividly social. As with many other of the eighteenth-century utilitarians, he was concerned about the community. This led to the beginnings of public health. Percival's scholarly and research interests were, as we have seen, very much oriented toward what we would call public health questions—immunization; the relation of disease to social conditions, poverty, and unsanitary urban conditions; and demographic data analysis. He was a central figure in the development of Manchester's infirmary, a social institution committed to providing health care for the lower classes—both for their benefit and that of the entire community.

This social ethic undoubtedly also reflects Percival's deep commitments to a kind of religious life that is loosely related to Judeo-Christianity. Judeo-Christianity is nothing if not social. Its ethic is one of the common good, of commitment to the welfare of the poor. Percival developed basic institutions for health care for the masses in a way not unlike John Wesley. Granted, Percival evolved religiously as a rational dissenter, a kind of unitarian, but, in contrast with twenty-first–century unitarians, he showed no explicit resistance to being called a Christian.

Thus Percival's consequentialism fits perfectly with that of Smith, Hume, and Paley. Although Jeremy Bentham does not appear to have been an influence on Percival, his thinking would also have fit with that of Percival. It is something of an accident that Percival's qualified social consequentialism can end up sounding like Hippocratic individual consequentialism, especially when Percival's focus is on the more isolated physician–patient relation. Percival's ethics, however, was undeniably social. He endorsed human experimentation when it was for the greater good:

Whenever cases occur, attended with circumstances not heretofore observed, or in which the ordinary modes of practice have been attempted without success, it is for the public good, and in an especial degree advantageous to the poor (who, being the most numerous class of society, are the greatest beneficiaries of the healing art) that *new remedies* and *new methods* of *chirurgical treatment* should be devised.

(Percival 1803, pp. 14–15, italics in original)[41]

Like Adam Smith, but very much unlike the Hippocratic author, Percival saw a convergence of the interests of the public and the individual. Although he finessed the distinction between the interests of the poor as a class and the interests of the poor patient on whom a new remedy might be tried, he nevertheless was of the belief that the individual patient could benefit from such an experiment. He went on, however, to impose some protecting limits: the "gentlemen of the faculty" should be "governed by sound reason, just analogy, and authenticated facts" and "no such trials should be instituted, without a previous consultation of the physicians or surgeons, according to the nature of the case" (Percival 1803, p. 15). His methods of protecting the patient were decidedly the paternalistic ones of the eighteenth century—peer review—rather than twentieth- or twenty-first–century ones such as informed consent, the right of refusal, government regulations, and interdisciplinary review boards, but his agenda of promoting the public good does incorporate some protections of the patient. Percival's protective mechanisms presumably also preserved the public's interest by eliminating bad science and risks to the reputation of the hospital. The possibility that the patient's interest and the public good could conflict was simply not on Percival's mind.

Percival and Hippocrates

Thus, although Percival was engaged in consequentialist reasoning, he was not under Hippocrates's spell. Percival had at most a passing interest in him. Hippocrates receives no significant mention in *Medical Ethics*. A passing reference appears when Percival discusses manslaughter. Here Percival shows that he knew that the Oath prohibits using a pessary to produce an abortion. Percival referred to Hippocrates as "the father of physic," mentioning "the oath enjoined on his pupils, which some universities now impose on the candidates for medical degrees" (Pervical 1803, p. 79), but even here Percival is critical. He notes that "even the pessary, so sanctimoniously forbidden by Hippocrates, has little of that activity and power, which superstition assigned to it" (p. 80).

Thus Percival lacked any real interest in Hippocrates. There is, at most, a convergence with Hippocrates on the subject of patient welfare, at least where more social utilitarian interests do not conflict. Percival was an eighteenth-century qualified social consequentialist in conversation with the Scottish and English utilitarians, held in check by his equally engaged conversations with anti-utilitarians like Gisborne and Price.

The historically remarkable feature of Percival is not where he ended up in the philosophical debates of late eighteenth-century Scotland and England; it is the fact that he was in the midst of them. Percival is a figure who worked with some agility among the major players of the day, absorbing and understanding the current controversies, then staking out his own nuanced position in an intellectually respectable if not creatively original way. Percival was, as Pickstone (1993, p. 174) has suggested, a full member of "a single, recognized social elite." Like Gregory in Edinburgh, Percival was in serious conversation with the elite humanists of his day, a role for a physician that cannot be demonstrated with comparable rigor again until some 170 years later.

4

ISOLATION OF
THE ENGLISH PHYSICIAN

EDWARD PERCIVAL AND THE BEGINNINGS OF ISOLATION

Thomas Percival died in 1804 just short of his 64th birthday. Like Gregory, he left a physician-son to carry on his work. Edward Percival (d. 1827), just like James Gregory, was not really up to the task. This should not be considered merely another example of a son failing to live up to the impossibly high accomplishments of his father. Rather, Edward Percival and James Gregory were the first generation of a new century and a new era. They were no longer living as eighteenth-century Enlightenment generalists who could strive to master all human knowledge, carrying out extensive oral and written discussions with the leading intellectuals of the world of philosophy, theology, law, and the arts. They exemplified the beginning of the era of scientific specialization.

Edward Percival carried the torch his father had lit. He collected his father's literary output, publishing it in four volumes (T. Percival 1807), and wrote a 262-page biography that served as a preface. But beyond the dissemination of his father's work, Edward's own accomplishments were more nearly those of mere modern mortals. He published *Practical Observations on the Treatment, Pathology, and Prevention of Typhous Fever* (1819) from the results of his experience in treating several thousand cases of fever, which he encountered while he was a physician at the Hardwicke fever hospital in Dublin.

If one wants to consult the important works in medical ethics from England in the first half of the nineteenth century, however, what one finds is successive new editions of Thomas Percival's *Medical Ethics*. An anonymously edited edition appeared in 1827, published in London, and a third edition edited by Greenhill appeared in 1849 in Oxford.[1] In England, as in Scotland, the more typical interests of the period are a more pragmatic agenda suggested by the title of the son's published volume.

EMERGENCE OF HIPPOCRATES

The shift from scholarship of the generalist in the latter part of the eighteenth century to more concrete, mundane, scientific interests took place quite dramatically at the beginning of the nineteenth century. Along with that shift came an increased interest in the Hippocratic Oath and the related Hippocratic literature. It is as if the Hippocratic Oath were all the medical ethics the nineteenth-century physician could handle.

As we have seen, the elite physicians of the Enlightenment were aware of the Hippocratic literature. But often they were not terribly interested in it and not terribly respectful of it either. For example, it is reported that:

In 1771, John Morgan, an Edinburgh graduate, speaking at the conferment of the first doctorate of medicine at the College of Philadelphia, declared that the *Oath* prescribed by Hippocrates to his disciples had been generally adopted in universities and schools of physic. *His* college, however, which was a free spirit among institutions, had no need of such oaths; it wished only to bind its sons and graduates by the ties of honour and gratitude.

(Nutton, 1995, p. 522, citing the *Pennsylvania Gazette* as quoted in Packard FR, *History of Medicine in the United States*. NY: PB Hoeber (1931, Vol. 1, p. 368)

In fact, as we have seen, the Edinburgh oath for medical students had its origins in an oath of loyalty to the king and the university that was required of all students and faculty. As far as I can tell, the claim that other schools adopted the Hippocratic Oath cannot be supported. To be sure, some lines adapted from the Hippocratic Oath were added when the Edinburgh oath was modified for medical students, but the primary function was not an initiation into a profession.[2] There is generally a sense that the Hippocratic literature was a quaint bit from history, not a foundational part of the medical ethics of the profession.

All of this changed in the early years of the nineteenth century; precious little medical ethics was being written. What remained demonstrates two important characteristics: a tendency to copy from Gregory or Percival and an elevation of Hippocrates and his oath. The primary example of this trend is the writing of English physician Michael Ryan.

MICHAEL RYAN

Michael Ryan (1800–1841) was a London physician who practiced at the Metropolitan Free Hospital.[3] In 1831 he published *A Manual of Medical Jurisprudence*.

A second edition appeared five years later (1836a). According to the title page, it was "considerably enlarged and improved."[4] It was enlarged, in part, by the addition of a chapter on American medical ethics. The chapter was actually written by a Dr. Godman, who was Professor of Anatomy and Physiology at Rutgers's Medical College (Ryan 1836a, p. 105). This lends support to the thesis of medical ethics historian Chester Burns, who claims that after medical ethics had migrated from Scotland and England to the North American continent, it moved back to England again, reversing the flow (Burns 1977b).[5]

Ryan's views make clear how radically medical ethics had changed in the years since Percival wrote, for he bemoans the almost total lack of interest in medical ethics in medical education.[6] That being the case, Ryan is forced to revert back to the works of Gregory and Percival, although he makes clear how inadequate they seem from the perspective of some three decades of history. He decries the situation: "Indeed, the only works we have on the subject are those of Dr. John Gregory and Dr. Percival; but these are not deemed authority, nor are they perused by medical students." Then, while claiming that "both Gregory and Percival [are] unsuited to the state of the profession at the present time," he proceeds to present a condensed summary of Gregory, as it is the only thing available to him. What is not happening is the generation of a new and more up-to-date literature.

While these late eighteenth-century figures were being belittled, the place of Hippocrates was being dramatically expanded. In contrast to the sparse and skeptical use of Hippocrates during the Enlightenment, Ryan moved the Greek physician into a position familiar to most of us. He devotes an entire chapter to Hippocrates' medical ethics, claiming that, "the duties and qualifications of medical practitioners were never more fully exemplified than by the conduct of Hippocrates, or more eloquently described than by his pen" (Ryan 1836a, p. 9). Borrowing the Oath's own words, he praises it, saying that it provides "the most religious attention to the advantages and cure of the sick, the strictest charity, and most inviolable secrecy about private or domestic matters, which might be seen or heard during attendance, and which ought not to be divulged" (Ryan 1836a, p. 9).

Ryan had no contact with contemporary philosophy and theology. He was reduced to reluctant copying of Gregory and Percival while placing Hippocrates in a new-found central position. Ryan was not, like Gregory or Percival, an eclectic Enlightenment scholar versed at least to a respectable degree in the humanities. He was a nineteenth-century applied scientist practicing medicine, editing a medical journal, and conducting much more mundane research on scientific topics of current interest. From 1832 until 1838 he was the editor of the *London Medical and Surgical Journal*. His medical writing addressed more trivial issues.[7] In one tentative foray into more philosophical topics he nevertheless managed to focus on genitourinary diseases and physiology.[8] Gone are the quaint moralizing examples of a father's advice to his children and the more profound philosophical inquiries.

As in Scotland, the physician of early nineteenth-century England was something more of a practical, modern medical scientist content to master narrow, technical topics, edit journals, write textbooks, and remain isolated from the broader, more philosophical culture. After Percival, the conversation with the humanities was suspended. Physicians lacking the humanities repertoire needed a brief, manageable account of the morality of their profession. The Hippocratic Oath took on a new, more central place.

ALFRED S. TAYLOR

During this period, an even more famous writer of medical jurisprudence flourished. Keeping in mind that Percival chose the words "medical jurisprudence" for the original title of his *Medical Ethics*, it is worth inquiring whether Alfred Swaine Taylor's work could be considered a source of medical ethics in the early nineteenth century. Taylor (1806–1880) was a medical jurist who produced successively three medical jurisprudence texts that all went through many editions (Taylor 1836, 1844, 1865).[9]

Taylor spent his professional life as a lecturer on chemistry at Guy's Hospital, London.[10] One might be encouraged by the similarity in title of his texts and Percival's orginal *Medical Jurisprudence* and by the fact that Taylor discussed practical medical ethical issues such as confidentiality, competence, and the like. Taylor's real focus, however, was on topics that today we would consider the main substance of medical law: child abuse, infanticide, analysis of poisons and wounds, and giving evidence in court. With one exception, there is no evidence of awareness or influence of the likes of Gregory and Percival, nor is the Hippocratic author present in these pages.[11]

Taylor represents the almost total bifurcation of medical jurisprudence and medical ethics. In his *Manual* (1844, p. v) he defines medical jurisprudence as "that science which teaches the application of every branch of medical knowledge to the purposes of the law." Gone is any of Percival's more philosophical or ethical agenda. Taylor was a fascinating man with eclectic interests, but none of them strayed in the direction of the humanities. His medical writing was pedestrian.[12] In the *Manual* he includes a long discussion of the precise cause of death when a person drowns. Instructions on testifying in court for murder and manslaughter cases and the speed of decomposition of bodies were typical of his topics. Taylor's other major interest was photography. He devised a new technique and published "The Art of Photogenic Drawing." He also edited Arnott's *Elements of Physics* and later editions of Pereira's *Elements of Materia Medica*. None of this, however, makes Taylor a serious student of medical ethics or even conversant with humanists on relevant subjects.

JUKES DE STYRAP

One final figure of nineteenth-century English medical ethics deserves attention. Jukes de Styrap (1815–1899) produced what Peter Bartrip has called "the only important code of medical ethics to be published in Victorian England" (Bartrip 1995, p. 145).[13] The code that Styrap produced was originally published in 1878. Enlarged editions appeared in 1886, 1890, and 1895.[14] When it appeared, it had the trappings of Percival's work, quite possibly mediated by Styrap's access to the American Medical Association's (AMA's) code of 1847, which was circulating in England soon after its appearance. Styrap makes explicit reference to the example of "our eminently practical American brethren" (Bartrip 1995, p. 146). The Styrap code is divided into four chapters, reminiscent of Percival's code, but even more directly parallels the three chapters of the AMA's document. Table 4–1 shows the chapter structure of the three works.

Styrap borrowed from the AMA even the linguistic distinction between "duties" (which are attached to professional roles) and "obligations" (which are the moral requirements of lay people). Major sections were copied virtually verbatim from the AMA, some of which the AMA had copied from Percival. For example, in the first article (titled "Duties of Physicians to their Patients" by the AMA, "Duties of Practitioners to the Their Patients" by Styrap, and untitled by Percival)

TABLE **4–1.** Chapter Structure of Three Codes of Medical Ethics

PERCIVAL	AMERICAN MEDICAL ASSOCIATION	STYRAP
I. In hospital practice	I. Of the duties of physicians to their patients and of the obligations of patients to their physicians	I. On the duties of medical practitioners to their patients, and the obligations of patients to their medical advisors
II. In private, or general practice	II. Of the duties of physicians to each other, and to the profession at large	II. On the duties of medical practitioners to the profession, to each other, and to themselves
III. In relation to apothecaries	III. Of the duties of the profession to the public and of the obligations of the public to the profession	III. On the duties of the profession to the public and the obligations of the public to the profession
IV. In cases which may require a knowledge of law		IV. "Medical" etiquette, or the rule of the profession on commencing practice, etc.

of Chapter 1, Styrap reproduced the AMA language almost exactly; the AMA had taken some of its sentences from Percival. The four famous virtues of Percival and the AMA (tenderness, steadiness, condescension, and authority) (Percival 1803, p. 9; American Medical Association 1848, p. 13) are repeated by Styrap, only he changes "condescension" to "urbanity" (Styrap 1995, p. 149). By the late nineteenth century, "condescension" had already undergone a change in meaning.[15] The fact that Styrap copied the AMA code without any engagement in contemporary philosophical or theological discourse with the likes of John Stuart Mill or F. D. Maurice suggests that he was, in the typical nineteenth-century pattern, a physician of more limited humanities ability.

We know relatively little about the life of Styrap. He was born in 1815 and attended Shrewsbury School, after which he was educated at Stourport in Worcestershire (Bartrip 1995, p. 146). He studied medicine at King's College, London. He practiced medicine in Ireland in the 1830s and 40s. There is no evidence of any involvement in broader humanities education. In the 1850s he set up practice in Shrewsbury, where he helped found the Salopian Medico-Ethical Society and became its secretary. The society merged with the Shropshire Branch of the British Medical Association (BMA), during which time Styrap was responsible for publishing two pamphlets: A Tariff of Medical Fees and Medico-Chirurgical Tariffs (Bartrip 1995, p. 147). The latter, which went through five editions, was a modest 28 pages and appeared in 1890. His only other published work I could locate has, at most, modest humanities interest: The Young Practitioner: with Practical Hints and Instructive Suggestions as Subsidiary Aids for His Guidance on Entering into Private Practice (1890b).

In 1864 Styrap suffered a "severe illness" that led to his retirement from clinical practice. It was during this prolonged retirement that he developed his editions of his code of medical ethics. He also designed a "urinary cabinet," a device containing test tubes, a thermometer, forceps, and other equipment. It was Styrap's hope that the BMA would adopt his code. He offered it to the group in 1882, hoping the BMA would distribute it to newly elected members (Bartrip 1995, p. 145). This never happened. There is some evidence, however, that it did exercise some influence within the professional association (Bartrip 1995, p. 145).

The pattern, once again, is one of a nineteenth-century physician who was clinically and pragmatically oriented and forced by circumstances to pursue professional ethics and code writing without much preparation in philosophy, theology, or any other humanities. He copied his predecessors, who, in this case, had copied from theirs. It is a pattern we shall see over and over in the next chapter when we examine the evolution of American professional medical ethics. These clinicians turned to existing documents that traced back, either directly or indirectly, to Percival and Gregory, producing an ethics literature that was divorced from the continuing philosophical debates of the day.

NINETEENTH- AND TWENTIETH-CENTURY ACTIVITY
OF THE BRITISH MEDICAL ASSOCIATION

In fact, the BMA had been considering the writing of a code of ethics since the 1850s. Two committees had been appointed, neither of which had completed their work (Burns 1977b, p. 304). Even before this time, professional organized medicine in England existed as the Provincial Medical and Surgical Association, which had, as one of its objectives, "the maintenance of the honour and respectability of the profession" (British Medical Association 1981, p. 10). It formed a Committee on Medical Ethics in 1849 and two years later, a committee to frame a code of ethical laws. When the Provincial Medical and Surgical Association became the British Medical Association in 1856, no code had yet been produced. At its Edinburgh meeting in July 1858, another committee was established with Charles Hastings as chairman and T. Herbert Barker and Alexander Henry as secretary (Burns 1977b, p. 305). At the 1859 meetings, Barker was given additional time to prepare the report, but it was never completed (*British Medical Journal* 1858, pp. 657–58; 1859, p. 631, as cited in Burns 1977b, p. 305). That set the stage for Styrap's unsuccessful attempts to have his edited version of the AMA's 1847 code adopted by the British association.

I have not been able to locate any additional evidence of the BMA's involvement in medical ethics in the late nineteenth and early twentieth centuries. The BMA had a central ethical committee chaired by Dr. C. O. Hawthorne, "who was one of the great personalities in the association during the inter-war years" (in British Medical Association 1963, p. 56).

By 1963 the BMA *Members Handbook* contained a chapter entitled "Medical Ethics," which was the precursor to their *Handbook of Medical Ethics* (British Medical Association 1981). This chapter begins with a reference to the Hippocratic Oath as the most celebrated expression of the ethic of the profession, proclaiming "the fundamental principles of professional behaviour have remained unaltered through the recorded history of medicine" (British Medical Association 1963, p. 54). Following this statement is an English translation of the Oath, then a statement that the Oath has "endured through the centuries, and whether or not the modern doctor formally affirms it at qualification, he accepts its spirit and intentions as his ideal standard of professional behavior" (British Medical Association 1963, p. 55). This is followed by the World Medical Association's Declaration of Geneva, which is described as "a modern restatement of the Hippocratic Oath." There is no hint of any references to any religious or philosophical ethical theories, and no awareness of the potential conflicts between this ancient Greek professional tradition and either secular liberal political philosophy or the various religious traditions. There is no reference to any modern or ancient philosopher or theologian, no reference to the great tradition of modern British utilitarianism.

The organization has even lost its recorded institutional memory of its non-Hippocratic Scottish Enlightenment ancestors, Gregory and Percival. The material cited above is reprinted verbatim, without any reference to the moral traditions inside or outside of British medicine, in the 1970 edition of the BMA's pamphlet, *Medical Ethics*, a reprinting of the chapter from the 1970 edition of the *Members Handbook* (British Medical Association 1970, pp. 1–3).

By 1981, that part of the BMA's institutional memory had been recovered. The introduction to *The Handbook of Medical Ethics* provides a short, explicit acknowledgment of Thomas Percival and his 1803 codification, but clearly shows no awareness of Percival's philosophical nurturing or his lack of interest in Hippocrates (British Medical Association 1981, p. 10). The same paragraphs still appear in the 1984 edition. In Britain the isolation of physicians persists.

The resistance to communication with philosophers and other humanists is symbolized by the response to my 1979 request to the BMA for a copy of the *Medical Ethics* pamphlet. The reply was that "the current booklet is part of the BMA Members' Handbook and therefore available only to Members of the Association."[16] In 1979, the ethical standards of British physicians were officially confidential information that could not be shared with laypeople.[17] This stance soon changed with the publication of the new *Handbook* (1981). The resumption of the conversation had officially been sanctioned.

THE BASIS FOR ENGLISH ISOLATION

In the chapters on Scotland, we saw that one possible explanation for the lack of interest in or knowledge of the humanities was the young age of entry into medical school. In Britain in the nineteenth century, students could move directly into medical school from secondary school, giving them no real exposure as young adults to great literature, history, philosophy, or theological thought.

Although some students also entered medical school at a young age in eighteenth-century England, Thomas Percival provides an important exception. He was born in 1740 and did not enroll in the medical course at Edinburgh until 1761. Prior to that he studied for four years at Warrington, where he had extensive exposure to more academic philosophy—both natural and moral.

More important than the age of entry to medical school was the change in social class of medical students in transforming the physician from an intellectual with eclectic interests into a skilled practitioner of an upper- to middle-class professional with more pragmatic interests and a more limited range of knowledge. Percival's social status as a member of the cultural elite was similar to that of Gregory, if not quite as spectacular. His father was engaged in commerce, but his paternal grandfather and uncle were both physicians. His uncle played a role as mentor and role model after the death of Percival's father and left a considerable library for him. According to the biographical account by Percival's son, that uncle had studied in Leyden under Boerhaave and was said to have "combined with his medical pursuits the study of various other branches of knowledge. . . . [F]ollowing the steps of his great master, he directed his attention to Natural History, Chemistry, Ethics, and theology" (E. Percival 1807, p. iii). In Chapter 3 we traced the critical influence of Percival's enrollment in the newly founded Warrington Academy in 1757 where, prior to entry into medical school, he gained a thorough introduction to the Scottish philosophers.

Likewise, the explosion of knowledge in nineteenth-century England meant a narrowing of scholarly interests. In the last years of the eighteenth century, Percival not only wrote *Medical Ethics* but also published volumes of more philosophical essays covering slavery, public health, and population. He also wrote "A Socratic Dialogue on Truth," and *The Discourse on the Divine Permission of Evil*. Percival's agenda as a physician was not all that different from Wesley's agenda as a clergyman. Both considered matters of philosophy, theology, and ethics, as well as medicine part of their domain.

By contrast, the nineteenth-century Englishmen were forced to limit their attention to narrower topics just to master some area of the exploding quantity of knowledge in the world. In jurisprudence, for instance, the focus was primarily on more technical legal issues. Ryan and Taylor had all they could manage to produce multiple editions of jurisprudence volumes that cataloged the state of the law and the technical medical tests needed for one to function well as a forensic pathologist. Apart from medical ethics, Styrap was concerned primarily about the local professional medical society, medical and surgical fee schedules, and advice to young practitioners.

Thus in England as well as in Scotland, social and intellectual forces conspired to force physicians into narrower and narrower domains. Physicians were pressed back into the recesses of their laboratories and libraries in their own areas of specialization and further away from scholars in other schools of the university. Similar forces were emerging in the new parts of the English-speaking world.

III

THE UNITED STATES, CANADA, AND NEW ZEALAND

5

PHYSICIAN–HUMANIST INTERACTION IN THE EIGHTEENTH CENTURY IN THE UNITED STATES

The close link between medicine and the humanities in late eighteenth-century Scotland and England provided the foundation for the emergence of a New World medical ethics. The Scottish medical schools, particularly Edinburgh, had far and away the greatest influence (Girdwood 1988, p. 39).[1] Some 650 medical students from North America graduated with medical degrees from the University of Edinburgh between 1750 and 1850. Lesser numbers attended Glasgow as well as Aberdeen and St. Andrews. Benjamin Rush, the physician who signed the Declaration of Independence, got his medical degree from Edinburgh in 1768, during the era of John Gregory, William Cullen, and Alexander Monro, Primus.

The predecessor of the University of Pennsylvania Medical School, called the College of Philadelphia, was founded in 1765 and was based on the Edinburgh model (Girdwood 1988, p. 40). Rush was elected professor of chemistry at the College of Philadelphia in 1769 (Rush 1948, p. 18). When the College of Physicians of Philadelphia was founded 1787, 8 of 24 fellows were Edinburgh graduates. In New York, John Jay, an Edinburgh graduate of 1763, proposed a medical school. In 1767 the trustees of King's College invited six physicians and surgeons, including Samuel Bard, graduate of Edinburgh in 1765, to found a medical faculty. That college closed, but in 1787 the Medical Faculty of Columbia College was opened. It had five professors including Bard and Nicholas Romayne, an Edinburgh graduate of 1779. Other U.S. medical schools arose under Edinburgh influence as well. Dartmouth's founders included Nathan Smith, who studied medicine at Edinburgh at the end of the eighteenth century. He became professor of surgery at Yale. Many Americans trained at William and Mary then spent a few years in Edinburgh or Glasgow. The colonies imported the Scottish Enlightenment through its intellectual elite, including its medical elite. A brief examination of the writing of people such as Benjamin Rush and Samuel Bard makes clear that American medical ethics has its roots in the early Scottish education of these medical leaders. As was true of their teachers, they were Enlightenment generalists, studying medicine in the context of contemporary Scottish philosophy.

COTTON MATHER

The communication moved in both directions in the United States, much as it had in Scotland and England. Humanists pursued medicine just as physicians understood the humanities. The most important example of the former was the remarkable theologian Cotton Mather (1663–1728).[2] Known for his involvement in the Salem witchcraft trials, he seems to have played a moderating influence and invited a supposedly bewitched child into his house to study her case. He flourished at the end of the seventeenth century and the beginning of the eighteenth and is a remarkable exemplar of the intellectual eclecticism of the elite. Mather wrote over 450 books and was an accomplished editor and compiler. He is described as "a well-bred amateur of many fields of knowledge" (Murdock 1957, p. 388), having written *The Ecclesiastical History of New England from its First Planting* (1702); *The Negro Christianized* (1706); *The Good Education of Children* (1708); *Fair Dealing Between Debtor and Creditor* (1716); *The Accomplished Singer* (1721); and, most importantly for our purposes, several medical volumes including *Sentiments on the Small Pox Innoculated* (1721) and *An Account . . . of Inoculating the Small-Pox* (1722).

Just as Wesley has been described as the most important medical figure of eighteenth-century England, so Mather has been called by medical historians Otho Beall and Richard Shryock (1954) the "first significant figure in American medicine." According to them, Mather's medical writing, including the small pox volumes and a booklet called "The Angel of Bethesda," as "pertinent to any comprehension of the medical thought of his time and place." His medical works were "the only instance of systematic medical writing in this country prior to the national period" (p. 6).

Medicine was for Mather a "second vocation." Believing a stammer would hinder him if he entered the ministry, he began the study of medicine when he graduated from Harvard. He returned to medicine periodically throughout his career. He was a recognized scientist and a leader in medicine, especially public health. This led to an invitation to membership in the Royal Society. "The Angel of Bethesda" was a small book of remedies that anticipated Wesley's *Primitive*

Physick[3] and boldly advocated combating small pox by inoculation (Mather 1954, pp. 160–186). During the eighteenth century, no clear differentiation between physicians and humanists existed, at least not in many of the great intellects.

BENJAMIN RUSH

The most significant of these figures at the end of the century was Benjamin Rush (1746–1813). It is impossible to understand Rush's contribution to the study of medicine and morality without examining his Edinburgh roots.

Nurturing an Enlightenment Man

In 1800, at age 54, Benjamin Rush began writing an autobiography, which is our best source on his life (Rush 1948). He never intended it for publication. It was, as the twentieth-century editor says, for his own satisfaction and his family's edification.[4]

Rush's father died when he was five years old, a beginning not unlike that of John Gregory and Thomas Percival (Rush 1948, p. 28). The boy was a student at West Nottingham Academy in what is now Rising Sun, Maryland, and was taught by Rev. Dr. Samuel Finley, who later became President of the College of New Jersey (what would become Princeton University). Finley married a sister of Rush's mother. Thus, Rush had links to a head of a college, as did Gregory. He became close to Finley, attending him at his death every other night for several weeks (Rush 1948, p. 33).

Rush left Nottingham in the spring of 1759 at 15 years of age to go to the College of New Jersey, receiving a Bachelor of Arts degree in September of 1760. He had decided to study law and applied for a position as an apprentice to a lawyer in Philadelphia when he paid a visit to his teacher, Dr. Finley, who urged him to study "physic." This led to his becoming a pupil of Dr. John Redman, the leading physician in Philadelphia. Redman was the founder and first president of the College of Physicians of Philadelphia (Rush 1948, p. 37 and note 31). That portion of Rush's education included the reading of Boerhaave and Sydenham. He attended the lectures of Dr. William Shippen (1736–1808) and John Morgan (1735–1789), founders of the University of Pennsylvania Medical School and the first professors of anatomy and medicine there. They had also studied at West Nottingham, Princeton, and Edinburgh, and Morgan had apprenticed under Redman. Rush was clearly moving in the right circles.

Rush set his sights on the best medical education he could obtain. He and a colleague, Jonathan Potts, set out for Edinburgh in August 1766. Benjamin Franklin had written letters of introduction to the eminent Edinburgh physician, Sir Alexander Dick, and to William Cullen, the professor of medicine who shared teaching duties with Gregory (Goodman 1934, p. 14). Franklin actually gave Rush a letter of credit for 300 guineas to use while in London. Rush had to use 30 guineas of the credit, which he paid back to Franklin's wife after returning to Philadelphia. Rush wrote, "I take great pleasure in recording this delicate act of paternal friendship in Dr. Franklin. It attached me to him during the remainder of his life" (Rush 1948, p. 74). He enrolled in the Edinburgh medical school on November 3 of that year (Rush 1948, pp. 42–43), thus arriving the same year that Hume returned to the city and Gregory assumed his professorship.[5]

The Edinburgh Connection

Arriving in Edinburgh, Rush realized that he needed to do some review and remedial education.

Finding myself less acquainted with classical and philosophical learning than was necessary to comprehend all that was taught in medicine, I employed the summer months in reviving my knowledge of the Latin language and in studying the mathematicks, under a private tutor, in each of which I advanced with a rapidity and pleasure I never had known before.

(Rush 1948, p. 42)

He was apparently a rapid learner. That summer and autumn he made himself master French and taught himself Italian and Spanish "so as to be able to read them both to this day (July 2, 1800)" (Rush 1948, p. 43).

The professors at Edinburgh were the team we met in Chapter 1: "Monroe [sic, i.e., Secundus], Cullen, Black, Gregory, and Hope" (Rush 1948, p. 42). The second winter Rush attended lectures on classics and philosophy as well as those of Dr. Gregory on the practice of physic and those of Dr. Hope on the materia medica (Rush 1948, p. 43). Thus he received Gregory's introductory ethics lectures that would soon be student published and would appear two years later as the crucial *Lectures* (Gregory 1772). In his own career as professor of medicine, Rush gave similar lectures, first published as *Six Introductory Lectures to Courses of Lectures upon the Institute and Practice of Medicine* (Rush 1801).[6] An expanded collection of these lectures appeared 10 years later as *Sixteen Introductory Lectures to Courses of Lectures upon the Institutes and Practice of Medicine* (1811).

Rush graduated as Doctor of Medicine on June 19, 1768, later saying, "the two years I spent in Edinburgh I consider as the most important in their influence upon my character and conduct of any period of my life." The public lectures and private conversations with professors "not only gave me many new ideas, but opened my mind so to enable me to profit by reading and observation" (Rush 1948, p. 43). This was the formative period in his intellectual life.

In his autobiography Rush makes clear that this stimulation was not limited to medicine. He recounts being first exposed to republican ideas and calling the authority of the king into question (p. 46): "For the first moment in my life I now exercised my reason upon the subject of government." He became a regular houseguest of the Rev. Dr. John Erskine, an evangelical clergyman who preached at Old Greyfriars Church in Edinburgh and was friendly with American clergy, including Jonathan Edwards.

Rush had at least one direct meeting with David Hume, at the table of Sir Alexander Dick (the man to whom Franklin had introduced Rush). He also ate at the table of John Gregory, having met there Dr. William Robertson, a distinguished clergyman and "principal" (head) of the University of Edinburgh. While in Scotland, Rush played a significant role in convincing Dr. John Witherspoon to accept an appointment as president of the College of New Jersey. When Witherspoon's wife was hesitant to move to the New World, he spent several days with the family, after which she changed her mind.

In London late in 1768, after leaving Edinburgh, Rush met Sir John Pringle, the moral philosopher/physician to whom Gregory's *Lectures* were dedicated. The meeting led to an invitation to a weekly "conversation party" in Pringle's home. Rush also went to Pringle's home another evening of the week and "often dined with him in large and highly polished companies" (Rush 1948, p. 53). He spent time in the home of Benjamin Franklin, who was then in London, where Rush met a number of Franklin's literary friends.

Another distinguished contact in London was George Whitefield, a one-time close associate of John Wesley, the founder of Methodism. Rush met him occasionally in Edinburgh and frequently in London. He was much impressed by both men, saying that "he and Westley [John Wesley] constituted the two largest and brightest orbs that appeared in the hemisphere of the Church in the 18th Century" (Rush 1948, p. 56). Although Rush claimed to have not been acquainted with Wesley, he heard him preach twice in Edinburgh, describing him as "more learned, but less eloquent than Mr. Whitefield" (Rush 1948, p. 57). Rush was a regular at Scottish and English churches, attending Anglican, Methodist, and dissenting churches alike.[7]

Rush also associated with artists such as the popular American Benjamin West, who helped organize the Royal Academy of Artists and eventually became the historical painter of the king. Through West, Rush met other distinguished artists and authors. He dined with Samuel Johnson (Rush 1948, p. 58) and attended a dinner with Adam Ferguson, the Edinburgh mathematician turned moral philosopher who occupied the Edinburgh chair between Pringle and Dugald Stewart. Rush's account of acquaintances in Edinburgh and London goes on and on with countless other figures less central to our story.

In February 1769, Rush left for Paris. He had received from Ben Franklin a letter of introduction to several of Franklin's philosophical friends in Paris. Among those of various professions that Rush met were the philosopher Diderot (who entertained Rush in his library) and others who were to become active participants in the French revolution. Diderot gave Rush a letter for Hume, which Rush says he delivered to Hume when he returned to London. On his return voyage to America, Rush borrowed books to read, having sent his own books back to America earlier. He read Blackstone's newly published *Commentaries* and Foster's *Crown Law*, which he credits with providing the "relish for political science which I felt in the beginning of the American Revolution" (Rush 1948, p. 77). He also read novels until he had exhausted all the books on board, at which time he says he would have lapsed into "inquietude of mind" had not a friend offered to teach him German. A young man in his early twenties, Rush was clearly being socialized into the multidisciplinary cultural elite of the late eighteenth century in France as well as in England and Scotland. Rush was transformed into the American version of the Enlightenment man.

Philadelphia Enlightenment Man

Variously described as "physician, patriot, humanitarian" (Sudds 1957, p. 227), a "gadfly" (Hawke 1971), "revolutionary physician," "educator," "controversial figure" (Binger 1966), and a "reformer and philosopher" (Goodman 1934, p. 272), Benjamin Rush associated with the likes of Thomas Paine, John Adams, and Thomas Jefferson. He claimed to have suggested the title *Common Sense* for Paine's tract, a term he surely held vividly in his mind from his Edinburgh days (Binger 1966, p. 100). He was a member of the Continental Congress, a signer of the Declaration of Independence, and instrumental in developing a new constitution for the State of Pennsylvania. He served as treasurer of the United States Mint. He established the first free dispensary in the country, served as President of the Society for Promoting the Abolition of Slavery, and was instrumental in the creation of the American temperance movement. He was a regular correspondent with John Adams and Thomas Jefferson, mediating their famous feud and serving as something like Adams' personal psychiatrist. In medicine, he began teaching at the University of the State of Pennsylvania in 1780, was elected professor of the theory and practice of medicine at the College of Philadelphia in 1789, and, after the two schools merged in 1791, became professor of the course referred to as the "institutes of medicine and clinical practice."

The Empirical Science of Morality

Some of the most vivid evidence of the influence of the Scottish Enlightenment on Rush is in his theory of the science of morality. He wrote about the *moral sense* as early as 1774.[8] His position is developed at great length in his 1786 lecture, "Enquiry into the Influences of Physical Causes upon the Moral Faculty" (Rush 1786, reprinted in Rush 1947, pp. 181–211), his lecture "On the Study of Medical Jurisprudence" (Rush 1811, pp. 363–96), and his *Lectures on the Mind*, which plays less of a role in nineteenth- and twentieth-century Rush scholarship than it should because it was not published until recently (Rush 1981).[9] The editors of this volume, Eric T. Carlson, Jeffrey I. Wollock, and Patricia S. Noel, stress what is apparent from these primary sources: the enormous dependence of Rush's thought on his Scottish teachers.

Rush's debt to the Edinburgh scholars is conspicuous. He specifically mentions Gregory, but Cullen was even more influential.[10] Rush noted that "Dr. Gregory's lectures abound with excellent practical observations, but are by no means equal to the unrivaled Dr. Cullen's, whose merit is beyond all praise" (Rush 1768, p. 51).[11] Cullen advocated a "system" that focused on the role of the nervous system rather than the humors. Developing a variation on the system of John Brown, another of Cullen's students, Rush attempted to attribute all diseases to a single cause: excessive excitability or spasm in the blood vessels (Sudds 1957, p. 229; Goodman 1934, pp. 229–32). This was the theoretical foundation for his near-universal remedy of bleeding and purging. He used it widely during the yellow fever epidemic of 1793, leading a vitriolic critic who observed the relation between Rush's treatment and increasing mortality to describe it as "one of the great discoveries . . . which have contributed to the depopulation of the earth" (Cobbett, William. *The Rush-Light*. New York: Feb. 28, 1800, p. 49, cited in Sudds 1957, p. 230).

Rush continued the project of Cullen and Boerhaave before him of attempting to understand the relation of the mind to both neurophysiology and morality. He was clearly beginning the process of differentiation of physiology and philosophy. Consider, for example, the passage in his lectures where he discusses the "internal and external senses." Reconstructed from a hand-edited manuscript, Rush's text includes, in various versions, the following:

Chemistry has been adulterated by its mixture with alchemy, astronomy has been adulterated by its mixture with astrology, religion has suffered from its mixture with mysticism, [and phrenology has shared the same fate from its union with all the trash known by the name of metaphysics. In imitation of the illustrious reformers who have separated the above sciences from their unnatural mixtures, I shall endeavor to separate phrenology, from all the Scholastic and unintelligible jargon of metaphysics.] [bracketed material crossed out in Rush's final manuscript].

(Rush 1981, p. 406)

Nevertheless, as Carlson points out in his introduction to the *Lectures*, Rush was still heavily under the influence of such metaphysics and was an admirer of Locke, Reid, and Beattie (Rush 1981, p. 27). Rush followed Beattie and Reid in thinking of the mind as a system of faculties and operations (see Rush 1981, p. 29). The senses were localized as "faculties," which were conceptualized as having a locus physiologically as organs. Thus, like his Edinburgh predecessors, Rush conceptualized the mind and morality physiologically. He came to advocate a "unitary system of knowledge" in which "truth is an unit, and the more we discover of it in one branch of knowledge, the more we shall discover of it in others. Physiology and medicine, above all other sciences, lead to just principles in theology, religion, morals, and metaphysics" (p. 193, *cf.* Carlson's introduction, p. 30).

In the *Lectures*, Rush developed the concept of *sympathy* (Rush 1981, pp. 238–44), by which there is communication from one body part to another, and explored the senses that a twentieth-century person would think of as physiological (touch, taste, smell, sight, and sound) (pp. 244–351). He then turned to the faculties and operations of the mind (p. 403ff.), in which he viewed the moral faculties as critical. The moral faculties (pp. 460–76) are three in number: "1. the moral faculty properly so called, 2. the sense of Deity, or the theosophic faculty, . . . and 3. conscience" (p. 461). These are innate faculties of the mind that receive certain sensory impressions. They are senses precisely analogous to the external senses of sight and sound, etc.

The moral faculty per se is a term borrowed from James Beattie (Rush 1981, p. 461, n. 3). He explains in the 1786 lecture, "The Influence of Physical Causes Upon the Moral Faculty" (Rush 1947, p. 182), that the moral faculty has received different names. In the *Lectures* he mentions "Dr. Hutchison" [*sic*] using the term *moral sense*; "Dr. Adam Smith," *the sympathy*; and Rousseau, *moral instinct*, but says he has adopted the term *moral faculty* from "Dr. Beattie." Rush differentiates it from the sense of the deity in that it "has for its objects the duties we owe to our selves and fellow creatures only" (Rush 1981, pp. 461–62). He differentiates it from conscience in that the moral sense is the legislator or governor of our moral conduct while the conscience is the judge (p. 462; also see Carlson and Simpson 1965, p. 25). He associates the moral sense with the will and differentiates it from reason. He thinks Locke is in error for confounding the moral sense with reason and Shaftesbury is mistaken for confusing it with "taste" (Carlson and Simpson 1965, p. 26).

Rush acknowledges taking his terms for the other moral faculties from Scottish philosophers as well. His "sense of the Deity" he says comes from "Lord Kaims," i.e, Lord Kames (1696–1782) (Rush 1981, p. 462). Rush's presentation of the sense of the Deity encompasses references to the German founder of phrenology Franz Joseph Gall (1758–1828), the explorer Captain James Cook (1728–1779), his correspondence with his friend President John Adams (1735–1826), as well as biblical sources. In his discussion of the "sense of conscience" he draws on "Dr, Clark," (Samuel Clarke, 1675–1729, a leading clergyman and metaphysician of England). Clarke influenced Samuel Price, Joseph Butler, Francis Hutcheson, and Lord Kames, who, in turn, influenced Rush (Rush 1981, p. 470 and n. 2).

More generally, the *Lectures* show the influence or working knowledge of the philosophers and theologians Aquinas, Augustine, Beattie, Berkeley, Butler, Descartes, Hartley, Hobbes, Hume (whom Rush described as providing "absurdities and nonsense" [Rush 1981, p. 356]), Locke, Lord Kames, Martin Luther, Increase and Cotton Mather, Newton, Thomas Paine, Price, Priestley, Reid,

Rousseau, Seneca, Socrates, Dugald Stewart, Voltaire, John Wesley, and George Whitefield, as well as the physician/philosophers Boerhaave, Cullen, and John and James Gregory. All of these lectures are part of a set of lectures on the theory of medicine focusing on neurophysiology.[12] Similarly, many of these figures surface in various free-standing lectures, including "Observations on the Duties of a Physician, and the Methods of Improving Medicine" (1789), where Rush says to his medical students, "The authors I would recommend to you upon metaphysics, are, Butler, Locke, Hartly [sic], Reid, and Beattie. These ingenious writers have cleared this sublime science of its technical rubbish, and rendered it both intelligible and useful" (p. 10).[13]

Contribution to Medical Ethics

Rush's immersion in Scottish philosophy was not restricted to his development of theory related to the moral faculties. He published widely in both abstract and practical topics in ethics. Some of these essays began as the annual introductory lectures for his course in medicine (Rush 1801, 1811), following the tradition of Gregory and Cullen.

Selected Writings of Benjamin Rush and Introductory Lectures

Many of the more influential of Rush's writings on ethical topics are now collected together in *The Selected Writing of Benjamin Rush* (Rush 1947). The volume contains moral reflections addressed to the general public.[14] His published collections of introductory lectures (1801 and 1811) included several that were explicitly devoted to topics in philosophy and ethics.[15] More of his writings directed at a more general audience were published in *Essays, Literary, Moral & Philosophical* (Rush 1798).

Lack of Interest in Hippocratic Ethics

As we might expect from what we have seen in the Scottish English physicians who were in conversation with the humanities, Rush shows a relative lack of interest in Hippocrates, especially Hippocratic ethics. There is no mention of Hippocrates in *Lectures on the Mind* and not a single mention in his autobiography. Neither the historical figure nor the Oath that bears his name is associated with Rush in the major secondary works on Rush (Goodman 1934; Hawke 1971;[16] D'Elia 1974; Binger 1966) (except as noted below). It is not that Rush and his Enlightenment predecessors were ignorant of Hippocrates; Gregory cited him for his eloquent use of Greek. It is more that they were not engaged with his philosophical and ethical thought (see D'Elia 1974, for observations about Cullen's dislike of Hippocrates). In the eighteenth-century Edinburgh tradition, Rush translated Hippocrates' aphorisms but is described as "turning away from the first principle of the Hippocratic tradition: the healing power of nature"(D'Elia 1974, p. 18).

Rush makes passing references to Hippocrates' skills as a clinician and as an observer of medical phenomena and Rush finds him wanting in both respects. He sees the reverence for the great medical figures of history as stifling medical science. In "The Progress of Medicine" (1801) he refers to an "undue attachment to great names:

Hippocrates, Galen, and Aaraeteus, among the ancients; Boerhaave, Cullen, and Brown among the moderns; have all, in their turns, established a despotism in medicine, by the popularity of their names, which has imposed a restraint upon free inquiry, and thereby checked the progress of medicine, particularly in the ages and countries, in which they have lived.[17]

(Rush 1947, p. 228)

There is one important exception to the observation that Rush pays only minimal attention to Hippocrates. One of his introductory lectures to his course on the theory of medicine, from the relatively late year of 1806 (when he was 60 years of age, seven years before his death), focuses on the Greek figure. That lecture, "On the Opinions and Modes of Practice of Hippocrates" (Rush 1811, pp. 274–293), is revealing. He is decidedly ambivalent, organizing his lecture into two sections: the first discusses elements in Hippocrates that Rush believes are correct, and the second, a longer section, mentions opinions that Rush believes are erroneous. What is striking is that, much as with Gregory, the entire focus is on Hippocrates as a clinician and medical observer of nature. He endorses Hippocrates' observations about the influence of climate and seasons on health and life, the influence of "water and situation" on the human body, and certain clinical practices. He endorses Hippocrates' use of "evacuations," "external caustics," venesection, "bleeding from parts that were diseased," purges, diuretics, and sudoforifics, as well as "exercise and labor." But he is critical of Hippocrates' ignorance of anatomy. He claims "his physiological opinions are fanciful" and "his pathology is many particulars is erroneous." He goes on to say that "the errors of Hippocrates appear chiefly in his treatment of diseases." From Rush's perspective, Hippocrates can be faulted on the forbidding of bleeding and purging in the early stage of fevers and in pregnancy. Hippocrates rejects the unity of diseases, making an expensive stock of drugs necessary for treatment. Along the way Rush does praise Hippocrates' moral character, seeing him as a man of "piety, charity, patriotism, benevolence, integrity, candor, and the highest degree of disinterestedness." But Rush concludes his lecture by damning Hippocrates as a clinician: "Were he to revive, and enter upon the practice of physic with no other stock if knowledge than that he has left behind him, he would not be equal, in a combat with a violent disease, to a common nurse who had for a number of years administered the prescriptions of modern physicians" (Rush 1811, pp. 292–93).

What is striking is that even when Rush mentions Hippocrates, he is not only critical but also focuses, as Gregory did, on Hippocrates skills as a clinical observer. There is not a single mention of Hippocrates' Oath or other deontological (ethical) writings except the aphorisms (which were the stock Greek translation exercise in Edinburgh).[18]

SAMUEL BARD

The Edinburgh Connection

Meanwhile, in New York another giant of early American medicine was emerging. Samuel Bard (1742–1821) was the son of another distinguished physician, John Bard (1716–1799), who was the first president of the Medical Society of the State of New York.[19] Bent on turning his son into a physician, John Bard entered him into King's College. After graduating in 1760, Samuel Bard departed for Britain to pursue his medical education. He first went to London where, having made contact with Drs. Hunter and Fothergill, he entered St. Thomas's hospital as a physician's pupil, and then to Edinburgh where he studied under Cullen, Whytt, the Monros, and Hope. (He graduated in 1765, and thus did not study with Gregory.) Bard developed a reputation as a good classical scholar. Thomas Percival was a student with him. He was particularly delighted with Cullen's lectures (McVicker 1822, p. 44), commenting that "Cullen has lately entertained me much, by some private lectures he gives to those who attend him for the second year. . . . I cannot help comparing him on these occasions, to some one of the ancient philosophers, surrounded by his admiring pupils" (McVicker 1822, pp. 55–56). In Edinburgh Bard was exposed to the aphorisms of Hippocrates, which were, as we have seen, part of the final examination.

Bard's New York Medical Practice

Upon graduation, Bard returned to New York where he practiced medicine with his father but soon became involved in the efforts to establish a medical school in New York on the pattern of the new school in Philadelphia. He became a founder, professor of the theory and practice of physic, and for many years its dean. Although Bard had loyalist leanings during the revolution, he returned to favor soon thereafter, becoming the private physician of the mayor of New York and eventually of George Washington.

Duties of a Physician

Although his inaugural dissertation at Edinburgh (1765) and his later publications tended toward medical topics (Bard 1771, 1788, 1807), one early address, a commencement address for the first medical degrees at King's College, gained Bard a reputation as a significant contributor to medical morality in American history.

Entitled "A Discourse upon the Duties of a Physician, with some Sentiments on the Usefulness and Necessity of a Public Hospital" (Bard 1769), it positioned Bard as second only to Rush in moral commentary on American medicine at that time.

The lecture is a rather modest undertaking. It admonishes the young graduates to be diligent in their pursuit of medical knowledge, impressing on them that "where the Object is of so great Importance as the Life of a Man; you are accountable even for the Errors of Ignorance, unless you have embraced every Opportunity of obtaining Knowledge" (p. 4). He extols several uncontroversial virtues of the physician: integrity and ability, honesty, delicacy, and compassion. He opposes secret nostrums (p. 10), a theme that was to become important in nineteenth-century American medical ethics. In this lecture, however, are several items of importance to our study. First, he makes reference to Hippocrates, but only in the same manner as that of his Edinburgh mentors and Rush: Bard praises his "unwearied Diligence in observing and collecting the Symptoms of Diseases, his Fidelity and Accuracy in relating them, his happy Facility in discovering their Causes, his almost prophetic Knowledge of their Events, and his successful Treatment of them" (p. 6). Like Rush and Cullen, Bard is ambivalent in his praise of the so-called father of medicine, saying, "do not affect the Pedantry of despising the Moderns; and carefully avoid that Rock, upon which most of the fond Admirers of Antiquity have split, a blind and slavish Attachment to its Opinions; the Bar where Truth has been so often Shipwrecked, and which more than the want of Ingenuity or capacity, stopped the Progress of Leaning for about twelve hundred Years" (p. 7).

What is striking is that, even though this is unlike any twenty-first century commencement address speaker, who would not be able to avoid reference to the Hippocratic Oath or other ethical writings when discussing the duties of the physician, Bard shows absolutely no interest in these writings. In fact, his focus is on matters of medical duty that are quite alien to the Hippocratic tradition: concern and compassion for the poor. In moving, graphic detail he recounts the suffering of the sick who are destitute, "the unhappy Victims, both of Poverty and Disease, claim your particular Attention; I cannot represent to myself a more real Object of Charity, than a poor Man with perhaps a helpless Family, laboring under the complicated Miseries of Sickness and Penery" (p. 14). He concludes with a plea for the creation of a public hospital as "one of the most useful and necessary charitable Institutions that can possibly be imagined" (p. 15). These concerns of compassion for the poor—for a social responsibility in ethics—is in keeping with the benevolence of Edinburgh.

Of note in Bard's address is his emphasis on use of simple remedies, which we saw in Wesley and again to some extent in Rush. According to Bard, "it is impossible to learn the true Virtues of Medicines, from compound Prescriptions; and Inelegance frequently disappoints us of their effects" (p. 12). We also begin to see a theme that first appeared in Bacon and became more important later in the century: the focus on the first priority for preserving life (pp. 3, 10)—another non-Hippocratic theme.

Bard is an interesting turn-of-the century transition figure. He clearly had a classical Enlightenment education and broad interests in humanities concerns, but he was not the virtuoso that Rush or his Edinburgh predecessors were. We see in Bard a late eighteenth-century gentleman maintaining his high status with dignity, but feeling pulled more toward narrower medical projects of research and administration. While Rush was president of the American Philosophical Society, a political philosopher, moral theorist, and founder of the horticultural society, Bard was for the most part content to be the long-term dean of Columbia's College of Physicians and Surgeons. Still, he was the New York area's moral voice, revealing that the well-educated physician of the time could still retain, at least to a moderate degree, a serious interest in broader, more humanities-oriented aspects of medicine. This trend toward narrower interests in the science and administration of medicine is a pattern that will accelerate in the coming decades, a story to which we turn in Chapter 6.

6

THE SCIENTIZING OF MEDICINE
IN THE UNITED STATES

One looks in vain for the successors of Benjamin Rush and Samuel Bard in American medicine. As in Scotland and England where William Alison and the rest of the Edinburgh medical faculty withdrew from the public discourse of the Enlightenment to a more aggressively discipline-bound medical science, so in the United States during the first quarter of the nineteenth century the "scientizing" of medicine went forward. As knowledge expanded, the breadth of the interest of medical practitioners contracted. Even the best academicians could no longer take the knowledge of the world as their domain. They became creatures of their discipline.

Looking for an examplar of academic medicine at its best in the first half of the nineteenth century, we cannot find a plausible example of a medical scholar whose interests roamed from political philosophy to the healing arts and on to ethics in anything remotely resembling the richness of a Rush or a Bard. The most interesting figure—because of the potential he had to be his generation's Rush and the connection he made to the succeeding developments in medical ethics of organized medicine—is Nathaniel Chapman (1780–1853).

NATHANIEL CHAPMAN

The Right Roots

The Philadelphia Elite

Born in 1780 to an Alexandria, Virginia, family of considerable distinction, Nathaniel Chapman married into the elite Biddle family in Philadelphia. Richman (1967, p. 185) describes this connection as "firmly establishing Chapman as one of *the* physicians to the Philadelphia elite." As the years passed, he became the unchallenged leader of American medicine in the first half of the nineteenth century.[1] Referred to as "a leader among followers," he was the founder of the *Philadelphia Journal of the Medical and Physical Sciences* in 1820 and became the first president of the American Medical Association in 1847 at the founding meeting that was to give rise to the first national, professionally generated American code of medical ethics (Richman, 1967, p. 5). The first half of the nineteenth century has been referred to as the "Medical Age of Chapman" (Richman 1967, p. 1).

Chapman began his medical training at age 15 in the apprenticeship system, first with relative John Weems of Georgetown and then with Elisha Cullen Dick of Alexandria, the distinguished private student of Benjamin Rush who attended George Washington at his death. Chapman eventually joined the faculty of University of Pennsylvania Medical School, becoming Professor of Materia Medica (in 1813) and then, like Gregory and several others we are following, being named to Professor of the Theory and Practice of Medicine (three years later). In Chapman's case, it was the same position held earlier by Rush.

The Rush Connection

In 1797 Chapman moved to Philadelphia to study at the Medical School of the University of Pennsylvania, where Rush was among the faculty. At the time, the same loose system of education that existed at Edinburgh could be found at the Pennsylvania medical school. Students had to take one course from each professor, for whom they bought admission tickets for a price of 20 dollars. In addition, Chapman became one of Rush's private students, a relationship that continued throughout Chapman's formal medical training. Since Rush generally limited his private students or apprentices to six, it was a prized position. The fee was the extraordinary sum of 100 pounds in cash (Richman 1967, p. 28). A hint of things to come, however, is seen in the mundane and scientific nature of Chapman's doctoral thesis, *An Essay on the Canine State of Fever* (Chapman 1801), i.e., rabies. Chapman's publications during his lifetime were essentially restricted to technical, scientific medicine. His books included *Discourses on the Elements of Therapeutics and Materia Medica* (1817–1819), *Essays on Practical Medicine and Surgery* (1841), and *Lectures on the More Important Eruptive Fevers, Haemorrhages and Dropsies: and on Gout and Rheumatism* (1844). He also edited a number of texts on scientific aspects of medicine used in his classes.

Port Folio and the Tuesday Club

On occasion, Chapman did stray beyond writing on scientific medicine. Under the pseudonym "Falkland," while still a student he published two short pieces of political opinion in letter format in the new local magazine, *Port Folio*, expressing his anti-Bonapartist views. The writers gathered together into an informal group, the Tuesday Club, reminiscent of the Wise Club in Aberdeen or the Philosophical

Society in Edinburgh, but there is no record of Chapman using this venue to develop his philosophical or ethical interests. Chapman's only other nonmedical publishing of note was his editing of five volumes of *Select Speeches, Forensick and Parliamentary with Prefatory Remarks* in 1807–1808, which he undertook in the early years of his medical practice when he was apparently underemployed as a physician. The topics were political and legal, including taxation and reservations about popular suffrage. Philosophy, religion, and ethics were not on his agenda, although he did attack the slave trade in his editorial comments on William Wilberforce's speech on the subject.

The Edinburgh Connection

Chapman's opportunity to continue the Enlightenment tradition of medicine in conversation with the intellectual elite in other disciplines was not limited to his Philadelphia connections. We know he was exposed to some other figures discussed in this book. He read Cullen and Percival's essay on hydrophobia (rabies) (Richman 1967, p. 29), which later was treated critically in his doctoral thesis.

Soon after obtaining his medical degree, Chapman followed in the tradition of Rush and left for Britain—with a letter of introduction from his mentor, much as Rush had relied on one from Benjamin Franklin. He studied first as a private student under a well-known medical teacher, John Abernethy, in England and then departed for Edinburgh Medical School. At the time of his arrival, just after the turn of the century, John Gregory and Alexander Monro, Primus, were gone, but James Gregory was there, and Chapman eventually made the acquaintance of Dugald Stewart, the Professor of Moral Philosophy we encountered in Chapter 1 (Richman 1967, p. 43). In summary, Chapman came close to the giants of the Scottish Enlightenment and their descendants, but never quite engaged their extravagant style of sweeping intellectual range, in which philosophers and other humanists co-mingled with the medical elite a few years earlier.

From the Philadelphia Clubs to American Philosophical Society President

It is not that Nathaniel Chapman was out of touch with some of the cultural elite of the day. Much as Monro, Primus, in Edinburgh, he seemed to be in contact without having the humanities stick to him. In addition to his role of private physician, he participated in a number of social and intellectual groups such as the Wistar Party (Richman 1967, p. 166). In 1798, Dr. Caspar Wistar and his wife began holding parties at their home that involved the local literati of Philadelphia. They continued at that venue on a regular basis until his death in 1818. At that time, the group formalized the gatherings, establishing the Wistar Party, which continued to meet at the homes of its members. The group would eventually evolve to the status of a group within the American Philosophical Society. The gatherings were remarkably similar to those of the Philosophical Society of Edinburgh, with one exception. Wistar was a professor at the medical school, which slanted the participation. The group included faculty from the medical school and members of the Board of Trustees.[2] Critically, however, it lacked clergy, philosophers, poets, and other humanists that peopled the clubs of Aberdeen and Edinburgh.[3] In 1830–31, 9 of the 24 members were physicians, none were humanists. This configuration had to shape the intellectual content of the gatherings.

A second Philadelphia group to which Chapman belonged had somewhat broader intentions. The Athenian Institute, formed in 1838, had as its purpose, "public Lectures on Moral Literary and Scientific Subjects" (cited in Richman 1967, p. 167). There was some overlap in membership with the Wistar Party.[4] In fact, sectarian religion and party politics were explicitly excluded as acceptable topics for lectures. The group sponsored an annual meeting, the intellectual content of which seems questionable. The reports focus on the "speeches and puns," concluding in one case that "nothing remarkable happened" (Richman 1967, p. 167). The group disbanded after eight years. There is no remaining record of any discourse that could be considered significant humanities conversation.[5]

Chapman was a member of other Philadelphia organizations: the Board of Managers of the Philadelphia Assembly, the Musical Fund, the Sons of St. George Societies, and the St. Andrews Society, but the most important was surely the American Philosophical Society, which he joined in 1807. His involvement was significant; he eventually became the society's vice president, a position he held from 1828 through 1846, before becoming its president, serving in that capacity until the first days of 1849 when, aging and in failing health, he declined a new term. The intellectual content of his involvement, however, resembled remarkably that of Monro's in the Philosophical Society. Specifically, there was not much of what we would call philosophy. His first responsibilities were reviewing scientific medical papers on light and longevity, not unlike Monro's contributions, but radically different from Gregory's six presentations to the Aberdeen Wise Club that gave rise to his philosophically oriented *A Comparative View*. Chapman contributed funds for purchasing a copy of Muhlenberg's *Herbarium*, signaling a horticultural interest that later would be manifest in his involvement in the Pennsylvania Horticultural Society. With a colleague he studied two South American medicines for the Society. He became involved in a project to develop a canal connecting the Chesapeake and the Delaware River, donated a portrait of ornithologist Alexander Wilson, helped write a condolence letter at the death of fellow-member Thomas Jefferson, proposed a resolution of regrets on the death of John Adams, and was deeply involved in the writing of bylaws and fundraising. His years as president have been described as "tranquil." As Richman (p. 175) summarizes, "his only actions were of a procedural nature."

What emerges is a picture of an engaging figurehead skilled in humorous oratory and willing to do committee work who got excited about technical scientific projects. What is lacking is any inclination to engage the deeper, more philosophical issues. In short, he is no Gregory or Percival. He is not even his generation's Benjamin Rush.

Chapman had the best possible credentials to continue the Edinburgh and Benjamin Rush tradition as an elite, upper-class, classically educated scholar of the Enlightenment with eclectic interests that connect medicine and the humanities. As with his Scottish and English counterparts after the turn of the century, however, Chapman's interests were more constricted. Like Monro, Primus, the prototypical medical scientist whose narrow interests represent the beginnings of the isolation of medicine from the humanities, Chapman's attention turned to commerce, industry, and horticulture (Richman 1967, p. 176).

Chapman as Scientific Era Physician (in the Monro Model)

Professor with Interests Limited to Mundane Medicine

The narrow focus of Chapman's interests can be seen in his doctoral thesis. As a student of Rush, he took up a dispute between Rush and Cullen about the theory of fevers. But what for these masters was a minor theme in a grand scheme of scholarship became for the student a major focus. In this project he attempts to prove (in support of his mentor) that various fevers, including rabies, are all manifestations of the phenomenon of "fever." He does this by means such as noting that the various conditions he is examining show similarities in pulse. The conclusion is support for Rush's prescription of bleeding and the purgative calomel. Richman describes him as "parroting . . . the ideas of Benjamin Rush" (Richman 1967, p. 36). Although later in life he would move away from Rush on some matters (Richman, pp. 55–62), he remained loyal with regard to valuing bleeding and purging. Here we have a less creative mind doing what Thomas Kuhn (1962, p. 35) calls the "puzzle-solving" of day-to-day science, rather than the more creative, imaginary minds of the previous generation who could move back and forth from medicine to philosophy, literature, and what we would now call the humanities. Like Monro, Chapman was more at home pursuing more technical, scientific problems in medical physiology and anatomy. At one point he performed experiments to confirm Monro's finding that maternal and fetal circulation were distinct. This is the kind of problem that challenged both Chapman and the older Edinburgh anatomist.

Sympathy: What Has It Come To? (Chapman's Medicalizing of Sympathy)

Perhaps the most vivid example of the narrowing of interests to medicine as a science can be seen by what has happened to the Enlightenment's concept of *sympathy*. While for Hume and others of that generation, including Benjamin Rush, sympathy was a critical concept integrating a physiological theory of the human senses with a broader social theory of morality, by Chapman's time, sympathy had undergone a very remarkable transformation into a theory of medical science and pharmacology.

Hume and his philosophical colleagues explored a grand theory of human moral conduct, drawing out the connections with current discoveries in sensory physiology. This, in turn, stimulated Rush to expound a physiologically based account of what was to become modern psychiatry that included an extended theory of the moral sense. These moral scientists were addressing the mechanism of how one person's suffering could be transferred to produce effects on the feelings of others. Their answer was to posit a sensory mechanism they called "sympathy," a capacity of one person to "feel with" another person's anguish. Rush was still bridging the gap between the physiological medical sciences and morality. Sympathy was a moral concept grounded in newly discovered sensory physiology.

By Chapman's generation the focus had shifted. He and his colleagues were now pursuing more technical medical questions. One problem of concern was the mechanism by which a drug (or chemical such as wine or opium) taken into the body could manifest effects so quickly on distant organs. Drugs reaching the stomach would exert their effect almost immediately on some other distant organ of the body—the kidneys or lungs, for example. It was, in fact, the problem that Chapman had originally planned to address in his doctoral thesis before his mentor pressed him to study the implication of rabies for the concept of fever (Richman 1967, p. 32). Drawing on others working on these issues, Chapman maintained, "my theory of the operation of medicines is of modern date, and alleges, that they all act by exciting a local impression, which is extended through the medium of *sympathy"* (Chapman 1823–24, Vol. 1, p. 42, quoted in Richman 1967, p. 92, italics added).

The early nineteenth-century physiologists and pharmacological specialists had proposed a neurological communication between the organs that directly paralleled the way the moral-sense theorists understood moral communication between those who suffer and those who identify with that suffering. This formulation is the linguistic origin of our modern notion of the "sympathetic nervous system." For Chapman, sympathy provided an explanation of drug action that is independent of the circulatory system of humoral theory. Can it be an accident that the moral term of Hume, Gregory, and the Enlightenment theorists that led Rush to construct a complex physiological psychology and moral theory surfaced a generation later in Rush's student, who had shifted his attention to the more technical, physiological workings of the body, totally divorced from the social and moral context of the earlier generation?

In fact, Chapman was apparently not the first to use the term *sympathy* in a narrower physiological and pharmaceutical way. It appeared in the text of John Murray, *System of Materia Medica and Pharmacy* (1815), that Chapman edited · for use as a text. In this context *sympathy* refers to a "nervous association of the parts," a suitable analogy to the relation between persons in the earlier use of the term. Later Chapman used the term *sympathy* to explain how semen reached the ovaries during conception.[6]

The American Medical Association's First President

While president of the American Philosophical Society, Chapman was further honored by being named the first president of the American Medical Association (AMA). He was at least 67 years old (there being some dispute about the exact date of his birth). Given his age and other responsibilities, his role in the AMA founding was rather marginal. He took no part in the organizational meetings. At the first association meeting in May 1847, he was elected the group's president. (Alfred Stillé was chosen as secretary and Arrangements Committee chair, and Isaac Hays was chosen to be treasurer, both of whom we shall encounter later in this chapter.)

JOHN REDMON COXE

A second Philadelphia figure deserves attention as a possible successor to Rush as a contributor to nineteenth-century medical ethics. John Redmon Coxe (1773–1864?) is the period's most serious student of Hippocrates. He studied in Edinburgh for 15 months, after which, in 1789, he attended courses in anatomy and chemistry at the London Hospital (Waterson 1912, p. 204). He then studied under Rush from 1790 to 1794, when he obtained his degree of Doctor of Medicine. He fought the Philadelphia yellow fever epidemic with Rush and was an enthusiastic advocate of vaccination.

Coxe was a professor at the University of Pennsylvania's Medical School from 1809 until 1835, serving as chair of Materia Medica. He was something of a linguist and classical scholar, publishing the first comprehensive English edition of Hippocrates' writings (Coxe 1846). While testifying to the popularity of Hippocrates and Galen by the early decades of the nineteenth century, he bemoaned the lack of serious knowledge of these authors: "Our books continually quote them [Hippocrates and Galen]; and yet, not one in a hundred of the Profession, at least in America, have ever seen them, and if interrogated, could not inform us of what they treat" (Coxe 1846, pp. iii–iv).

Coxe was an enthusiastic defender of Hippocrates as well as a scholar, but his interest was not in the Hippocratic ethic. Although Coxe included the Oath in his English translation of Hippocrates, he did not discuss it anywhere, nor did he discuss any other Hippocratic ethical writings. Rather, he was interested in Hippocrates as a prototypical empirical scientist, much as the eighteenth-century physicians were. The critical difference between Coxe and Rush is that Coxe defended Hippocrates' technical views on anatomy and physiology against attacks by Rush.

This much more sympathetic view of Hippocrates appears in Coxe's "An Introductory Lecture in Vindication of Hippocrates Delivered in the University of Pennsylvania,"[7] dating from November 3, 1829. He describes the development of his interest in Hippocrates and his disagreements with his mentor as follows:

Nearly 40 years have elapsed since, under the guidance of my much respected friend and preceptor, the late Prof. Rush, I imbibed the highest veneration to the character and writings of the illustrious Hippocrates; . . . [my enthusiasm for his work led me to prepare this lecture] . . . which is intended as a vindication of the great father of medicine, from aspersions thrown upon his fame, by Dr. Rush himself.

(Coxe 1834, p. 219).

Coxe's defense of Hippocrates continues: "The writings of Hippocrates can, however, I think, scarcely be consulted, without . . . tacit acquiescence in the opinion, that whoever wrote them, must have had a competent acquaintance with practical anatomy" (Coxe 1834, p. 221). Thus Coxe played a key role in the rehabilitation of Hippocrates from his eighteenth-century obscurity, but he is not the one who should be directly credited with resurrection of the Oath as the icon of medical ethics.

Aside from his unusual proclivities for classical scholarship in the history of medicine, Coxe's interests were quite mundane. As befitting a professor of materia medica (the study of medicinal plants), his best-known works were *The American Dispensary* and the *Philadelphia Medical Dictionary*. He published on combustion and yellow fever. His only nontechnical publications dealt with such obscure matters as recognition of friends in another world and phrenology in connection with the soul. In 1835 he was removed from his professorship by the university trustees following a four-year dispute over the quality of his teaching syllabus.

EARLY HISTORY OF ORGANIZED MEDICINE'S ETHICS

Boston

Philadelphia was not the only city in which the new century saw practitioners of medicine narrow their attention to more scientific medical concerns. It was not the only place in which medical ethics in communication with the fields of humanities was replaced with a more narrow focus on professionally articulated ethics for the medical profession. In fact, the first city, at least in modern times, in which a professional organization developed a code for its members was Boston.

Boston Medical Police

In 1807 the Association of Boston Physicians instructed a standing committee to propose a "Code of Medical Police," that is, a code of ethics for its members. That committee issued its report in March 1808, and the result was the adoption of the first professionally generated code by an organization of physicians (*Boston Medical Police* 1808; for a reprint see also Warren et al. 1995, p. 41). This was a modest document consisting of nine sections in 11 pages dealing essentially with relations among practitioners. The sections included issues related to the use of consultations, interference with other practitioners' patients, discouragement of quackery, fees, provision of medical care for colleagues and their families without charge, and seniority. The topics on patient care that late twentieth-century medical ethicists would consider central were not on the agenda.

The committee made clear what its method was. The group of three examined the publications of Gregory, Rush, and Percival and "selected from them such articles, as seemed most applicable to the circumstances of the profession in this place" (Warren et al. 1995, p. 41). They claim to have made alterations or additions to them as they thought necessary. This claim is hard to support, but, as Chester Burns (1977b, p. 302) has noted, "all of the precepts in the *Boston Medical Police* could be found in the second chapter of Percival's *Medical Ethics*, the chapter that discussed such situations in private practice as consultations, arbitration of differences, interferences with another's practice, fees, and seniority among practitioners."

Controversy over Links to Earlier Works

Late twentieth-century scholarship has produced something of a controversy over the intellectual and historical links between the *Boston Medical Police* and earlier works—not only those of Gregory, Rush, and Percival but also those with non-physicians such as Gisborne. The controversy relates to the question of whether the committee adopted the social contractarian position of earlier political philosophers and medical ethicists. The code of the *Boston Medical Police* referred explicitly to a "tacit compact, not only to submit to the laws, but to promote the honour and interest of the association, so far as they are consistent with morality and the general good of mankind" (Warren et al. 1995, p. 44).

This is language that can be traced to Percival and, from him, to Gisborne and ultimately to Locke, Hobbes, and Rousseau. Thus, the question is whether the *Boston Medical Police* reflects a moral theory with this impressive pedigree. Can the committee members be seen as standing in a long line of philosophers going all the way back to Locke, a philosopher who was also physician?

In the 1984 monograph *Physicians, Law, and Ethics,* Carleton Chapman, a physician who has an interest in the history of medicine, noted the contractarian language, but claimed that the compact mentioned "was in no way comparable to the social contract of the political theorists of the Enlightenment, from Locke and Rousseau. The closest analogue was the agreement between the medieval craftsman and his guild" (Chapman 1984, p. 86).

Robert Baker, a philosopher/historian from Union College, took issue with Chapman (Baker 1995b, pp. 25–31). He traced the conceptual and historical roots of the contract notion, emphasizing the tie between Gisborne and Percival. He then showed that the Association of Boston Physicians confronted a problem of social cooperation, in which physicians' short-term self-interest could lead them to competitive actions against colleagues that were, in the long run, contrary to the interest of all the association's members—a problem similar to that commanding the attention of the earlier contractarians.

I suspect, however, that Chapman and Baker are talking past each other and, in the process, may be missing an important point. While Baker shows both the historical and conceptual links of the Boston document to the eighteenth-century works, Chapman wants to emphasize the crucial difference between a hypothetical social contract involving an entire society and a cooperative agreement among members of a guild who pursue a common interest against others in society outside the professional group. Thus for Chapman it is important that the *Boston Medical Police* does not address physician–patient relations. What is critical is the conceptual discontinuity between broad societal compacts and narrower compacts among professionals to pursue a common interest against outsiders. Baker's interest, by contrast, is in showing that, whatever the differences, both the Boston compact and the earlier ones are addressing what he calls the "cooperative dilemma."

From my point of view, the critical issues are not whether the *Boston Medical Police* and earlier documents were historically linked and whether they addressed similar problems—certainly they did. For me, the real issue is whether the committee members and the full membership had any real understanding that they were entering a long-standing dispute in political philosophy, taking a position that placed them in a long line of social contractarians. While Percival and certainly Gisborne did have such knowledge, I see no evidence that the committee members who drafted the *Boston Medical Police* did. These later authors were not continuing an ongoing philosophical discourse in political theory—in fact, they probably had neither knowledge of nor interest in such theory—but were borrowing from the most philosophically sophisticated literature *within medicine* they could find that was relevant to the problem they were addressing. The writings of Gregory, Percival, and Rush were treatises written by physicians who were among the last of their profession who understood the philosophical ideas of their day. While these three documents would surely not have been the only philosophically informed writings that dealt with these issues, they were apparently the only literature available to the committee members.

Background of the Committee

To support this claim, we need to examine the makeup of the committee that developed the Boston list of precepts. The three members were John Warren, Lemuel

Hayward, and John Fleet. None of them had the interests or skills that would enable them to understand or knowingly adopt the social contractarian ideas of their
time. Proving this may be impossible, but the available evidence points to this
conclusion.

JOHN WARREN. John Warren (1753–1815) was the first committee member
listed and the most distinguished one.[8] John Warren was a surgeon, born in
Roxbury, Massachusetts, in 1753, a generation after Gregory and 13 years after
Percival.[9] He graduated from Harvard in 1771, may have taken part in the Boston
Tea Party, taught courses in dissection, and became professor of anatomy and
surgery. He was, however, much more in the style of Monro than of Gregory. Like
Monro he was a surgeon and was the first professor of anatomy at a distinguished
medical school (Harvard). He was a man of practical, concrete interests. He es-
tablished a smallpox hospital (with future *Boston Medical Police* co-author Lemuel
Hayward), studied yellow fever, helped organize the local medical society in
Boston, and became the president of the state medical association, a position he
held from 1804 to 1815.

Outside of medicine his interests were in neither philosophy nor politics.
Rather, he served as president of the Humane Society and the Agricultural Society and as grand master of the Massachusetts lodge of Freemasons. He was a
member of Brattle Street Church, which was, at the time evolving from Trinitar-
ian to Unitarian doctrine, but left no evidence of his participation in the theological debate. His publications were in medical science, dealing with febrile
diseases and comparative anatomy. Like Chapman, he was in demand as a public speaker. In short, there is not a single trace of evidence of any interest or
skill in philosophy or the other humanities that would prepare him to enter the
tradition of moral and political philosophy of the three physicians whose works
the committee used in developing the *Police* code. The text of the *Boston Medical Police* makes clear that his attention was narrowly focused on the practical
problems of interaction among physicians. While the problem was similar to that
of Percival, the philosophical preparation for writing the first medical ethical code
of the Americas was nonexistent.

LEMUEL HAYWARD. Lemuel Hayward (1749–1821) was also a surgeon.[10] He
apprenticed under Joseph Warren, John's father. Four years older than John Warren, he was still of the new generation of more narrowly focused physicians. He
was eminent for his treatment of smallpox and was an original member of the
Massachusetts Medical Society, serving for some time on its executive council
and as a counselor, chairman of the censors, and member of a prize committee.
While well known as a surgeon, he was not as eminent as John Warren and certainly leaves nothing in his biography that would suggest skills or interest in ethics,
philosophy, or other humanities.[11]

JOHN FLEET. John Fleet (1766–1913) was the youngest of the three (Farlow 1928). He was a student of John Warren's and in 1793 was appointed his first assistant. Fleet was the first to receive a degree from Harvard Medical School. He was also a surgeon, leaving two published works. Both were technical discourses on medical matters.[12] Neither left much of a mark on medicine, let alone the broader society. Together the two publications total 36 pages. Fleet was a founder of the Medical Improvement Society and the Boston Medical Library, for which he served as the first librarian. He was also librarian and secretary of the Massachusetts Medical Society. There is no evidence of any interest or publications in the humanities.

Nothing symbolizes the radical turn-of-the-century transition from physicians who were legitimate scholars in humanities to a group of physicians narrowly focused on medical science more than the emergence of these three surgeons in Boston in 1808. While Gregory was a legitimate scholar in philosophy in dialogue with non-physician humanists, these Boston practitioners' only foray into something resembling philosophy or ethics was the production of the *Boston Medical Police*. Baker is correct in stating that they worked in the tradition of Gisborne, Percival, Gregory, and Rush, in that they appear to have done a quick study of these sources (indirectly getting a hint of Gisborne through Percival). What is important and new, however, is not that they read these late eighteenth-century giants, but that they appear to have read them as strangers, as pragmatic medical technicians and bureaucrats of a medical professional organization called upon by the local professional group to produce a document that would help solve the immediate problem of physician criticism of colleagues. The Monro model, with its virtues of affirming the all-consuming complexity of medical science and technique, had won out, pointing to a future of real progress in medical science and a dark night of professionally isolated and amateurish medical ethics. For nineteenth-century medical ethics code writers, Gregory, Percival, and Rush—and eventually the ancient physicians such as Hippocrates and Galen—became not gateways to the best contemporary philosophical minds but end points, final sources of ethics as it applied to medicine, detached from their mentors and colleagues as well as the cultural contexts in which they worked. Gregory and Percival were no longer conduits for greater understanding of the Scottish Enlightenment thinkers struggling with the questions of empiricism, skepticism, moral-sense theory, and the nonconforming church's challenge to the Anglican or Catholic authority; they were now timeless, ultimate authorities on matters moral in the isolated world of medicine.

Role of John Ware

While we are considering Boston medicine of the early nineteenth century, we should pause to say a word about another distinguished Boston physician, John Ware (1795–1864).[13] In the style and language of Gregory, he gave an introductory address to the medical class at Harvard University, October 16, 1833, with the title, "Duties and Qualifications of Physicians" (Ware 1833). The lecture was incorporated into Ware's 1847 book, *Discourses on Medical Education, and on the Medical Profession*, which, in turn, became part of the return migration of medical ethics from the United States back to England when the English edition appeared in 1849.

Ware was the son of Rev. Henry Ware, a famous clergyman and Hollis Professor of Theology at Harvard College. He practiced dentistry for 10 years before becoming a medical editor, educator, and researcher. He was one of the editors of the *Boston Medical and Surgical Journal* in the 1820s before joining the medical school faculty and eventually becoming the Hersey Professor of the Theory and Practice of Physic. In his role as editor, we can see evidence of broader humanities interests. He also edited the *Boston Journal of Philosophy and the Arts* between 1823 and 1826 and edited editions of William Smellie's *Philosophy of Natural History* (1824) and William Paley's *Natural Theology* (1829). Thus, like the early nineteenth-century sons of Scottish humanists, Ware had the opportunity to continue the dialogue between the humanities and medicine. But, just as in the case of John Gregory's son, James, Henry Ware's son never developed these humanities roots very far, instead moving his in the direction of more narrow and technical nineteenth-century medical science. Among his publications are such titles as *Contributions to the History, Diagnosis and Treatment of Croup* (Ware 1850a), *On Haemoptysis: Its Different Species, and the Method of Treatment Adapted to Each* (Ware 1818), and *Medical Dissertations on Hemoptysis or the Spitting of Blood, and on Suppuration* (Ware 1820a). Nevertheless, like Alexander Monro, Primus, his interests clearly ranged beyond medicine. What is important for our purposes, however, is that when they strayed from medicine they did not move toward matters of contemporary ethics. They included such matters as peace (Ware 1825), midwifery (Ware 1820b), and advice to "young men" (Ware 1850b). He also wrote poetry and a biography of his brother (Ware 1846). Ware was no more a philosopher than Warren, Hayward, or Fleet.

If the Bostonians did their ethics by means of a quick study, virtually copying their new-found mentors, the leaders of other American professional medical organizations were even more dependent on that mode of code generating. As Burns points out, the *Boston Medical Police* (itself a secondary document orphaned from its intellectual origins) became the model for codes of medical ethics in the period between 1817 and 1842 in at least 13 professional societies in 11 states (Burns 1977b, p. 302).

Medical Society of the State of New York

The local professional group that seems to have extended the *Boston Police* furthest was the Medical Society of the State of New York. It adopted *A System of Medical Ethics* in 1823 (Medical Society of the State of New York 1823).[14] As Burns (1977b, p. 303) notes, the New York group went beyond Boston, incorporating Percival's forensic obligations, but also endorsing Gregory's view that challenged a rigid separation between physicians and surgeons.

For our purposes, what is critical is that the committee that proposed the New York *System* relied exclusively on physician authors as their ethical authorities. While Gregory, Percival, and Rush freely cited philosophers such as Locke, Bacon, Newton, Reid, Beattie, and (occasionally) Hume, the New York authors limited their explicit references exclusively to physicians: Percival (Walsh 1907, p. 150) and Gregory (Walsh 1907, p. 147) as well as Boerhaave (Walsh 1907, p. 146). For the first time in a professional code, Hippocrates was introduced as a moral authority. The New York authors refer to the Oath's pledge requiring physicians to support their teachers. The New York authors relay that they are aware that such an obligation is imposed on medical students who are candidates for graduation in the United States and elsewhere.[15] These authors appear to ignore the fact that Hippocrates held surgery in low esteem, reserving this practice for others.

The New York *System* was authored by a three-person committee: James R. Manley, John H. Steele, and a Dr. Pascalis. All three were physicians, two were to become presidents of the New York Medical Society, and the third had already been a prominent member. Drs. Manley and Steele left very little record of their intellectual interests, apparently having no scholarly impact outside of medicine. Presumably Dr. Pascalis was Felix A. Ouvière Pascalis (1750?–1833), about whom more is known (Packard 1928–1936; "Pascalis-Ouvière, Felix" 1968, p. 667). A native of France, he practiced medicine in Santo Domingo for a number of years before being driven out in a slave insurrection in 1793. After practicing in Philadelphia, he moved to New York in 1810 where he lived until his death.[16]

Although a follower of Benjamin Rush, Pascalis' interests were apparently limited to more narrowly medical issues, such as Rush's theory of the origin of disease. Except for whatever role he played on the committee responsible for the *System of Medical Ethics*, his writing was also exclusively in medical science.[17] Outside medicine his interests were not academic. In 1801 he was vice president of the Chemical Society of Philadelphia; later he was president of the New York branch of the Linnaean Society of Paris. Whatever contacts he had with Rush (who was approximately four years his senior), they did not influence him in the direction of Rush's interests in the philosopher/theologians of the Scottish Enlightenment.

Thus it appears that, while the New York authors went further than copying the Boston code, they did not cast their nets beyond the world of physician authors. They were not philosopher–physicians in conversation with humanists of the day, but practical practitioners temporarily leaving the clinic and scientific interests to respond to an intraprofessional crisis by writing something they called ethics. Their sources were exclusively other physician writers, but, unlike their sources, the writers of the New York *System* appear to have had only cursory understanding of the philosophical or theological systems upon which a "system of ethics" might be built. By 1823, physician-generated ethics was isolated from wider intellectual discussion.

Philadelphia

Similar professional ethical activity arose in Philadelphia. An edition of Gregory was published there in 1817. Hugh L. Hodge, an obstetrician who studied with Wistar and was a member of the Wistar Party, gave an oration to the Philadelphia Medical Society reflecting on Gregory's views (Burns 1977b, p. 302). He had also read Percival, an edition of which was published in Philadelphia in 1823. Two years later, a code patterned after the *Boston Medical Police* was adopted in the city.

The transition from the eighteenth-century humanist physicians to the more isolated craftsmen of the nineteenth century is illustrated dramatically in Philadelphia. In the same medical culture in which Chapman operated, many other elite physicians were beginning the establishment of a more isolated, formally organized medical ethics. The center of that activity was a mysterious, secret medical society called the Kappa Lambda Society of Hippocrates. Often it was referred to simply as Kappa Lambda, though this full title was also used and is revealing. It had branches in New York, Washington, Baltimore, and Lexington, but the Philadelphia chapter's activities were particularly substantial.[18]

The Kappa Lambda Society existed from about 1819 until 1835. A good number of the prominent physicians of Philadelphia belonged to the society. Potential members were not informed if they were up for membership, and each member had to be unanimously elected. There was a formal induction ceremony, at which the new member swore an oath that the society seemed to believe was very close to the Hippocratic Oath. The group published a code of ethics for its members, which was a version of Percival's medical ethics, adopted for use in the United States; it set the range of fees that its members were allowed to charge for services; and it published the *North American Medical and Surgical Journal*. The society's connection with the journal was kept secret for the first four years of the journal's publication. The society seems to have become less secretive as the years went on, at least the Philadelphia group did. The New York group seems to have kept itself in the shadows longer.

The records of Kappa Lambda make clear that by the 1820s, physicians had lost their ties to the broader philosophical culture and organized themselves to promote their profession by drawing exclusively on fellow physicians for moral guidance. The preamble to the Kappa Lambda constitution makes use of the "social compact" language of Percival (Kappa Lambda 1825, p. 4). Its announced purpose was to "engraft medical ethics on moral precepts, and sedulously cherish that friendly feeling and courteous conduct, in our professional and social intercourse, which can alone confer happiness on individuals and promote the welfare of mankind" (Kappa Lambda 1825, p. 5). Article 14 of its bylaws provides "those articles of the Medical Ethics of Dr. Percival, which have been published by this Society [and] shall be adopted as rules of government for its members" (Kappa Lambda 1825, p. 19). This is followed by a fee schedule, such as "for a single visit and advice in a case" ($1–10) or "for rising at night, and a visit ($5–10). Midwifery cases were $8 to $20; vaccinations were a fixed $5 (Kappa Lambda 1825, p. 23).

Along with the constitution and bylaws pamphlet are hand-written pages pertaining to the society's initiation ceremony. The ritual existed in three different versions, the last of which appears to be circa 1824–26. It is titled, "Formula to be observed at the Initiation of a member elect, together with the Address to be delivered on this occasion." The "address" to be presented to the initiates after they took their oath boldly connects Kappa Lambda to the society of Hippocrates:

The venerable Hippocrates of Cos may be considered as the remote founder of this Society and the [oath/affirmation] which you have just taken is in substance the same as was administered to its members. The influence of this Society on the moral and professional demeanour of the physicians of that period is attested by the most respectable authorities.
(Kappa Lambda [1824–26])[19]

The emergence of Hippocrates as the symbolic figurehead at almost the same time that he assumed a similar role in New York is more than mere coincidence. This is surely the influence of the communication of ritual and symbol between two branches of the fraternity for the medical elite.

Quite remarkably, even though the members seemed to believe they were replicating "in substance" the same oath administered to members of the ancient Hippocratic group, the actual text of the Kappa Lambda oath bears almost no resemblance. It is administered in the second person (not the Hippocratic Oath's first person), it contains none of the Oath's wording, and it is focused on the welfare of the professional organization, not on that of patients:[20] The text, which has not been published previously, was obtained from the original Kappa Lambda hand-written records in the Philadelphia College of Physicians archives. It is reprinted here in full:

Oath or Affirmation

You do [swear/affirm] that you will endeavor to exalt the character of the Medical profession by a life of virtue and honour—that you will keep the secrets, guard the reputations, and advance the interests of this Society and each of its members; and that you will never encourage any one to devote himself to the study of Medicine whose learning, talents, and honourable qualities are not such as to render him respectable in his profession, and worthy to be distinguished as a member of this Society.
(Kappa Lambda [1824–26])

The medical ethics that the society set out to promote was thus associated with the historical figure, with little evidence that the nineteenth-century members really had much knowledge or understanding of either the historical Hippocrates or the Oath attributed to him. Hippocrates had become a timeless symbol of an ageless profession, a replacement for the rich interdisciplinary philosophical discourse of the Enlightenment.

Aside from Hippocrates, their only other source of medical ethics was another physician—Percival. In an earlier version of the initiation ritual, carrying the date 11-27-22 in the College of Physicians catalogue, the society announced its intention "at some future period to publish a code of rules and regulations for the government of its members. For the present, however, we have adopted such parts of the medical ethics of the illustrious Doctor Percival, as are adapted to the state of the profession in this country" (Kappa Lambda [1822]). It is this excerpt from Percival that appears in the society's bylaws. It appears that no other code was ever written. None is in the collection of materials at the College of Physicians.

In addition to the provisions in the bylaws, the society published "Extracts from the Medical Ethics of Dr. Percival" (Kappa Lambda 1829). It provides about 25 pages of Percival with considerable attention to matters of professional relations: avoidance of "officious interference" with a case under the charge of another, courtesy when calling on a patient formerly under a colleague's care, consultations, and relations between junior and senior physicians.

The Philadelphia society appears to have been something of a promoter of Percival. In an 1823 letter from Ansel Ives of New York to Dr. Franklin Bache of Philadelphia, in which Ives informs Bache that a Kappa Lambda Society has been established in New York, Ives writes:

I beg leave also to acknowledge on behalf of the NY KΛ the receipt of twenty copies of "Percival's Medical Ethics" which accompanied your letter to Dr. Stevens [Alex H. Stevens is listed earlier in the letter as President of the NY society], this [2 words illegible, "gift from" would make sense] your [cross-hatched box[21]] was highly appreciated and the books have been advantageously distributed.

Bache wrote back on December 19, 1823, in response to Ives's letter. He gave Ives a list of the names of officers and members of the Philadelphia society, as Ives had given him the names of officers and members of the New York society.[22]

Apparently, the society's version of Percival's medical ethics was never made public—at least not in the *North American Medical and Surgical Journal*. It is worth noting that the journal contained nothing concerning ethics or debates about conduct, etc. It contained very technical descriptions of procedures, case histories, reviews of literature, and the like.

The adoption of excerpts from Percival as the society's code of ethics was an issue when the group was forced to examine its functioning as a secret organization. In 1827 a committee was formed to deal with the secrecy policy. It consisted of Bache, John Bell, and George B. Wood. (Bell will emerge as a key player in the adoption of the American Medical Association's code of ethics to be discussed below. Isaac Hays, the other key player in the AMA's code, was also a member of Kappa Lambda.) The committee report endorsed a policy of permitting members to disclose their membership in Kappa Lambda, its connection with the *North American Medical and Surgical Journal*, and the commitment of its members to the society's scale of compensation for medical services. At the same time, it said that members were permitted "to acknowledge the printed Extracts from Percival's medical Ethics, and the amendments and alterations thereof duly adopted, as the Code of the Society, for the regulation of Medical etiquette, and that by which he, as a member, agrees to be governed." However, "the Constitution, By-Laws, matters of government, discussions past and future, and other matters not enumerated" were to be kept secret.

While there is no evidence that outsiders raised the issue of whether the society in Philadelphia should remain secret, it appears that its sister group in New York was so challenged. A pamphlet entitled "Some Account of a Secret Society in New York entitled the 'Kappa Lambda' in A Letter to Alexander H. Stevens MD LLD by a Retired Physician" (Douglas 1859) appeared in 1859. The author name given is Sholto Douglas, MD, although this is clearly an alias. The author bitterly attacked the New York Kappa Lambda, claiming it had acted "not for the purposes of mutual improvement of the science, art, and practice of Medicine,—but with the (not undisguised) sole object of promoting the pecuniary interests of its members by depreciating the reputations of others." It then proceeded to name physicians who had been injured.

The 1831 "Report of the Committee of the Medical Society, of the City and County of New York, Appointed to Investigate the Subject of a Secret Medical Association" was appended to the letter, thus indicating that the controversy had existed since 1831. The committee investigating the New York society in the name of the Medical Society included Felix Pascalis, one of the physicians responsible for writing the New York code. According to the report, about 30 of the New York City and County Medical Association were members of New York's Kappa Lambda. This is described as an "uncomfortable proportion."

In Philadelphia there was considerable overlap between the Wistar Party and its Kappa Lambda chapter. Among those with dual membership were Bache, Dewees, Harris, Hodge, Horner, James, LaRoche, Meigs, and Mitchell. Conspicuously absent from this list is Nathaniel Chapman.[23] A report of the Committee on Medical Ethics dated 7-5-1826 notes that the members of that committee were William Dewees (chair), Joseph Hartshorn, and Harry Nevill (Neill?). Also in the records is a note from C.D. Meigs accepting the presidency of the society, dated 11-25-1826. Bache had served earlier as president. Meigs and LeRoche were involved in the writing of the Philadelphia code adopted in 1825. Meigs was a physician and professor, also in obstetrics. He read French, German, Latin, and Greek, and published on yellow fever. Outside of medicine his writing, other than the code, was in history and ethnography. Rene LaRoche was an associate of Meigs and Chapman, but has left little record of interests outside of medicine.

Isaac Hays certainly held various offices in Kappa Lambda, as there is some official correspondence for the society addressed to him. We shall return to the role of Bell and Hays after filling in the regional picture in Baltimore and Washington, D.C.

Baltimore and Washington, D.C.

If Boston and New York represent medical ethics in isolation from the broader stream of philosophical discourse, the isolation was even more severe in the city medical societies that were to adopt ethical codes in the following years. The Medico-Chirurgical Society of Baltimore adopted a code in 1832 that Burns (1978) describes as being under the "obvious influence" of New York. It also drew on the code of the Connecticut Medial Society, which had been based on the *Boston Medical Police*. Likewise, it included a synopsis of Rush's list of duties for patients, which R. E. Griffith had appended to the American edition of Ryan's *Manual of Medical Jurisprudence*. Once again, the physician organizations were passing medical ethical material back and forth among physicians who indirectly traced their philosophical education back to Gregory, Percival, or Rush. The nineteenth-century physicians who wrote codes could not count on the same elite classical education and rich familial nurturing that were available to the eighteenth-century physician-scholars. The shift in social class of the student entering medicine and the poor quality of education in the classics meant that, while they might have had rudimentary knowledge of Greek or Latin, they were not equipped to carry on extended analysis. The new-found interest in the Hippocratic literature, especially the Oath, provided a one-page version of a medical ethic that sounded both profound and distinguished. These nineteenth-century physicians were not equipped to process the moderns—Kant, Hume, or Bentham—let alone the ancients.

The story in the District of Columbia was similar. The city had had a Medical Society chartered by Congress in 1817, but the charter prohibited codes of ethics, as well as what were called "fee bills," or schedules of minimum fees that members could charge (which suggests that such codes were recognized at the time as being controversial, functioning as conspiracies in restraint of free trade). By the 1820s the conflicts within the profession were severe and the Society lost its charter (Rothstein 1972, p. 80). In 1833 a group of physicians formed an unchartered organization that did form fee bills and a code of ethics (Medical Association of the District of Columbia 1833). Like its predecessors, its code was a short document (15 pages) when compared with the monographs of Gregory, Percival, and Rush.

AMERICAN MEDICAL ASSOCIATION CODE OF 1847

All of this state and local activity (in which distinguished physician–scientists in state and local medical societies were diverted from their clinical and scientific interests to write codes of ethics by drawing on the work of equally non-philosophical precursors) continued up to the creation of the American Medical Association's 1847 *Code of Ethics* (American Medical Association 1848).[24]

In the background at the time were intense struggles among competing schools of medical thought (with Thompsonians, homeopaths, and other "irregular practitioners," as well as all manner of quacks and charlatans) and efforts to govern consultations and licensure. Added to this were disputes over medical education (Rothstein 1972, p. 114). Short, poor-quality education flooded the market with unqualified practitioners. Reform was almost impossible because, if one school or jurisdiction attempted to improve quality, students would simply move to another school. During this period in the history of American medicine, what we now think of as "orthodox" or "allopathic" medicine was carving out its territory and staking its claim to be a "profession." One of the fundamental characteristics of the claim to being a profession is attempting to establish that the group is self-regulating and capable of acting ethically. Hence, the writing of a code of ethics was a critical early task for advocates of legitimizing medicine in this particular direction. In fact, writing of the code was undertaken and it was endorsed before adoption of the AMA constitution (Baker 1995a, p. 50).

The evidence shows that this was primarily the work of two men: Isaac Hays and John Bell. They were both students of Nathaniel Chapman, both ophthomologists, both primarily editors of medical literature rather than independent scholars, and deeply committed to establishing what we would today call orthodox, allopathic medicine as the victor in its battles with other forms of medical practice. Neither had the experience in the humanities to do much more than copy once again the work of their eighteenth-century predecessors.

Isaac Hays

Hays's Role in the American Medical Association Code

The story of the founding of the AMA and the central importance of the writing of its first code of ethics has been told many times (see note 24). Here we are primarily interested in the relation of that activity to the broader stream of philosophy and religion of the day.

Hays's role and interests are transparent. He attended the first national meeting of medical societies in New York in 1846. That meeting proved premature since only 16 societies from 14 states attended. Hays introduced the resolution to reconvene in Philadelphia the following year (Baker 1995a, p. 49). It passed unanimously. The content of the resolution makes Hays's concern clear. The focus of the new group was to create an association of the "Medical Profession of the United States," for the "protection of their interests, for the maintenance of their honour, and respectability, for the advancement of their knowledge, and the extension of their usefulness."[25] The group was to promote a "uniform and elevated standard of requirement for the degree of M.D." To achieve this, "it is expedient that the Medical Profession in the United States should be governed by the same code of Medical Ethics, and that a Committee of Seven be appointed to report a code for that purpose, at a meeting to be held in Philadelphia, on the first Wednesday of May, 1847" (text in Baker 1995a, p. 49).[26]

Hays's concerns were, in part, practical. He had recently lost a lawsuit in which as editor of the *Medical News*, he had been accused of harming the financial interests of the producer of a remedy by claiming it inefficacious (Baker 1995a, p. 50). Thus the problems of approaches to medical practice, consultation, criticism of nostrums, and medical education—all problems of the shaping and control of financial aspects of the practice—were joined in a project that demanded a code that would help a group gain respectability.

This agenda, which was a widespread concern of physicians of the time, is reflected in the text of the code. A brief initial chapter spells out the duties of physicians to their patients and the obligations of patients to their physicians. The perspective is practical and totally alien from the Kantian and utilitarian perspectives of the broader societal ethical discourse. The paternalism seen in Percival remains in the 1847 text. According to this code of ethics, the physician should be "imbued with the greatness of his mission" and "reasonable indulgence should be granted to the mental imbecility and caprices of the sick." Physicians have a "duty" to avoid making gloomy prognostications. (The code even endorses breaching confidentiality by giving the patient's friends timely notice of danger.) "The opportunity which a physician not unfrequently enjoys of promoting and strengthening the good resolutions of his patients, suffering under the consequences of vicious conduct, ought never to be neglected" (American Medical Association 1848, Chapter 1, Art. 1). A patient, by contrast, has as his "first duty," selecting "as his medical adviser one who has received a regular professional education." (Thus it was the patient's moral duty to avoid dealing with the unorthodox practitioners who were the competitors of the AMA members.) "A patient who has thus selected his physician, should always apply for advice in whatever may appear to him trivial cases, for the most fatal results often supervene on the slightest accidents." While physicians were allowed to withhold diagnostic information from patients, "patients should faithfully and unreservedly communicate to their physician the supposed causes of their disease." The text goes on to caution, however, that "a patient should never weary his physician with a tedious detail of events or matters not appertaining to his disease" and "the obedience of a patient to the prescriptions of his physician should be prompt and implicit. He should never permit his own crude opinions as to their fitness, to influence his attention to them."

The overriding concern for controlling competition among physicians then surfaces in the initial chapter: "A patient should, if possible, avoid even the *friendly visits of a physician* who is not attending him—and when he does receive them, he should never converse on the subject of his disease" (American Medical Association, Chapter 1, Art. 1).

This is followed by a second, and longer, chapter on the duties of physicians to each other and to the profession at large and then by a chapter on the duties of the profession to the public and of the public to physicians. The central theme is that, since the public benefits greatly from the "unwearied beneficence of the profession," the public ought to show proper appreciation of the differences between "true science" and "ignorance and empiricism," i.e., should recognize the difference between those who are members of the medical societies and those who practice outside that framework, competing with the members for business.

In short, the focus of the first AMA code is on protecting the special status of "real" physicians and avoiding deviant practitioners who jeopardize the status of the membership (Rothstein 1972, pp. 170–74). To be sure, the text of the code reflects a commitment to service to patients, but gives no hint that the creators were engaging any of the real ethical questions of the day.

The reasons are apparent in the statements of the members of the committee that created the code. All seven committee members were physicians. Five of them were sufficiently obscure that no record can be located today of their scholarly interests outside of the advancement of their professional association.[27] Only Hays and Bell left their mark, and that mark is narrowly defined within medicine.

The preliminary "Note to Convention" (Bell et al. 1995) from the committee makes clear how dependent the committee was on the sources with which we are, by now, so familiar:

On examining a great number of codes of ethics adopted by different societies in the United States, it was found that they were all based on that by Dr. Percival, and that the phrases of this writer were preserved, to a considerable extent, in all of them. Believing that language that had been so often examined and adopted, must possess the greatest merits for a document such as the present, clearness and precision, and having no ambition for the honours of authorship, the Committee which prepared this code have followed a similar course, and have carefully preserved the words of Percival wherever they convey the precepts it is wished to inculcate. A few of the sections are in the words of the late Dr. Rush, and one or two sentences are from other writers.

(Bell et al. 1995, p. 73)

In other words, the words are Percival's and Rush's. The committee admits to "changing a word, or even a part of a sentence," but it is clear that the authors (or more rightly, editors) followed the same path as that of the local medical society code writers. They sought out the two (or, in the case of the earlier, more local codes, three) physician–philosophers who were capable of communicating with the humanists of their day, and they copied them. The blind copied from the blind until they finally got back to the three students of the Scottish Enlightenment (Gregory, Percival, and Rush), who could be considered serious, if amateur, philosophers. The complex texts of these three were abstracted and edited until they were totally isolated from the philosophical problems that had commanded the attention of their predecessors, and then conscripted into service of the insulated professional problems of control of medical education, consultation, quackery, intraprofessional communication, and income. The problems of deism, skepticism, empiricism, moral-sense theory, and the relation of the Scottish national covenant to the English king were replaced by the problems of differentiating physicians from charlatans, control of income, and secret nostrums. Just as surely, the code writers, as physicians and medical society enthusiasts, were divorced from the philosophical and theological problems of their own generation. They were practicing physician–scientists with little or no interest in or knowledge of the humanities who were called temporarily to the task of constructing a professional code. The process of isolation was complete.

Hays's Other Publications and Interests

Although John Bell was named chair of the committee that drafted the code, there is reason to believe that Hays played a key role. He not only introduced the resolution that created the committee but is also credited in the introductory "Note to Convention" as presenting the committee's report and is listed second under the chair, out of alphabetical order. Baker, attributing major responsibility for the code to Hays, argues that Hays regularly took on the role of facilitator and editor rather than one who would take credit of authorship (Baker 1995a, p. 55). This "habitual diffidence," Baker suggests, may be attributed to the fact that Hays was a practicing Jew in a gentile America who preferred to speak through the words of distinguished deceased gentiles.

Regardless of the correctness of this hypothesis, Hays surely left no trace of being a talmudic scholar. He played the role of a modern, secular leader of organized medicine, capable of isolating his medical contributions from any religious convictions he might have had.[28] Hays began his medical studies at the University of Pennsylvania in 1812, which placed him there during Rush's tenure. Nevertheless, he was an office pupil of Nathaniel Chapman. Indeed, one author describes him as a Chapman "protégé" (Richman 1967, p. 195). Hays developed a special interest in ophthalmology, and his work in this field has been called his chief contribution to medicine (McCrae 1957, p. 462). He studied astigmatism and color blindness and invented a special knife for cataract operations. He was eventually appointed surgeon at Wills Eye Hospital in Philadelphia. He thus takes his place as another surgeon/code-writer without other medical humanities interests. Other than his work with the committee that drafted the code, he served the AMA as treasurer and chair of its publications committee. He became a fellow of the College of Physicians where, again, his contribution was technical. He chaired the building committee. He also worked often as an editor, bringing out an edition of William Lawrence's *Treatise on the Diseases of the Eye* and working as an editor of the *Philadelphia Journal of the Medical and Physical Sciences*, founded by Chapman. Hays then assumed editorship of the *American Journal of the Medical Sciences*, a position he held until his death. He also edited *Medical News* and the *Monthly Abstract of Medical Science* and many other technical medical texts. His modest list of authored papers include titles such as "The Forces by which the Blood is Circulated" and "Observations on Inflamation of the Sclerotica," interests reminiscent of Monro's. Hays did no writing or editing in the medical humanities, jurisprudence, or ethics.

Nor were his interests outside medicine directed toward the humanities. He edited an edition of Alexander Wilson's *American Ornithology*, was a member and eventually president of the Academy of Natural Sciences, and was a founder of the Franklin Institute as well as the American Medical Association. He was a member of the American Philosophical Society, which, as we have seen, evolved in the nineteenth century as a broadly encompassing academic and scientific institution, not a philosophical society in the modern sense of the term.

John Bell

Bell's Introduction to the American Medical Association Code

Hays recruited John Bell (1796–1872), a fellow University of Pennsylvania graduate who had also been a student of Chapman and was a fellow member of the surgical staff at the Pennsylvania Institute for the Relief of Diseases of the Eye and Ear, to chair the committee that drafted the AMA code. Bell wrote a long introduction to the code, which was adopted at the May 1847 meeting along with the code (Bell 1995). Bell gives some hints that he realized that a medical code of ethics must be grounded in some underlying philosophical or religious normative framework. He opens his introduction with a surprisingly bold statement:

Medical ethics, as a branch of general ethics, must rest on the basis of religion and morality. They comprise not only the duties, but, also, the rights of a physician: and, in this sense, they are identical with Medical Deontology—a term introduced by a late writer, who has taken the most comprehensive view of the subject.

(Bell 1995, p. 65)

This would be a controversial statement now, at the beginning of the twenty-first century, when many physicians writing on medical ethics insist that the profession of the physician has an "internal morality" of its own, one not dependent on external sources.[29] By contrast, Bell seems up front about the dependence of physician ethics on some broader system. He even talks about the "rights of a physician" (Bell 1995, p. 65). This may not appear to be unusual to the twenty-first–century reader, but I know of no other document generated by organized medicine in the nineteenth or twentieth century before 1980 that uses the language of rights. The 1847 code does not use the term and no other codification does until the AMA's 1980 revision, published the following year (American Medical Association 1981). Physicians writing during this period were more inclined to use the language of benefits and harms, that is, the language of the consequentialists, rather than the language of rights.

Rights language reveals the influence of the liberal tradition of political philosophy, the language of Locke, Hobbes, and Rousseau as well as the Bill of Rights of the U.S. Constitution. It is a language that is quite alien to physician discourse, yet another sign that physicians of this period were quite isolated from the philosophical thought of the broader culture. It is striking that, although Bell speaks of the rights of physicians, he does not speak of the rights of patients. Bell picked up the term, but was not tainted by liberal political philosophy sufficiently to imagine that patients might be the possessors of such entitlements.

Bell's Philosophical Sources

Although Bell observes that physician ethics must be dependent on religion and ethics outside of medicine, he shows little other evidence that he was a student of such thought. After the bold statement that medical ethics must rest on religion and morality from general ethics, he mentions only one source, and that author is a writer on medical ethics, M. I. Simon, to whom Bell attributes the term *medical deontology*, from Simon's *Deontology Médicale, ou Devoirs et Des Droits Des Médecins Dans L' État Actuel De la Civilization*. It is presumably from Simon's reference to the rights of physicians that Bell adopted his rights language. There are clearly no references to the eighteenth-century philosophers who introduced the terminology or even a mention of the American founding fathers' use of the concept.

After this opening reference to Simon, Bell immediately grounds his ethics in Hippocrates. This is completely consistent with the pattern we have seen: physicians who are in communication with their humanist colleagues struggling with contemporary issues have little interest in Hippocrates (except perhaps as an exemplar of a good observer and an eloquent writer of Greek). Only when the physician is out of communication with his surrounding culture does Hippocrates emerge as a kind of timeless ancient symbol of physician conduct. As Bell puts it, "the duties of a physician were never more beautifully exemplified in the conduct of Hippocrates, nor more eloquently described [than] in his writings" (Bell 1995, p. 65).

Bell's "Introduction" includes an aggressive attack on quackery, on "medical empirics," for their use of nostrums (Bell 1995, pp. 68–69). He had prepared for this role by serving on an 1827 committee of the Medical Society of Philadelphia to study the medical value of quack remedies (Richman 1967, p. 136). He urges "veracity," but makes clear that this is in the context of claims about treatments.

Hence, the concern is not honesty to patients but opposition to unscientific medicine. In fact, he urges that physicians associated together voice a "general harmony in doctrines and practice" so that "neither students nor patients shall be perplexed" (Bell 1995, p. 70). He even seems to be claiming that development of such harmony is one of the functions of professional organizations such as the AMA.

In short, Bell did not address any of the subjects of the medical ethics of Gregory, Percival, or Rush, and certainly not any of the topics of a more general theory of ethics, whether religious or secular. Rather, he was concerned about the idiosyncratic intraprofessional feuds and interpersonal relations among physicians as the "regular" physicians attempted to establish themselves and overpower their competitors.

Bell's Other Publications and Interests

That Bell was a physician and not an ethical analyst is made clear by his other publications and interests. After graduating from the University of Pennsylvania, he lectured on the institutes (that is, theory) of medicine at the Philadelphia Medical Institute and then was a professor of the theory and practice of medicine at the Medical College of Ohio. His graduation dissertation was published as *An Inaugural Dissertation on the Liver: Its Influence over the Animal Economy in Health and Disease* (1817). His writings focused on medical topics, often on mineral baths.[30] He also had an interest in public health[31] and wrote and edited basic texts in medicine such as *A Treatise on Physiology Applied to Pathology* (Bell 1826). He was editor of several medical journals, including *The Eclectic Medical Journal* (Bell 1836–40). What is absent is any other writing that would have prepared him to expound on the ethics of the practice of medicine.[32] Aside from his membership in the American Philosophical Society—an honor that, as we have seen, does not signify philosophical interests as much as good Philadelphia connections—Bell's career was one of a medical scientist and editor.

7

SOME PHYSICIANS WHO ALMOST CONFRONT THE HUMANITIES

At this point, the thesis I am arguing may begin to sound too simplistic. With the turn of the nineteenth century and the increasing specialization of medicine as a scientific endeavor, all the physicians who wrote codes of ethics (which was essentially an American activity) for their state, local, or national medical societies were surgeons with an interest in journal and textbook editing as well as organizational politics, but no prior interest or ability in ethics, theology, philosophy, or any other humanities discipline. If they had accomplishments outside of medicine, they were in mundane social organizations dealing with ornithology, agriculture, or engineering. For their medical ethics, they simply turned to the physicians who preceded them at the end of the eighteenth century—in particular Gregory, Percival, and Rush—and copied the sections that appealed to them, especially the sections relevant to the interprofessional feuds of the day.

For the most part, that is indeed the picture of Anglo-American, professionally generated code writing. The story is a bit more complex, however. There were a small number of academically gifted, intellectually curious physicians whose education and interests extended to the humanities. We must consider Worthington Hooker, Alfred Stillé, Austin Flint, Lewis Pilcher, and especially William Osler and Richard Cabot—all physicians with something of a reputation for delving into the humanities. In each case, however, we will see that their abilities in the humanities were modest and their involvement in organized medicine marginal. They did not serve as connectors between the two disciplines because they were not as firmly attached to either, as their reputations suggest. They are exceptions to the general pattern we have found, but exceptions that do not seriously challenge the thesis of this book.

WORTHINGTON HOOKER

The first challenge to this thesis comes from a person who, after graduating from Yale College in 1825, began his medical studies in Philadelphia and then received his M.D. degree from Harvard in 1829. Worthington Hooker (1806–1867) established a medical practice in Norwich, Connecticut, where he stayed for 23 years.[1] A lineal descendant of the Rev. Thomas Hooker (1586–1641) (Walker 1891), the Puritan divine who was influential in the founding of the Connecticut colony, Worthington Hooker comes as close to the eighteenth-century model of physician–humanist as any nineteenth-century American physician.

In 1844 Hooker read an essay before the Connecticut Medical Society that signaled his interests in medical morality. Entitled *Dissertation on the Respect Due the Medical Profession, and the Reasons that It is not Awarded By the Community* (Hooker 1844), it anticipates his best-known work, *Physician and Patient; or A Practice View of the Mutual Duties, Relations, and Interests of the Medical Profession and the Community*, which appeared in 1849. This work shows that Hooker had more than a casual understanding of the philosophical issues of the day. Nevertheless, over half the book deals with the great nineteenth-century interprofessional feuds among different schools of practitioners. Chapters are devoted to quackery, Thompsonianism, homeopathy,[2] and natural bone setters as well as the means of removing quackery. Two additional chapters address tensions over consultation, "undue attentions to the patients of others," reckless attacks upon professional character, and the familiar controversies of a young profession trying to establish harmony and a common front to present to the public.

The remaining chapters, however, discuss subjects that we would classify as philosophy of medicine. Some of the issues were the ones on the minds of Gregory and his colleagues: the nature of cause, empirical observation, erroneous attribution of cure based on case reports, and so forth. Hooker repeats the physiological notion of "sympathy" as the mechanism of communication among bodily organs that we saw in Chapman. Then he confronts a major moral issue about which physicians have often disagreed with moralists outside of medicine. In Chapter 17, "Truth in our Intercourse with the Sick," Hooker puts forth a classic utilitarian argument in favor of truth telling to patients. In opposition to the widespread defense by physicians of benevolent deception of the sick, he points out that it is erroneous to assume that concealment can always be done successfully (Hooker 1849, p. 361) and argues that deception, if discovered, is even more harmful (p. 362). Moreover, it destroys confidence (p. 365). Reflecting an acquaintance with the incipient rule-utilitarian moves of the philosophers of his day, Hooker points out that deception will have the general effect of tainting the perception of the medical profession in the eyes of the community. "If it be adopted by the community as a common rule, that the truth may be sacrificed in urgent cases, the very object of the deception will be destroyed" (p. 375). He points out that, once the door is opened to deception, one cannot define its limits. His conclusion is: "I think it perfectly evident, that the good, which may be done by deception in a *few* cases, is almost as nothing, compared with the evil which it does in *many* cases" (p. 378).

Nevertheless, Hooker makes it clear that he is not a Kantian. He bases his defense of honesty with patients on the harms of deception, concluding that "the truth should not be withheld unless there be a reasonable prospect of effectually preventing discovery of it" (p. 381). In developing his utilitarian philosophical argument for truth telling, Hooker shows that he is familiar with Percival's treatment of the subject, quoting him at length, suggesting that he is even more in favor of truthfulness than Percival in his careful mediating between Gregory and Gisborne. The question is, however, to what degree did Hooker depend on Percival in his analysis? Was he capable of independent philosophical analysis or did he merely rely on Percival?

First, it appears that Hooker was unaware of how useful Gisborne's *Enquiry into the Duties of Men* would have been to him. Hooker makes no mention of it, even though Percival refers explicitly to Gisborne (Percival 1803, pp. 156–57, 163). Hooker does refer to Hutcheson, but hardly in a way that suggests familiarity with the philosopher of the early Scottish Enlightenment, referring to him as "Dr. Hutcheson of Glascow, as quoted by Dr. Percival" (Hooker 1849, p. 379), thus revealing that he has no direct knowledge of the man.[3] The only other authority discussed by Hooker in the chapter is Puffendorf (p. 361), but Puffendorf is also cited by Percival (Percival 1803, p. 161), who also refers to Grotius (p. 160), to Boswell (p. 164), and then "Grove's Ethics; Balguy's Law of Truth; Camray's Telemachus; Butler; Hutcheson; Paley; and Gisborne" (p. 165). None of these figures appear in Hooker. Likewise, there is no appeal by Hooker to Kant (either in support of his strong endorsement of truth telling or to contrast his own rule-utilitarian arguments with Kant's formalist approach). There is no reference to Hume's consequence-oriented ethics, to Smith or any of the other Scottish moralists, or to Gregory's rather more traditional paternalism regarding truth telling. There is no reference to Jeremy Bentham (1748–1832) or any other philosophical commentators. In short, Hooker seems to be a quick thinker, but one rather isolated from the most profound philosophers of his day. His view of truth telling appears to be based solely on his reading Percival. He was able to think independently, challenging the mainstream of his profession and even deviating from the most important ethical authority within Anglo-American medicine, but he was no longer part of a grand conversation across disciplinary boundaries. He was doing the best he could within a discipline that had lost its intellectual connectedness.

Hooker returned to the subject of the ethics of medical communication the following year, publishing *Lessons from the History of Medical Delusions* (1850), but by his own admission this repeats much of what is in *Physician and Patient*. Aside from these three works oriented primarily toward the ethics of truth telling, Hooker's interests were in medical science, clinical practice, research, and organized medicine.[4] He was, after all, a product of the nineteenth century.

ALFRED STILLÉ

Another place to search for nineteenth-century American physicians who were in serious communication with contemporary humanists is in the work of Alfred Stillé (1813–1900), the friend of Isaac Hays who compiled his memoir (Stillé 1881). Stillé also was responsible for revising, correcting, and adding material to *A Treatise on Medical Jurisprudence*, written by Francis Wharton (1820–1889) and Alfred's brother, Moreton Stillé (1822–1855) (Wharton and Stillé 1860). Since it is under the rubric of medical jurisprudence that Percival originally made his contribution to medical ethics, Alfred Stillé's interest in the area is promising.

There is a hint, however, that Stillé is not the philosopher–humanist we are seeking, in his statement that his contribution to the jurisprudence volume was to revise the "medical part." Moreover, as we have seen in the British nineteenth-century literature of medical jurisprudence, the term by this time had ceased to refer to medical ethics, taking on a narrower, legal-medicine meaning.

Stillé's other writings provide no further evidence of interest in the humanities. He helped produce *The National Dispensary* (Stillé and Maisch 1879) and wrote on cholera (Stillé 1885) and meningitis (Stillé 1867). He also published a number of texts on medical science (Stillé 1848, 1860).

AUSTIN FLINT, LEWIS S. PILCHER, AND THE NEW YORK SOCIETY

Somewhat later in the century the American Medical Association's ethical code, originally adopted in 1847 in part to solidify the orthodox practitioners' claim to legitimacy, became controversial because of its rigorous opposition to physicians cooperating with those practitioners considered unorthodox. The third edition of the AMA code exacerbated these tensions by opposing cooperation with other kinds of healers (American Medical Association 1879). Austin Flint (1812–1886), who was president of the AMA in 1883, published a text of the code together with commentaries defending the organization's strict opposition to cooperation (Flint 1883).

The AMA's position generated a strong backlash, particularly from physicians in New York, who were much more willing to cooperate with these unorthodox practitioners. A group calling itself the "Society for the Prevention of the

Re-enactment in the State of New York of the Present Code of Ethics of the American Medical Association" organized a symposium to which some of the leading medical figures of the day contributed (Post et al. 1883). Claiming to represent medical ethics from "the liberal standpoint," this volume carried the slogan "Why is my liberty judged by another conscience" on its title page. The papers carry equally provocative titles, such as "Reasons for Preferring a Larger Liberty in Consultations than that which is Allowed by the Code of Ethics of the American Medical Association" and "A Plea for Toleration." One of the best known authors, Lewis S. Pilcher (1845–1934), can serve as a representative for the others and a contrast to Austin Flint.

Flint is sometimes is referred to as the "father of cardiology." Educated at Harvard and Jefferson Medical College, he practiced medicine in New York and served as professor of theoretical and practical medicine at the College of Medicine at Bellevue Hospital from 1861 to 1886. While Flint was a very distinguished physician, he was not a specialist in medical ethics. His involvement with the ethical code stemmed from his long-term participation in organized medicine.

Flint's modest commentary on the AMA's code reveals the work of an AMA loyalist. He was clearly aware of the code's dependence on Percival, but in this he was apparently following Hays (Flint 1883, p. 5). His comments are interspersed with the AMA code over 97 small pages, but there is not a single reference to any significant moral controversy, theory, or author outside medicine. His focus is on legal interpretations and especially on the duty of the regular physician to abstain from interaction with "steam doctors, or Thomsonians," "botanical or herb doctors," "eclectics," and the like (p. 45). The volume concludes with an account of the action of the New York State Medical Society, which had adopted an alternative code in February 1882. Based on the national code, it omitted the sections on duties of physicians to patients and obligations of the public to physicians. The real controversy, however, was over a provision in the New York code that authorized consultation with "legally qualified practitioners of medicine" (p. 96). Flint pointed out that, in New York, homeopaths were legally qualified practitioners. This authorization, Flint claimed, was a "great disaster" and a "concession of honor." The internecine medical professional wars were at their apex. Medical ethics had nothing to do with ethical discourse outside medicine and everything to do with professional turf fights. Flint wrote nothing else on ethics.[5]

The response of the New Yorkers who were part of the "Prevention of the Re-enactment" symposium was predictable in its hostile reception of Flint's defense of the AMA and intraprofessional quibbling. Lewis Pilcher's paper is typical. After claiming that ethics is a matter of conscience, Pilcher turns immediately to the ethics of his profession without a hint of any engagement with basic philosophical issues. He begins by making the case that physicians are not to treat their professional code as a set of rules. "Of all classes of men," he maintains, "physicians are certainly least in the condition of children that need paternal watch guard and rules of conduct" (Pilcher 1883a, p. 44). Pilcher is righteously indignant that Flint and the AMA would have the gall to tell a member of a learned profession what constitutes ethical conduct. He grants that, however much one "may question the taste and dignity of the proceeding" (p. 47), members of the AMA have the right to impose these rules on their own members, but he cannot tolerate the suggestion that other members of the profession who refuse allegiance to the AMA's code are unworthy of professional recognition (p. 48).

Although Pilcher, like Flint, acknowledges his indebtedness to Percival, he was no more deeply engaged in scholarship outside medicine than Flint was. That is understandable when one views the pattern of his career. He published widely on topics in surgery,[6] but was largely a man of organizational identity. A decade after voicing his support for the New York position in the feud with the AMA he served as president of the Medical Society of the State of New York. He was deeply involved in the Grand Army of the Republic (the organization founded to commemorate the veterans of the Union army of the Civil War). He served as commander of the U.S. Grant Post No. 327, of the Department of New York, during the year 1913. By 1921 he was the national commander-in-chief of the organization. A photograph shows him decked out in uniform with a chest full of battle ribbons. To the extent that Pilcher had humanities interests at all, they were directed toward medical history, particularly the history of military medicine.[7] He was also a collector of medical books (Pilcher 1918). Aside from the battle with Flint over the authority of the AMA, he was not oriented toward ethics, and this is true of all the other contributors to the volume.

WILLIAM OSLER

About the same time that Flint and Pilcher were carrying out this intraprofessional debate, a giant of North American medicine appeared on the scene who had a stronger claim to engagement in the intellectual debate within the humanities. William Osler (1849–1919) continues the line we have been tracing. He was widely read; indeed, among medical writers alone he made reference to many of the people we have encountered, including Percival, Mather, Rush, Bard, Chapman, Warren, and Stillé.[8] He possessed works of each of these authors and substantial holdings of the writings of Gregory and Wesley in his wonderfully eclectic and massive library, now housed at McGill University (Osler 1929).[9] He once wrote in a letter to his collaborator, Thomas McCrae, about attending a meeting of the Royal Medical Society in Edinburgh at which he "met" (in his imagination) Rush and Bard and a number of other notables connected with Edinburgh, although he does not mention the Gregories, Cullen, or any of the late eighteenth-century faculty (Cushing 1940, p. 766).[10] These are just the medical authors whose works he read. I will explore his knowledge of the remarkably wide range of writers outside medicine below.

A Lifetime Coming Close to the Humanities

Born in Canada, William Osler was the son of an Anglican clergyman, Rev. Feather-stone Lake Osler.[11] He attended grammar school and Trinity College School at Weston, Ontario, where he came under the influence of its founder and warden, Rev. W. A. Johnson, as well as its medical director, James Bovell. Although a priest, Johnson was fascinated with biology and the natural sciences. Bovell would later become a priest. These two provided models for Osler to combine his interests in the ministry and medicine. Through Johnson, he became interested in the seventeenth-century physician–philosopher Thomas Browne (1605–1682), the author of *Religio Medici*, who would eventually become an enormous influence on him and be another role model for combining medicine and religion. This volume was, in fact, one of the first two books Osler ever owned (Cushing 1940, p. 50).[12]

In the autumn of 1867, Osler enrolled at Trinity College, an institution in Toronto affiliated with the Church of England, with the intention of studying for the ministry. Many of the faculty were clergy who had a significant interest in the natural sciences. Bovell helped to organize the medical department, serving as Dean and as Professor of the Institutes of Medicine as well as lecturing in physiology and pathology. Osler's June 1868 examination papers indicate that he studied algebra, Euclid, Greek, the catechism, trigonometry, Latin prose, Roman history, classics, and something called "pass Latin." Clearly, this was preparatory education, not yet formal study for the ministry. Osler was still a teenager. Already, however, his interests were straying toward the sciences. He spent many hours gathering samples of algae and other specimens from the waterways in the area.

After returning for his second year of study in the arts, young Osler announced his intention to study medicine. He entered Toronto Medical School that fall, attaching himself even more closely to Dr. Bovell, who was by then on that faculty. It is an interesting question whether Osler should be understood as a repressed theological and philosophical scholar or, alternatively, as one who developed his religious and philosophical interests only at an amateur level.

After two years, Osler enrolled at McGill's Medical School, which was patterned closely after Edinburgh (Cushing 1940, pp. 71, 84; Barker 1957, p. 84). Over the next few years he adopted the style of the medical scholar, publishing clinical cases, visiting clinics in Britain, Berlin, and Vienna, and working in histology, physiology, and experimental pathology, focusing on the study of the antagonistic action of atropine and physostigmin on white blood corpuscles.

The details of his life during this period show that he had traveled a considerable distance from his earlier interests in theology and the classics. Returning to Canada in 1874 at age 25, he was soon appointed professor of the institutes of medicine at McGill and then pathologist at the Montreal General Hospital. He maintained detailed records of his autopsies and worked in comparative physiology and histology at the Veterinary College.

In 1884 he was offered a professorship in clinical medicine at the University of Pennsylvania, bringing him into contact with another of the schools with historical importance to medical ethics (albeit decades after these schools' famous professors had made their contributions to professional ethics).

In 1888 he was appointed physician-in-chief of Baltimore's Johns Hopkins Hospital, where, over the next 16 years, he went on to become professor of medicine and one of the country's most famous and respected medical educators. During this period he prepared the critically important medical text, *The Principles and Practice of Medicine* (Osler 1892). He was an active researcher studying typhoid fever, malaria, pneumonia, amoebiasis, tuberculosis, cardiovascular disease, and cyanosis with polycythaemia (Vaquez-Osler disease).

In 1900 Osler came close to establishing a link to the figures we have been examining. He was intensively recruited for the position of professor of medicine at Edinburgh, the chair that had been occupied by the Gregories and Cullen (Cushing 1940, pp. 515–520). In a letter Osler admitted, "I would rather hold a Chair in Edinburgh than in any School in the English speaking world" (Cushing 1940, p. 516).[13] He was assured the appointment, but repulsed by the method of recruitment, which required that he formally apply for the position in response to a public announcement. He found the process unseemly and feared offending several friends with closer ties to Edinburgh. Nevertheless, he submitted his application on March 12, only to withdraw it two weeks later after experiencing enormous pressure from his Baltimore colleagues to remain where he was. In 1905 he accepted the Regius Professorship of Medicine at Oxford where he served until his death in 1919.

While producing an enormous amount of scientific research and scholarship, Osler was at the same time an inspiration to others, promoting efforts in public health, stimulating medical students, lecturing, and becoming a world-class bibliophile. He was famous for his literary style. In contrast with Warren, Bell, Hays, and the other nineteenth-century figures we have encountered who strayed into the humanities only as a temporary, almost accidental, deviation from their careers as more mundane, if high-status medical scientists, Osler was a prodigious writer of nontechnical lectures and homiletic advice. Nevertheless, it had been over 30 years since he left the formal study of the humanities.

Osler's Lifelong Interest in Classical Figures

Throughout his life many of Osler's writings reflected his lasting interest in the classics. This undoubtedly traced back to his Anglican clergyman father, his parents' directing him toward a classical education, and the courses he took at Trinity College. Nevertheless, he was still a teenager when he left his arts education and plans for the ministry to become a medical student. Like the classically educated physicians of the previous century in Edinburgh, he carried from his early education a remarkable orientation that penetrated his writing throughout his life. At various times he cited Thucydides, Marcus Aurelius, Epictetus, Lucretius, Lucian, Pythagorus, Seneca, and Protagorus[14] as well as Plato[15] and Aristotle.

Osler read the ancients as a historian, a classicist, and a public speaker, noting quotable lines and profound thoughts.[16] He never pursued the issues of Platonic or Aristotealian scholarship, however. I have found no place where he struggled with even the most central questions, such as Socrates's notion of obligation to the state, even to the point of suicide, Plato's theories of the forms, or Aristotle's discussion of the mean. In contrast to Gregory, and to some extent Percival, Osler was not deeply engaged with the ideas of the philosophers. He was an admiring auditor, not a participant in the conversation.

Osler's Relative Lack of Interest in Modern Philosophy and Ethics

In contrast with this ongoing interest in the classical figures in philosophy (at least in the details of the texts if not their overarching ideas), Osler was relatively uninterested in the moderns. We get a hint of this in his mature reflections on his early school days when he visited Bovell's library:

> One corner of the library was avoided. With an extraordinary affection for mental and moral philosophy, he had collected the works of Locke and Berkeley, Kant and Hegel, Spinoza, and Descartes, as well as those of the moderns. He would joke upon the impossibility of getting me to read any of the works of these men, but at Trinity, in '67–'68, I attended his lectures on natural Theology, and he really did get us interested in Cousin and Jouffroy and others of the French School.
>
> (Osler 1929, pp. xvi–xvii)[17]

This lack of interest in modern philosophers continued throughout his career. It helps explain why Osler did not actively enter into conversation with the philosophers of his time and could not therefore break through the barrier that prohibited any significant medical ethics discussion during this period. There are, as would be expected among those with such eclectic interests and vast knowledge, occasional allusions to philosophers of the modern period, at least in brief references. He apparently had read Haldane's *Life of Descartes* while waiting to move into his permanent residence after moving to Oxford (Cushing 1940, p. 745). Soon thereafter, he made a passing reference to Descartes in a lecture ("The Growth of Truth," in Osler 1958c, p. 215).[18] He made an occasional reference to Francis Bacon (Osler was not a fan), but with nothing like the interest shown by Gregory or even Percival (Osler 1958b, pp. 1–7). George Berkeley (1655–1753) got casual mention in a lecture in 1897 ("British Medicine in Greater Britain," in Osler 1905b, p. 170). Likewise, Joseph Butler (1652–1752) was the subject of a brief reference (Osler 1905d, p. 348).

Missing from Osler's philosophical cadre are the Scottish philosophers. There is no mention of Hume, Adam Smith, Hutcheson, Beattie, or Reid[19] in his writings, even though Osler was the most philosophically sophisticated physician of the late nineteenth and early twentieth centuries. The contrast with the leading English-speaking philosopher–physicians of the end of eighteenth century is dramatic. These references to modern philosophers, meager as they are, exceed the working vocabulary of any other nineteenth- or early twentieth-century physician. But they are nothing compared to Osler's constant and detailed references to classical figures.

Osler's Interest in Theologians

Given Osler's original inclination toward the ministry, one might expect that he would have been interested in humanists oriented toward theology and religion. Indeed, there are numerous mentions of ancient and medieval theological figures in his writings. He once wrote a friend with great joy that he had bought a fourteenth-century manuscript of Albertus Magnus (Cushing 1940, p. 957). He made a passing reference to both Albertus Magnus and Thomas Aquinas in his Classical Association presidential address ("The Old Humanities and the New Science," in Osler 1958d, p. 19). On several occasions he made reference to Thomas More's *Utopia* (Cushing 1940, pp. 407, 539). In a note to Dr. Henry Viets, who was serving in the occupation forces in Europe, Osler recommended the study of Nicholas de Cusa, noting that he had founded a hospital in Trèves. Referring to a number of Cusa's manuscripts, he mentioned having recently acquired an original edition of one of his works (cited in Cushing 1940, p. 1323). There are frequent references to Erasmus, whose biography by Froude Osler read on his 1900 European trip (Cushing 1940, p. 534).[20] Calvin was mentioned unfavorably in conjunction with Servetus. Osler possessed rare editions of both Calvin and Servetus in his library (Cushing 1940, p. 843).[21] He appears not to have mentioned Martin Luther.

Osler's interests were not limited to Christian writers. He made reference to Paracelsus, Confucius, Averroes, and Avicenna.[22] In this list we discover what may be a clue to Osler: all of these figures had medical as well as philosophical and religious interests. Often, however, Osler's motive was to obtain manuscripts and rare editions for his or others' libraries. All of these figures are well represented in the *Bibliotheca Osleriana*.[23]

This ecumenical scholar of Anglican origin referred to Cotton Mather, another religious leader in the Puritan/Calvinist tradition, but merely to describe his mentor, James Bovell, with the phrase "angelical conjunction of medicine and divinity," which he attributed to Mather (Osler 1905c, p. 370).[24] Mather, himself, represented this conjunction, and it is a phrase that could apply to Osler as well.

It is striking that the theologians who interested him were historical figures. Osler's concern was biographical, bibliographical, and literary, not with the intellectual content of the authors' works. In the same way, he cited many literary figures: Whitman, Wordsworth, Voltaire, Tennyson, Shakespeare, Milton, Molière,

Lamb, Samuel Johnson, Henry James, Horace, Keats, Samuel Butler, Chaucer, Samuel Clemens, Coleridge, and Oliver Wendell Holmes (about whom he gave a full lecture [Osler 1894]).

Osler's Interest in Physician–Humanists

Osler was particularly intrigued by humanists who had also been physicians or at least had had a serious interest in medicine, such as Cusa (who founded a hospital), Mather, and Keats, who had worked as a surgical assistant or apothecary (Osler 1908c, pp. 37–54). The most conspicuous of these figures is Sir Thomas Browne, the author of *Religio Medici*.

Sir Thomas Browne (1605–1682)

Not only was Browne the subject and author, respectively, of the first two books Osler ever owned; his favorite copy of *Religio Medici* was placed on his coffin when he died (Cushing 1940, p. 1372). Along with Plato, it was on his short list of texts he wanted read to him in his final moments (Cushing 1940, p. 1370). It was also on his list of works that he recommended to medical students for bedside reading (Osler 1905, p. 389).[25] He included references to Browne early and often in his writing and in October 1905, the week of the 300th anniversary of Browne's birth, Osler lectured on him before the Physical Society at Guy's Hospital, London (Osler 1908e).

An important clue to answering the question of the extent to which Osler was a serious philosopher is that, aside from Osler's extravagant admiration of Browne, the critics do not think as much of Browne's philosophical and theological abilities as they do of his literary skills.[26]

John Locke (1632–1704)

While Browne was the first physician–philosopher Osler encountered, he was not the only one. Among modern philosophers, Osler clearly was most interested in John Locke, who also happened to be a physician. Osler devoted a long essay to Locke,[27] but, as the title suggests, it was devoted to medical rather than philosophical thought. He dwelt at length on Locke's influence on Sydenham and on Locke's medical treatment of Lord Shaftesbury. He reviewed Locke's medical writings. What he did not pursue was Locke's philosophical ideas (except insofar as they affected medicine and medical science), and there is no mention of Locke's theories of property and of natural rights, or of Locke's notions of personal identity—all ideas that have been discussed by late-twentieth-century medical ethicists. Locke is a first-class exemplar of Osler's ideal: one who, like Browne, Johnson, Bovell, and Osler himself, combined the humanities and medicine.

Thomas Linacre (1460–1524)

Thomas Linacre, the Catholic physician to Henry VIII and founder of the Royal College of Physicians, was also an exemplar of this ideal and was one of Osler's heroes. Linacre showed up in Osler's lectures and writing, beginning with the obituary address he gave at the death of Oliver Wendell Holmes (Osler 1894) and in a 1901 lecture at the Boston Medical Library (Cushing 1940, p. 568). In 1908 he gave the Linacre lecture at St. John's College, Cambridge, choosing Linacre himself as his topic (Osler 1908f). Only 6 of the 64 very brief pages of the lecture deal with Linacre's medical humanism. The other pages discuss Linacre's life, his role as a grammarian, and the foundations he established for lectureships.

Servetus (1511–1553)

Another physician–humanist that fascinated Osler was the theological rebel Michael Servetus, to whom the discovery of the "lesser circulation" is attributed. Servetus wrote *Christianismi Restitutio*, in which circulation theory is described, in 1553, the same year in which he was burned at the stake for heresy. He had Unitarian tendencies that offended both the Catholic church and John Calvin. Osler described his interest in Servetus in an article in the *Journal of the American Medical Association* that gives an account of Osler's visit to Vienna where he was able to see one of the two existing complete copies of the work.[28] The following year he reviewed Servetus's trial record and lectured on him before the Hopkins Historical Club.[29] Soon thereafter he helped arrange an exhibit that included a collection of books relating to Servetus (Cushing 1940, p. 871). In a light-hearted 1913 letter to James J. Welch, he showed his bias, saying, "why don't you take Bacon and that old rascal Calvin who burned my friend Servetus?" (letter excerpt reprinted in Cushing 1940, p. 1077).

These are only a few examples of physician–humanists that interested Osler.[30] He was interested in the virtuous life, not what contemporary philosophical ethicists would call an ethics of actions. The ancients provided models of the character traits that he found virtuous. In contrast to Hooker, Percival, and Gregory, Osler showed no interest in the problem of what to tell the dying patient. He never discussed the ethics of utilitarianism.[31] Nor did he pursue the earlier nineteenth-century problems of intraprofessional relations: consultation, quackery, and relations with practitioners of other schools.

Osler and Hippocrates

Thus Osler combined interest in the classics with a lack of interest in modern philosophy and theology (especially modern ethics). Without a modern source for a medical ethic, Osler had to turn elsewhere. In contrast to Gregory, Percival, and

Rush, who had modern philosophical tools for thinking about ethics, Osler looked to Hippocrates, the ancient who could plausibly fill this void.

Through Osler and his colleagues, Hippocrates finally emerged as the great hero figure at the center of the pantheon of historical figures in medicine with an interest in the humanities. Osler gave unlimited praise to Hippocrates, who was "the father of physic, the great Hippocrates, [who] came to excel, his theory being no more than an exact description or view of nature" (Osler 1921, p. 190). Whenever Osler wanted to offer the highest praise to some modern physician, he would refer to him as the "_____ Hippocrates" (filling in the name of the physician's country) as in "Boerhaave, the Dutch Hippocrates" (Osler 1921, p. 190; also see Cushing 1940, p. 765). Similarly, he described Sydenham as one "who took men back to Hippocrates" (Osler 1921, p. 190).

The Johns Hopkins Historical Club, which involved many of the medical staff, committed a portion of the 1891–92 year to the systematic study of the Hippocratic writings (Cushing 1940, p. 370). Osler presented his paper, "Physic and Physicians as Depicted in Plato" soon thereafter, having participated in the detailed study of Hippocrates.[32]

When Osler published his lecture on Elisha Bartlett, he appended an essay of Bartlett's taken from his *Discourse on the Times, Character, and Writings of Hippocrates*.[33] This is further evidence of the place Osler gave to Hippocrates.[34]

Lectures on The History of Medicine

In 1913 Osler gave a series of six lectures at Yale University, published later as *The Evolution of Modern Medicine* (Osler 1921). They revealed the depth of his interest in the history of medicine. The second lecture, "Greek Medicine," was expanded into a 50-page chapter when it was published. The published version contains a 14-page section (including two photographs), "Hippocrates and the Hippocratic Writings" (Osler 1921, pp. 58–71).

Osler and the Hippocratic Oath

Although Osler was interested in the entire Hippocratic corpus, he gave particular attention to the Oath. The Oath commanded his loyalty as a moral authority to the end of his career (Osler 1929, p. xvii). In an unpublished lecture in 1910, entitled "The Lessons of Greek Medicine," Osler revealed his admiration:

> But the high-water mark in research in that remarkable document, the Hippocratic Oath, which has been well called a monument of the highest rank in the history of civilization (Gomperz). For twenty-five centuries our 'credo', it is in many universities still the formula with which men are admitted to the Doctorate.[35]

He repeated this claim in virtually the same words in his Yale lectures three years later.[36] It is, of course, completely at odds with what we found in Edinburgh.

Medical students at Edinburgh did not take the Hippocratic Oath; they took a modified version of the same oath that other University of Edinburgh students had taken for 200 years, one dealing with loyalties to the king, the Scottish national covenant, and the university.

Osler was simply guilty of reading his current enthusiasm with the Hippocratic Oath, perhaps a spillover from his more general fascination with ancient Greece, back on 2300 years of the history of medicine, seeing it as a timeless, all-commanding core of the profession of medicine. The story is much more complex. There were, of course, periods when the Oath was given attention, but certainly through much of that history the Oath did not have the dominance that Osler attributes to it.

Osler certainly had the reputation of a good doctor with a saintly character, an exemplar of the virtues of the nineteenth- and early twentieth-century gentlemanly physician. What seemed to motivate his reading in philosophy was the quest for inspiration, for character strengthening, for lessons that could be applied to daily life. His philosophical wisdom was more pop-philosophy laced with classical references that would serve to inspire the reader. This pattern is suggested in his advice to medical students to "cultivate peace of mind, serenity, [and] the philosophy of Marcus Aurelius" (Barker 1957, p. 87). He was no Browne or Locke or Gregory, not even a Percival or Rush, who were in sophisticated conversation with the philosophers and theologians of their day—the Humes, Smiths, and Reids, the Wesleys and Gisbornes.

Osler is a complex case. He was not a simple, isolated medical scientist. If his interests had been more contemporary and more in the direction of medical ethics, he would be the one clear-cut exception to the pattern we see in the nineteenth century of physicians isolated from those doing medical ethics. As it is, he was not isolated from the humanities, but he was surely isolated from contemporary medical ethics.

RICHARD CABOT

One final early twentieth-century American physician must be considered. In contrast with Osler, Richard Clarke Cabot (1868–1939) had a clear interest in ethics.[37] He wrote several books on ethics (Cabot 1914, 1926, 1936, 1937, 1938) in addition to many in medical science, including classic texts on physical diagnosis (Cabot 1905)[38] and differential diagnosis (Cabot 1911–14). He was not only professor of medicine at Harvard, attending physician at Massachusetts General Hospital, and founder of its Social Services Department[39] but also chair of the Department of Social Ethics at Harvard College. Cabot was the first person to hold professorial positions in both medicine and ethics since Gregory.

Cabot's Interest in Religion, Ethics, and Medicine

Cabot's father was a philosopher, the biographer of Emerson, and an overseer of Harvard College, where his son was educated. Richard Cabot majored in philosophy and planned (shades of Osler) to enter the ministry (Unitarian in Cabot's case), but chose medicine instead.

Cabot's wife taught at a private girls' school and wrote two books for this purpose. Of them Cabot wrote, "in these books and in her teaching she has followed the principle that one way to teach ethics (and not merely to teach about ethics) is to practice pupils in the formation of good habits of thought" (Cabot 1926, p. 101).[40]

This summary of pedagogy reveals Cabot's interest in ethics—to build the character of his students.[41] He did this with almost no contact with the great ethics scholarship around him. He lived next door to Episcopal Theological School in Cambridge. At the request of the dean, he taught a weekly class for seminarians. But his subject matter was entirely practical. His topics included visiting the sick, attending on the dying, consoling the bereaved, advising on marriage and parenthood, and similar topics (Cabot 1926, pp. 4–5). His books on ethics are almost entirely devoid of reference to any of the contemporary debates of philosophical or theological ethics.[42] His ethics is platitudinous, as seen in his endorsement of the Boston School Committee's list of "laws" that he borrowed from William J. Hutchins' morality code for children (Cabot 1926, p. 109). These included self-control (tongue, temper, thoughts, acts), good health (hygiene, body and mind clean, skill, strength), kindness (in thought, word, act), sportsmanship, self-reliance, duty (not shirking, or living on others), reliability, honesty, good workmanship, teamwork, and loyalty.

In a chapter on business ethics, Cabot generates a list of principles by consulting a book of codes of ethics compiled by one Edgar L. Heermance.[43] The codes "concern every conceivable trade, such as ice-cream dealers, tailor, hairdressers, undertakers." Cabot had his secretary tabulate the principles to generate a list based on the number of codes in which a stated principle or practice was mentioned (justice = 62, service = 36, public welfare = 29, veracity = 16, responsibility = 12, other principles[44] = 3) (Cabot 1926, pp. 80–81). His efforts must have been an embarrassment to the two institutions in his Cambridge neighborhood (the Episcopal seminary and Harvard, both its philosophy department and its Divinity School). This is certainly a far cry from the complex scholarship in theological and philosophical ethics that had to have been occurring in these settings.

Cabot's Interest in Truth Telling

Cabot's naive and pietistic understanding of ethics had a surprising outcome. His simple commitment to the virtues included *veracity*, or truth telling.[45] Apparently unaware that his colleagues in medicine—Gregory, Percival, and especially Hooker—had struggled with the paternalistic justification of failing to disclose diagnoses truthfully to patients, Cabot became one of two physicians (along with Hooker) who devoted extensive efforts to arguing for the moral necessity of honesty.

Early Treatment of Truth Telling

An essay of Cabot's on truth telling first appeared in the *British Medical Journal* in 1903 and then in *Social Service and the Art of Healing* (Cabot 1909).[46] Later in life he devoted a full monograph to the subject (Cabot 1938). In the earlier essay, which is usually reprinted under the title "The Use of Truth and Falsehood in Medicine," he claims he is using an "experimental method." He considers two hypotheses, submitting them to the "test of experience." He begins with the hypothesis in which he was trained as a medical student, when his teacher had instructed him as follows:

When you are thinking of telling a lie . . . ask yourself whether it is simply and solely for the patient's benefit that you are going to tell it. If you are sure that you are acting for his good and not for your own profit, you can go ahead with a clear conscience.

(Cabot 1978, p. 189)

This was the standard, paternalistic position taken not only by physicians in the Hippocratic tradition but also by Hutcheson and Sidgwick, along with many other utilitarians. Cabot proceeds to illustrate the consequentialistic reasoning, by citing examples of lying that not only benefit the patient but set the mind of a wife of a patient at ease.

Cabot presents a case from his own experience in which he attempted to tell a benevolent lie to the wife of a patient. He had been told that she was "too delicate and too unstrung by neurasthenia to be capable of bearing the truth about her husband" (Cabot 1977, p. 244). He, however, got caught by her in his deception, causing the woman even more distress. Moreover, once he got caught, he proceeded, the only way he could, to tell her the unvarnished truth. Much to his surprise, the woman, who was supposed to collapse from the unbearable shock, held up well. Cabot wants us to conclude that his experiment proved that truth telling does not produce bad consequences. Cabot has, of course, committed the medical scientist's unpardonable sin of reasoning from the single case, but, forgiving him that flaw, he essentially suggests that the consequences of lying are worse than those of speaking the truth.

His argument is a simple version of Hooker's: deceit is likely to fail, causing the patient more agony than a straightforward statement of the truth. (It is simpler because Hooker at least develops a more complex rule-utilitarian version of argument.) However, neither Hooker nor Cabot follow Kant's more deontological claim for the duty of honesty—the position that it is one's duty to speak truthfully regardless of the consequences.[47] They both could have borrowed from Bentham or Mill or Sidgwick to provide a more sophisticated case for veracity based on consequences. They would then have had to confront, as Sidgwick did, the case in which, even taking into account the disutilities of dishonesty, the consequences still seem better with the lie.

The troublesome feature of Cabot's account (and of Hooker's) is that, at least in his early writing, he appeared to be oblivious to the existence of a rich philosophical literature exactly on his subject and from which he could have drawn to make his case more sophisticated. Cabot was a physician who had been exposed to simpler versions of morality from his deep, but unschooled commitment to a Christian (or Unitarian) ethic. He correctly intuited that much of Christian ethics is at odds with Hippocratic paternalism on the subject of truth telling. He failed, however, to analyze the tension, much less the possibility, that different ethical theories would explain the tension differently. Cabot blundered into a challenge to the received paternalism in his profession by absorbing a simple pro–truth-telling Christian ethic and by having the good fortune to have his one vividly remembered case steer him in that direction. He never seemed to appreciate, however, that discourse with moral theorists would have helped him understand why he took the stand he did or why that stand was in tension with the Hippocratic tradition.

Later Truth-Telling Writings

In the next publication, the relatively early *Social Service and the Art of Healing* (1909), Cabot's position was still that of a naive utilitarian. By 1938, shortly before his death, when he published *Honesty*, his knowledge of the philosophical literature had grown only modestly. In an introductory chapter he mentions A. E. Taylor, Leslie Stephens, Richard Baxter, R. L. Stevenson, and Newman Smyth (Cabot 1938, pp. 5–6). Later there are passing references to Sidgwick (p. 248), Emerson (p. 292), and Royce (p. 303). He mentions Kant quite a few times, without reference to texts.

It certainly seems that he understood these works, although the tone of his book is quite different from a text attempting to engage these authors in the arena of philosophical and theological ethics, where the above works would generally reside. *Honesty* is more single-minded, representing an attack on lying in all forms and all professions. In some sense, this could be seen as an early work of "practical" or "applied" ethics. The 11 chapters of Section II discuss problems of honesty in various contexts: Chapter 6, In War and Crime; Chapter 7, In Government; Chapter 8, In Industry; Chapter 9, In Science; Chapter 10, In Education. He attempts to show how lying is problematic in all sorts of situations. However, the last 80 pages (Section III, "The Philosophy of Honesty," containing Chapters 17–22) is the most theoretical. In spite of his clear appeals to consequences, he casts this section as an attack on utilitarians.

He begins by noting that "first cousin to intuition is 'common sense,' the philosopher's stone of the English Utilitarians, who have put up, I think, the best arguments in defense of occasional 'sensible' and well-meant lies" (Cabot 1938, p. 247). He expresses his objection to such lies, including lying to murderers, by arguing that "such fibs are known to be exceptions; our general sense that men are trustworthy is not impaired by them. Common sense (for Henry Sidgwick) decides the who, the when, and the where of our occasional lies. *But common sense does not hand down the same decisions in every sensible person*" (p. 248, emphasis his). Furthermore, "any candid person who looks over the literature of utilitarian ethics on the subject of Honesty will be led to the conclusion that common sense varies in the exceptions which it allows to the rule of veracity" (p. 249) He claims that instead of this intuitionism, "what we need is a rule that can be applied with average intelligence and good will on the basis of data reasonably clear" (p. 249). He then proceeds to analyze what he takes to be the mistakes of utilitarians:

Writers like Henry Sidgwick who ask us to make sensible exceptions to the rule of honesty seem to me to be oblivious of two essential truths about human nature: (1) that we are all in imminent danger of self-deceit. (2) That lies which do no appreciable harm to society may work serious mischief in the liar. . . . But if the utilitarian is unaware of the temptation to self-deceit in us all he is writing about a subject—human nature—of which he is densely ignorant.

(Cabot 1938, pp. 254, 256)

Cabot makes an odd mistake about Kant. In his objections to utilitarians, he quotes someone he refers to as "Johnson," interrupting the quote in mid-sentence to label Johnson as working in "Kant's spirit": "'You have no business with consequences, you are to tell the truth. Besides' (he goes on, very much in Kant's spirit), 'you are not sure what effect your telling him that he is in danger may have'" (Cabot 1938, p. 249).

Now the first half of this Johnson quote would seem to be "in Kant's spirit" but the second half certainly is not. Kant's objections to lying concerns contradictions of will and contradictions of conception, not the unpredictability of unintended consequences from lying. Thus, when the philosophers put in an appearance in even the most mature work of Cabot, he still does not get them exactly right. As he did earlier in life, he seems to assume that anyone—both Kantians and the utilitarians—will base their ethical norms on consequences. To him the difference is that those he calls "utilitarian" make case-by-case exceptions, whereas the consequences of lies in every case make it clear that there needs to be a more exceptionless rule against lying. He makes "utilitarians" what today would be called "act-utilitarians." To him the alternative is something very close to what we would call "rule-utilitarianism." The actual Kantian position (and the actual Protestant Christian position that underlies much of Kant's view) is not on Cabot's radar screen.

Cabot, like Osler, is a complicated case. If there are exceptions to the generalization that nineteenth- and early twentieth-century physicians working on issues

in medical ethics were out of touch with contemporary philosophical and theological discourse, these would be the best examples we could find. However, even
in his most mature work, work that shows some signals of familiarity with the
ethics scholarship of the humanities of his day, Cabot, like Osler, seems to be more
a distant observer than a participant in the conversation. He lacks insights into the
real controversies of the day.[48]

Cabot's Interest in the Hippocratic Oath

That Cabot lacked these insights can be gleaned from his simple and lavish em-
brace of the Hippocratic Oath. Contrary to his views on truth telling, the Oath
expresses cautious views about disclosure to patients. It departs from the Christian ethic that Cabot espoused, not merely in its reference to Greek gods and
goddesses but, more importantly, in the notions of keeping medical knowledge
a secret from those outside the Hippocratic group and in the closing lines that
link fulfillment of the oath to divine reward. None of this would be acceptable
to Christians. In fact, the medieval physicians who adapted the Hippocratic Oath
insisted on rewriting it to deal with these objectionable features. Cabot did not
grasp these tensions the way physicians more thoroughly schooled in one of the
major religious or philosohical traditions would have.[49]

Cabot devotes a considerable portion of his chapter "Ethics and the Medical
Profession," in *Borderlands*, to the Hippocratic Oath and the AMA codes, both
the original 1847 version and the 1912 revision. To his credit, he was moderately aware of at least one of the Oath's more glaring problems—the prohibition on surgery (which Cabot calls "trade unionism," apparently not recognizing
the possibility that its basis lay in archaic concerns about blood contamination
and ritual impurity). He says nothing about the way the Oath treats medical
knowledge as cultic *gnosis* too dangerous for lay people, the archaic virtues of
purity and *holiness*, the ambiguous prohibitions on euthanasia and abortion, the
Pelagian ethic of rewards and punishments, or the references to Greek gods and
goddesses. He says nothing about its theory of moral epistemology (that knowledge of moral right and wrong is lodged with the professional authority rather
than with traditional religious sources, such as the religious texts or the Pope,
or secular sources—reason or empirical observation).

On balance, however, Cabot's assessment of the Oath is reverent. He claims
that it contains "sound sense valid for all time" (Cabot 1926, pp. 35–36). Regarding the Hippocratic confidentiality pledge, not recognizing that it acknowledges
that some medical secrets may be disclosed, Cabot opines, "one wishes that such
an anti-gossip rule were in force today" (Cabot 1926, p. 36).

Whatever one thinks of Cabot's endorsement of the Oath, he did not place it in
relation with either ancient or modern moral theories outside of medicine. He did

not consider the tension between the Hippocratic ethic and other moral systems, either religious or secular. He never discussed these other traditions and clearly did not know much about them.

This is not to suggest that the isolation was entirely the fault of the physicians. As we shall see in the next chapter, the religious ethicists were equally unaware of the efforts in ethics of their physician colleagues.

REVISIONS OF THE AMERICAN MEDICAL ASSOCIATION'S PRINCIPLES

The AMA code revisions that Cabot took up in his *Borderlands* volume were organized medicine's attempt at fixing some of the problems in the original 1847 version. Unfortunately, the AMA did not hear even the gentle concerns of Cabot, much less the more challenging tensions that could be gleaned from the religious and philosophical theorists of the day.

Throughout the remainder of the nineteenth and the first half of the twentieth century the AMA was essentially content with its codification functioning in isolation from the world of ethics. Revisions were undertaken periodically. A second edition appeared in 1871 (American Medical Association 1871) and a third in 1879 (American Medical Association 1879). Additional revisions appeared in 1903 (American Medical Association 1975a), 1912 (American Medical Association 1975b), 1947,[50] and 1957 (American Medical Association 1957). These, however, constituted tinkering at the edges of a narrowly professional document without any evidence of contact with ethics outside of medicine. The revisions were introduced as commitments that the writers perceived as tracing directly back to the Oath of Hippocrates. According to the AMA in 1971, "the Oath of Hippocrates . . . has remained in Western Civilization as an expression of ideal conduct for the physician (American Medical Association 1971, p. iv). The AMA also insisted on linking its ethical tradition with Percival, apparently not aware of Percival's relative lack of interest in Hippocrates or his differences with the Hippocratic ideal. The AMA presented the revisions as modest changes in what it perceived as a timeless tradition. For example, in 1903 the restriction on consultation with practitioners outside the association was eliminated. In 1957 there was a significant format change, reducing the longer, discursive paragraphs to a list of 10 general principles. The Judicial Council went out of its way to emphasize that the 1957 edition was "not intended to and [did] not abrogate any ethical principle expressed in the 1955 edition." It insisted that "the basic ethical concepts . . . are identical" (American Medical Association 1971, p. v). It was not until the revision of 1980 that we saw real evidence that the AMA was coming out of its century and a half of being walled off from moral and philosophical debates of the outside world.

REASONS FOR ISOLATION IN THE UNITED STATES

As we bring to a close our exploration of the experience in the United States of gradual separation of physicians and secular humanists and before we consider the relation of religious ethicists, we should pause to see how the American experience compares to that of Britain. When examining the reasons for isolation of British physicians from their humanist counterparts, I suggested that the young age of entry into medical school could have been a factor. The most significant American contributor to medical ethics of the eighteenth century seems to support that observation. Benjamin Rush, like Thomas Percival, entered medical school at a relatively old age. Born in 1745, he entered the medical course at Edinburgh in 1766, having completed his arts degree at the College of New Jersey. He had an apprenticeship in law, and had begun an apprenticeship in medicine prior to enrolling at Edinburgh. Thus two of the three giants of eighteenth-century Anglo-American medical ethics were relatively late enrollees into medical school and had had a relatively prolonged academic adolescence with rich exposure to philosophical and other humanities perspectives.

Nevertheless, the age of entry into medical school by itself does not seem to account for the lack of interest in the humanities. If that were so, the nineteenth- and twentieth-century American medical students, who were forced to complete a baccalaureate education prior to entry to medical school would have shown a richer knowledge of or interest in the humanities, like their eighteenth-century counterparts.

In the United States, some early contributors to our story, such as Cotton Mather, began their college study early. Mather entered Harvard at the age of 12, but, as with Gregory, his family clearly gave him a head start and intellectual orientation. His father, Increase Mather, was President of Harvard. Cotton Mather was "schooled partly at home and partly at the Boston Latin School, but the greatest influence in his early years was that of his family" (Murdock 1957, p. 386).

Benjamin Rush had a somewhat less auspicious family background. His father was a gunsmith and farmer, but his uncle, Samuel Finley, became a scholar of some note. When Rush's father died, he came first under the influence of Presbyterian clergyman Gilbert Tennent, and then, at age eight was sent to board at Finley's academy at West Nottingham, Maryland, where Rush received a classical education. From there Rush went, at age 15, to the College of New Jersey, now Princeton, where he came under the influence of its president, Samuel Davies. Davies was succeeded by Finley, placing Rush in the best of intellectual circles. This was followed by a medical apprenticeship with Philadelphia's leading physician, John Redman. By the time Rush was ready to study medicine at Edinburgh, Rush was very well connected. As we saw in Chapter 5, Benjamin Franklin wrote him a letter of introduction. Thus in the late eighteenth century the three key physicians that were to shape medical ethics all had outstanding connections to elite academic families and associated in the highest intellectual circles of their day. They learned the classics, including what we would consider philosophy and ethics, at home.

Insofar as William Osler counts as something of an exception to the nineteenth-century pattern, his exceptional status can be traced to his family influence. His father, an Anglican clergyman, had a library of 1500 volumes. This influence undoubtedly played a role in orienting Osler toward the ministry, for which he began studying before medicine, and biology captured his attention. At grammar school and then at Trinity College School at Weston the influence of its founder and warden, Rev. W. A. Johnson, as well as its medical director, James Bovell, further shaped his interests. Nevertheless, this unusual familial and educational influence was not sufficient for Osler to completely break through the nineteenth-century isolation. At least when it came to contemporary philosophical and theo-logical study of ethics, Osler was, at best, an amateur. Insofar as he had any humanities interests, they leaned toward the classical Greek and Latin period and even here he was more a bibliophile than a serious student of the philosophy of the period.

Being born into a family of the cultural elite was not sufficient to overcome the tremendous power of the explosion of the quantity of knowledge to force schol-ars to become more and more specialized. The increasing rigor of science that made such enormous strides possible seems to have had an unanticipated side effect of cutting scholars off from their colleagues in other disciplines.

In North America, eighteenth-century figures such as Rush and Bard published on a wide range of topics. Rush, the "physician, patriot, humanist," wrote and worked on the anti-slavery movement, temperance, capital punishment, and ex-ercise, as well as his theory of the moral sense. He published an entire volume of essays on literary, philosophical, and moral topics as well as his *Observations on the Duties of a Physician*. The Philadelphia physicians of the next generation wrote on eruptive fevers and rheumatism. The best medical ethical mind of the AMA at its founding (John Bell) wrote on the liver, hydrology, and mineral bathers when he was not writing ethics. His partner in the writing of the AMA's code of ethics was a journal editor more than a scholar in any medical field. Even the physicians of this period who stand out for their work in humanities—people like Hooker and Osler—cannot claim real scholarship in philosophical subjects. Hooker's ethics is a one-note song resting heavily on Percival. Osler's bibliographic and histori-cal interests did not lead to any real scholarship in contemporary ethics.

The nineteenth-century U.S. experience makes clear that an additional factor contributed in a surprising way to the isolation of physicians from humanities scholars studying ethics. New scholarship on Hippocrates made the Hippocratic literature available to physicians at just the moment when they had lost a working knowledge of the more complex and sophisticated alternatives in philosophy and theology.

When physicians are not as well educated in the humanities, they need a short version of ethical theory and they need it applied as closely as possible to medicine. The Hippocratic Oath in one page is much more convenient than a lifetime of humanities scholarship for a physician whose education is consumed with the natural sciences and clinical application. Fortunately, new scholarship in the classics made Hippocrates available as never before.[51]

The nineteenth-century physicians such as those associated with Kappa Lambda did not have any real knowledge of the Hippocratic literature or its cultural context. They saw themselves as part of a worldwide, timeless brotherhood with an ethic that could be reduced to a page. Since they did not have real knowledge of Plato, Aristotle, the Talmud, or early Christian ethics, let alone various modern moral theories, they were unaware of the potential contradictions and tensions we have identified—treating the ethical code as a secret not to be revealed to lay people, stigmatizing surgery for its conflict with the Hippocratic virtues of "purity" and "holiness," and the reward-and-punishment ethic so fitting for a Greek, but so alien to a Christian.

Scientifically trained, but philosophically isolated nineteenth-century physicians could be good practitioners by touting a platitudinous page-length oath. They had no idea of the moral traditions and their unique perspectives behind the page. To scientist/clinicians, "benefit your patient according to your ability and judgment" was good enough for an ethic. As long as they stayed in the clinic or doctor's office and didn't converse with humanists who spent careers worrying about these differences, they were protected from serious moral conflict.

Thus, in the United States, as in Scotland and England, the changing social class of the physician and the explosion of medical information made specialization both comfortable and necessary. It remains to be seen whether the religious inclinations of people like Osler and Cabot led them to retain their links with the humanities by turning to the religious leaders of the day.

8

DIVERGING TRADITIONS: PROFESSIONAL AND RELIGIOUS MEDICAL ETHICS OF THE NINETEENTH CENTURY

While nineteenth-century physicians, for the most part, were not in close com-munication with philosophers and the philosophical controversies of the day, philosophers also were not contributing to the debate within organized profes-sional medicine. It could be that physicians were having their medical ethical thought shaped by humanists who worked more in theological ethics. Of par-ticular interest is the relation of the religious communities to the AMA code and other professional activities to articulate a medical ethic. This chapter explores that relation.

RELIGIOUS TRADITIONS IN MEDICAL ETHICS

It is widely assumed that the Hippocratic tradition has been the sole or at least dominant view in Western medical ethics. Some scholars have hypothesized that, although there were clearly competing schools of Greek medicine, including medical ethics, there was a convergence of Christian thought with Hippocratic medical ethics soon after Constantine that led to the dominance of Hippocratic ethics (Edelstein 1967, p. 62, n. 45; Carrick 1985, pp. 66, 159; Verhey 1984, pp. 157, 170). However, there are important substantive differences between the religious ethical traditions and Hippocratic medicine. The Oath is the product of a school of Greek philosophical thought having links with Pythagoreanism. It serves as a symbolic oath of initiation into a closed group that treats secret knowledge as too powerful to be in the hands of the ordinary lay person, a view radically at odds with Christian theology. It maintains a ritualistic separation of surgery from medicine. It incorporates a reward-and-punishment system that is alien to Christian thought. Early Christians paid little attention to Hippocratic medicine and its ethics. There is almost no evidence of contact between them, at least during the first eight centuries of the Christian era. I could find only two explicit references to Hippocratic ethical writings in writings of the church fathers Jerome and Gregory of Nazianzus of the fourth century).[1] Both of these consciously distinguish between Hippocratic and Christian medicine.

From about the eighth to the twelfth centuries there was a much more complex intermingling of religious and medical roles than in the earlier period. A Christianized version of the Oath was produced with the earliest manuscripts dating from the tenth century, entitled "Oath According to Hippocrates in so far as a Christian May Swear It" (Jones 1924). This version is sometimes taken as evidence for convergence, but it can at least as well be taken as evidence that medieval Christian writers were unable to accept many provisions of the Hippocratic writings.

By about the twelfth century a secularization and professionalization of medicine had begun. Priests were forbidden from practicing medicine (Kelly 1979, p. 51). It can be argued that the Enlightenment brought on the final stages of secularization and professionalization of medicine. McCullough (1985, pp. 88–89) has suggested that with Percival's Manchester code, written in the 1790s and published in 1803, we have a "radical shift" from Gregory's approach and a "major shift in kind" in Anglo-American medical ethics. There is a less clear connection between the dominant religious and philosophical scholarship of the day (including that of Hutcheson and Hume) and a more isolated, independent concern with intraprofessional matters of physician authority and power. I have suggested that Percival was still very much in conversation with not only contemporary philosophical debates but also theological perspectives. Clearly, however, soon after Percival the professionalization of medical ethics that began with him left physicians of the next generation; they were out of touch with both philosophers and theologians, so that the professionally generated ethics was out there on its own.

Kelly (1979, p. 14) claims that by the early modern period, secularization and professionalization of medical ethics among organized medical professionals generated a backlash among religious scholars, who perceived a greater need for an explicitly religious moral framework to differentiate their positions from the matters of concern to medical professionals. While Kelly is concerned specifically with the development of Catholic medical ethics in North America, the same point could be made with regard to Judaism and Protestantism as well. All three groups have long had ethical traditions with at least implicit medical ethical implications.

The roots of Jewish medical ethics are in the Talmud and responsa. Jakobovits (1978, p. 792) points out that Judaism never had a Jewish version of the Hippocratic Oath, relying instead on its own long medical, ethical heritage including the Oath of Asaph, the writings of Jewish rabbi–physicians, and more recent medical ethical documents such as the eighteenth-century prayer attributed to Maimonides. Although no specific research has been done on Jewish treatment of medical ethical issues in the nineteenth century, there is no evidence that Jewish scholarship took cognizance of the AMA Code at mid-century. While talmudic scholarship has shown respect for secular work in medicine, it would be totally out of keeping with this tradition of scholarship to credit the consensus of a group of primarily gentile physicians meeting in Philadelphia in May 1847 with insights worthy of attention to rabbinical scholarship.

Likewise, Protestant thought in the mid-nineteenth century showed no concern about the ethics activities of the AMA. American Protestantism was dominated primarily by other, more timely matters: first the Great Revival of 1830 and then the voluntary charitable societies and abolition movement that followed.[2] The dominant theme related to medical ethics was the emphasis on diet, temperance, and simple, natural remedies. This continued the significant contribution of John Wesley as seen in his phenomenally successful and influential *Primitive Physick* (Wesley 1747; see also Vanderpool, unpublished).

The influence of Wesley particularly manifested itself in the nineteenth-century American movements of sectarian Protestantism. Mormonsism, Seventh Day Adventists, Jehovah's Witnesses, and Christian Science were all mid- to late nineteenth-century sectarian movements with significant medical components emphasizing the link between disease on the one hand, and diet and life style on the other. Although all but Christian Science made use of orthodox medical knowledge, their unique doctrines relating healing to their religious beliefs made them less interested in the authority of the AMA on matters moral. They all used specialized healers or practitioners and, in varying degrees, incorporated moral positions that would have been incomprehensible to those outside the faith. For members of these groups, the source of moral authority and knowledge was within their sectarian communities, not in the AMA (Fuller 1989; Jones 1985).

The detailed histories of the medical ethics of Jewish and Protestant groups in the nineteenth century cannot be developed here. Rather, as a way of exploring my hypothesis in detail, I want to pursue Roman Catholic moral theology and its treatment of what we would call medical ethics. I have chosen this focus both because its history is so rich and because Roman Catholicism generally seeks ways of integrating with the surrounding culture. If Catholicism was willing to be integrated into the Greco-Roman world of thought, then it is the most promising candidate for a religion that would be in communication with the secular world of medicine.

ROMAN CATHOLIC MEDICAL MORALITY

In spite of the tradition of integrating into the surrounding culture, the Roman Catholic tradition in the United States increasingly differentiated itself from the medical ethics of organized medicine during the nineteenth century. It is not that there was an overt, hostile reaction to the development of local, state, and national codes of ethics such as those of the AMA. Rather, the methodology and substantive normative ethical concerns of Catholic theologians and physicians writing on the subject simply took them in significantly different directions. As far as I can tell, there was no public response to or even acknowledged awareness of the AMA's adoption of its code in 1847. There was, however, a rich tradition of continuing pursuit of the morality of the physician's role. At the beginning of the century, this was based primarily on use of Catholic materials from Europe. By the end of the century, American materials in the same tradition were common.

There is a perception, at least by later commentators, that with the increasingly professionalization of medicine, the concern of organized Anglo-American medicine turned to problems of power, authority, and particularly relations among medical professionals and their competitors (Kelly 1979, p. 14). It is even suggested that Catholic commentators refused to use the term *medical ethics* for their work for fear of confusing "real" morality with the questions of intraprofessional etiquette being addressed by professionals.[3]

Three closely related genres of Catholic moral literature spoke to issues of medical ethics during the nineteenth century.[4] First were the moral-theology manuals, which had their origins in the seventeenth century, but the nineteenth-century works evolved from the 1785 expanded edition of Alfonso Liguori's *Theologia moralis*. Works throughout the nineteenth century following this model have been described as "nearly carbon copies of their predecessors" (Kelly 1979, p. 30).[5] None of these works is exclusively a medico-moral work, but certain important issues for medicine were covered.

A second group of writings approached medical ethical issues under the rubric of *casus conscientiae*, or cases of conscience. They followed the same organizational structure as the manuals of moral theology, but based their conclusions solely on "natural" human reason (Gury 1881; Lehmkuhl 1907; Villada 1885–87).

Finally, an important genre of Catholic writing in the nineteenth century was what was called "pastoral medicine" (Capellmann 1879; Scotti 1836). These volumes were designed to serve two purposes: to provide medical knowledge for pastors and theological and ethical preparation for medical practitioners. Carl Capellmann's *Pastoral Medicine* was the first to appear in English at the time when Catholic moral theology was just beginning to be written in the vernacular. It appeared in English one year after the original publication and explicitly acknowledged its dependence on the moral theology of Gury, Liguori, and Scavini (Capellmann 1879, bottom of table of contents page).

The authors of these documents operated in a different world from that of the professional medical ethical literature of the time. It would be understandable if some of the Europeans were not familiar with the Anglo-American professional ethical literature, but the problem was the same for the American authors. They were working in an ethical tradition that was not in communication with the medical professional organizations. Still they positioned themselves to provide authoritative advice for physicians and patients—at least those within the Catholic tradition.

COMPARING THE ETHICS OF ORGANIZED
MEDICINE AND THE CATHOLIC CHURCH

The significance of the existence of multiple medical ethical systems, each ignorant of or indifferent to the existence of the other, cannot be overstated. It would seem that this would be a matter of concern for Catholic physicians who are simultaneously loyal members of the AMA or for Catholic patients who obtain their health care from physicians guided by AMA ethics but who are not Catholic. A similar concern would be plausible for Jews, Seventh Day Adventists, and others of some specific religious medico-moral tradition who are subject to the AMA perspective either as physician members or as patients getting care from an AMA physician.

The critical question, then, is the degree to which the religious and professional medical ethical frameworks are different. We will look briefly at their methodologies and their normative concerns.

Medico-Moral Methodologies

We know how the AMA went about writing its code of ethics. As we have seen in previous chapters, the AMA committee writing the draft took whole sections verbatim from Percival either directly or mediated through intermediary documents and incorporated material from Benjamin Rush as well, as had been done in earlier state and local codes such as those in Boston in 1808, New York in 1823, and Philadelphia in 1825. The working assumption was that a profession was responsible for articulating its own code of ethics. It drew on other medical professional writing, but there is no evidence of any interest in the major philosophical or theological schools of thought of the day.

The opening sentence of the 1847 code claims that medical ethics (the term used by the physicians) "as a branch of general ethics, must rest on the basis of religion and morality" (American Medical Association 1848, p. 5), but that is the only reference to the fields of ethics, morality, or religion. The project is clearly one belonging to the profession, not to the theologians, philosophers, or the general public. The AMA's professional medical ethics is detached from the foundations of ethics, whether secular or religious.

By contrast, the Catholic medico-moral literature we have examined saw medical ethics as derivative from a more general moral theology. Any claim of moral authority by a medical professional body was appropriately viewed with skepticism. In the moral theology manuals, the organizational structure was primarily around the Ten commandments and the sacraments (Kelly 1979, pp. 24, 30). An alternative organizational structure used the classical virtues—the Christian virtues of faith, hope, and love or the Greek virtues of wisdom, temperance, courage, and justice (Kelly 1979, p. 38). Some manuals had a special section on the obligations of medical personnel. Regardless, we can assume that there ws a general framework for doing moral theology. It included presuppositions about methods of justification and sources of authority. Once that framework was in place, the implications for medical roles could be established derivatively. Thus most questions of interest to medical analysis arose under the rubric of the fifth or sixth commandments (the commandments against killing and committing adultery). Under the heading of the fifth commandment (which in the Catholic version is the prohibition on killing) was abortion, euthanasia, suicide, castration, and mutilation (Kelly 1979, p. 31). Under the sixth commandment (the prohibition on commiting adultery) the issues of fornication, rape, adultery, incest, coital positions, contraception, homosexuality, and masturbation were treated Additional questions arose under the heading of the sacraments, particularly matrimony, under which some of the sixth commandment issues were sometimes covered.

Normative Ethical Issues

The differences in moral methodology thus led to important differences in substance between the AMA and other professionally articulated medical ethical codes on the one hand, and the medico-moral framework of the theologians on the other. It is striking that the substantive issues developed ad nauseam in the Catholic literature were scarcely mentioned in any of the professional codes. Jonsen and Hellegers (1974, pp. 3–20) have argued that the professional codes emphasized the development of virtues rather than the norms of right conduct (duties or obligations) that are the focus of the Catholic medico-moral literature.

Much of the emphasis was indeed on the character of the physician, including the oft-quoted, controversial virtues of the gentleman: tenderness, firmness, condescension, and authority. Even as virtues they were strangely at odds with the cardinal virtues that provided the structure for the virtue manuals in Catholic moral theology. Even though the 1847 AMA code included some talk of duties, the handling of the duties differed from that of the Catholic medico-moral tradition of the nineteenth century as much as treatment of the virtues did. In sum, none of the dominant duty themes of one tradition was comparable to those of the other. Using Capellmann as an example, we can see the difference by summarizing the main themes of the Catholic literature, starting with abortion and then risky surgery, sexual ethics, terminal illness disclosure, and the social ethics of medicine.

Abortion

As we have noted, the Catholic medico-moral discussions were often structured mainly around the fifth and sixth commandments. Capellmann (1879, pp. 10–20) followed this standard approach, devoting the first 10 pages of his work to abortion and "perforation of the living fetus." It comes as no surprise that the Catholic literature gave substantial attention to this issue. In fact, through the nineteenth century the Catholic concern about abortion actually heightened, leading to Pope Pius IX's 1869 Constitution *Apostolicae Sedis* (Pope Pius IX, 1923, pp. 24–31, esp. p. 28.), which eliminated any lingering doubt about the moral difference between formed and unformed fetuses and made excommunication the penalty for abortion. The AMA, by contrast, was silent on the subject of abortion.

Risky Surgery

Immediately following the treatment of abortion in Capellmann's work (1879, pp. 20–28) is an equally detailed nine pages on "operations attended with risk to life." This detailed discussion led to the conclusion that "no one is obliged to undergo a severe operation involving risk of life, although affording, at the same time, a hope of its preservation" (Capellmann 1879, pp. 21–22). In fact, Capellmann specifically made the point that excessively risky operations were morally forbidden.

The AMA treatment of this subject was much more shallow. The focus seemed to be on the possibility that a physician would abandon a patient in a hopeless condition. Patients should not be abandoned, we are told, because, if the physician stays with the patient, pain and mental anguish may be relieved. There was no awareness of the possibility that the burden to the patient of treatment might be overwhelming and provide a moral justification for foregoing further care.

Capellmann's discussion of the fifth commandment includes a long discussion of morphia, chloroform, and animal magnetism, all dealing with the issue of whether these were so dangerous that they were morally prohibited. He concluded that "the physician should always make use of such remedies as are regarded *safe* in the existing state of medical science" (Capellmann 1879, p. 29). Nothing remotely similar can be found in the 1847 AMA code.

Sexual Ethics

Capellmann's even longer discussion of the sixth commandment occupies over 40 pages, covering such topics as masturbation, "pollutions" (nocturnal emissions), and the uses of marriage. Under the latter topic the questions of ethical and unethical copulation, contraception, and coitus interruptus are addressed in great detail. William Dassel, the American priest who translated Capellmann, obviously struggling with these delicate subjects, explained in his preface that although he favored the use of the vernacular, he attempted "to lessen the disgust necessarily provoked by unavoidable details, but putting them into a Latin disguise" (Capell-mann 1879, p. iv).

By mid-century, the pope had put to rest any doubt about the Catholic view on contraception. On May 21, 1851, the Holy Office issued the following decree:

The Apostolic See is asked what theological note is to be applied to the following proposi-tions: (1) a married couple may practice contraception for morally good motives; (2) this form of marital intercourse is not certainly against the natural law. The Holy Office answers: the first proposition is scandalous, erroneous and contrary to the natural law of marriage; the second is scandalous and implicitly condemned in proposition 49 of Innocent XI.

(Cited in Jonsen and Toulmin 1988, p. 271)

By contrast, the AMA in 1847 made no mention of contraception and related ethical problems of marital relations. One would think that the AMA would at least have been aware that these were a potential issue for its Catholic members and for Catholic patients, but the AMA did not have these subjects on its horizon.

Terminal Illness Disclosure

Two additional normative themes are worth mentioning because of the contrast between the Catholic and AMA positions regarding them. First, Catholic moral theology has long emphasized, in cases of terminal illness, the need to disclose to patients their diagnosis. As early as the fifteenth century Antonius of Florence (1477) taught of the necessity of the physician to warn patients of their impend-ing death so that they might adequately prepare their souls (Kelly 1979, p. 26). The same theme appeared in the nineteenth century manuals and pastoral medi-cine texts (Capellmann 1879, pp. 167–69). This is, no doubt, in part, because of the Catholic belief in the importance of preparation for death—an issue of no concern to the professional association.

In 1847 the AMA, influenced by Gregory and Percival, provided a much more Hippocratic, paternalistic reading of the physician's duty regarding truth telling. The physician "should not be forward to make gloomy prognostications, because they savor of empiricism, by magnifying the importance of his services in the treatment or cure of the disease. But he should not fail, on proper occasions, to give to the friends of the patient timely notice of danger, when it really occurs; and even to the patient himself, if absolutely necessary" (American Medical Assciation 1848, p. 14). The conflict with the traditional duty of confidentiality appeared to be overlooked. Certainly, there was no awareness of the possibility that the patient might need this information to make preparation—secular or religious—for his or her death.

Social Ethics of Medicine

Finally, there was a difference, at least in emphasis, in what might be called the social ethics of medicine. In 1847 the AMA departed from Hippocratic tradition in including an explicitly social dimension. The third chapter dealt with "duties of the profession to the public, and of the obligations of the public to the profession" (American Medical Association 1848, pp. 23–24). These duties and obligations concerned, however, newly emerging matters of public health—"medical policy, public hygiene, and legal medicine"—and the duty of the physician in an epidemic, rather than questions concerning the right of access to the poor.

Catholic moral theology, by contrast, had long emphasized a social ethic for medicine that includes a duty to treat the poor without fee. Kelly (1979, p. 26) traced this Catholic medico-moral theme back as far as Antonius of Florence in the fifteenth century.

Thus it seems clear that both in moral methodology and in substantive normative issues, the tradition of Catholic moral theology and that of organized professional medicine in the United States were operating in different worlds. Their sources of authority were different; the issues they were worried about were different; and even their concept of ethics was different. It is understandable that the AMA might not address itself to the Catholic agenda; it is less clear why the Catholic writers felt comfortable ignoring the AMA.

A CONCLUDING PUZZLE

In this section I address a final question that I have not been able to answer. During the nineteenth century in American medical ethics, positions were crystallizing. The AMA had to deal with what we now call nonorthodox practitioners. Much of their energy was devoted to clarifying how physicians should relate to the nonorthodox healers (King 1982). They seem to have formulated a code of ethics in part to convey that they were a profession with autonomy in matters of ethics. In doing so, however, the AMA took stands on some matters that should have made those in the Catholic tradition uncomfortable—on disclosure to patients and on the source of authority in ethics, for instance. More importantly, the AMA did not address what to those in the Catholic tradition was central—abortion, contraception, mutilation, the care of the dying, and social responsibility for the poor.

How can it be that Catholic physicians were not in a terrible crisis, caught between two competing claims on them for loyalty? Why weren't Catholic laypersons equally troubled, worried that they would get medical care from a physician who subscribed to the new code of the AMA and submitted himself to the AMA's authority on questions that could easily have been perceived as matters only resolvable (for Catholics) through the tradition of moral theology?

It appears that the two traditions simply were not in communication throughout the nineteenth century. Was it that they perceived no conflict?—a hypothesis that seems incredible given the obvious disagreements, especially on matters of authority. Or was it that each group really did not know what the other group was doing?—a hypothesis equally incredible given the visibility of each of the traditions. I see only one other possibility: that by the nineteenth century the world of physicians and the world of humanists were so far apart that the two groups could not grasp that they ought to collide on moral matters of medicine. It was as if the world of religious moral belief and the world of professional moral belief were so distinct that one could profess to be concerned about one while remaining totally ignorant or disinterested in the other. Hence, Roman Catholic physicians might find themselves feeling that, "as a medical professional," they could believe one set of moral norms applied while "as a Catholic" another set prevailed. Since religious physicians were, theologically speaking, laypeople, they tended not to venture into the realm of moral theology. At the same time, the theologians kept their hands off matters of professional medical morality—at least if it was not directed to the physicians who were confessing members of their religious community. If physicians were willing to subordinate their own religious authority to a priestly or rabbinical hierarchy when expounding on the special sectarian perspective, then the theologians would abstain from venturing into the territory of the profession when it commented secularly on matters of medical ethics for the profession as a whole.

This is a pattern strikingly similar to what psychiatrist Robert Lifton (1986) found in his profound and fascinating study of German physicians who cooperated with the atrocities of the Nazi era. Lifton coined the term "doubling" to refer to the seemingly paradoxical practices of Nazi physicians who could function as apparently devoted, compassionate providers of care for certain patients and family members and then, without hesitation, shift to a new and different, vicious personality as ruthless torturer of concentration camp inmates. Like schizophrenics, but without the gross ignorance of the simultaneous and contradictory personalities, these physicians were psychologically capable of functioning in two different worlds simultaneously without grasping the paradoxical position they were in. So, likewise, perhaps nineteenth-century physicians who were seriously religious were able to function simultaneously as medical professionals, getting their moral authority from their professional group and as members of a religious community, getting their theological authority from their religious sources. As long as professional medicine and theology or philosophy were seen as isolated and distinct worlds, a doubling was apparently mentally tolerable. What seems clear at this point is that there were separate medical ethical traditions in the nineteenth century, traditions apparently oblivious to the methods and conclusions of others, traditions that did not converse with one another.

9

MEDICAL ETHICS IN NEW ZEALAND AND NOVA SCOTIA: TEST CASES

> We are left with the chastening reflection that some of our predecessors were greater men than we are if width of interest and a higher level of culture are any guides. Perhaps they had more leisure and a better early education in an older civilization, and perhaps we can take a little comfort and excuse in the greater complexity of the medicine of our period, which, regrettably for most of us, makes it all-absorbing.
> —Sir Charles Ernest Hercus, Dean, University of Otago Medical School 1937–1958 (writing in 1964)

NEW ZEALAND: A NINETEENTH CENTURY SCOTTISH CASE

For my claim that physicians and humanists in the English-speaking world had quit talking with each other by the nineteenth century to hold, we should find a pattern like that of the United States in other nations that were the product of British emigration. The founding of the University of Otago in 1869 and the plan for a new medical school there soon thereafter provides a test case for dissemination of British medical ethics. No other medical schools were successfully established until the University of Auckland in the 1960s, so the Otago story is the nineteenth-century history of ethics education in New Zealand medical schools.[1] Dunedin, the town where the University of Otago is located, was founded by Scottish immigrants in 1848. The links with Edinburgh were close and have remained so to this day.[2] In fact, the name Dunedin is simply Scottish for Edinburgh. The

University of Otago had a chance for either Monro or Gregory models to emerge. As we have seen, by the mid- to late nineteenth century, any medical ethics to emerge at all in a new medical school would probably be Hippocratic rather than deriving from contemporary Scottish philosophy. The Otago school, however, was heavily influenced by the Scottish Presbyterians who were leaders of the community. Rev. Thomas Burns, the first minister of the central First Presbyterian Church, was named university chancellor. Scottish, and more generally, European philosophy was taught and was crucial in the early days of the university.

Founding of the Medical School

The Four Original Professors

When the school was founded, four professors were appointed. The first three were professors of Classics and English Language and Literature (Professor Sale), Mathematics and Natural Philosophy (Professor Shana), and Chemistry (Professor James Black) (Jones 1945, p. 43). The fourth is important to our story. Duncan Macgregor was named professor of Mental Philosophy and Political Economy (as this position was traditionally titled in Scotland). This last chair came to be maintained by the Presbyterian Synod as a chair of Mental and Moral Philosophy (Jones 1945, p. 43; Thompson 1920, pp. 7, 38, 286). Macgregor was educated in Scotland (M.A. [Aberdeen]; M.B., C.M. [Edinburgh], Ferguson Scholar in Mental and Moral Philosophy, University of Edinburgh) (Thompson 1920, p. 38).

Duncan Macgregor: Physician–Moral Philosopher

At the time, Macgregor was in favor with the Presbyterians. Moral philosophy being done in the university then was very much mainstream. The exam for the arts degree at the university was based on the typical Scottish curriculum, relying on Calderwood's *Handbook of Moral Philosophy* as the textbook. Calderwood was a Hume scholar of renown.

Macgregor was not only a moral philosopher of distinction but also a physician.[3] Later in his career, Macgregor took charge of the asylum and became successively Inspector of Lunatic Asylums and Institutions and Inspector of Hospitals (Jones 1945, p. 58). In 1872 he was included in the select committee created to look into setting up law and medicine classes in connection with the university (Jones 1945, p. 49).

A plausible scenario would have been for Macgregor to emerge in the leadership of the new school. He would have nurtured the links between medicine and the humanities. Those links would have been revived in the tradition of Gregory. Thus, seeing whether Macgregor, the philosopher with deep involvement in medicine, would re-establish the bridge between the two disciplines is important to test our claim that the two had become isolated from each other by this time.

In fact, Macgregor and the medical school had almost no contact. The closest he came to the medical school was when John Halliday Scott, who eventually became the first long-term dean of the school, was asked to share an office with Macgregor when Scott first arrived in Dunedin (Hercus and Bell 1964, p. 14). Perhaps Macgregor himself did not see the relevance of moral philosophy to medicine. For whatever reason, even the sharing of offices did not lead to a re-establishing of the link between the disciplines.

Emergence of the Monro-type Anatomist Physicians

The university Council decided on December 9, 1873, to advertise in Great Britain for a Professor of Anatomy and Physiology (Jones 1945, p. 51). The successful candidate was Dr. Millen Coughtrey, an Edinburgh graduate of 1871 who had held teaching posts in anatomy there (Hercus and Bell 1964, p. 11). He had been junior demonstrator in anatomy in Edinburgh and, before that, in Liverpool. His first classes were held in May 1875. The offerings were: Anatomy, general and descriptive; Anatomical Demonstrations; Practical Anatomy; and Anatomical Dissections. In addition, Chemistry, Theoretical and Practical, was taught by the chemistry professor, Professor Black, M.A., D.Sc, and Natural History was taught by Captain Hutton, F.G.S., C.M.Z.S. Clearly, no interest in the humanities existed in this curriculum.

Coughtrey's inaugural address from May 31, 1875 (Coughtrey 1875) and his later address to the first graduates in 1887 (Coughtrey 1887) verge on boring. (For the early years, only the first two years were offered at the University of Otago. Students then went to Britain, usually Scotland, for the rest of their study.) These addresses have no humanities content at all. Even at the commencement address where one might hear grand moral advice to the young doctors, there is nothing but discussion of technical developments at the new medical school. Likewise, in 1875, Coughtrey gave lectures that were open to the public on such technical topics as "The Organ of Hearing" and "The Brain and Organs of Sense" (Jones 1945, p. 65).

Coughtrey resigned after two years, partly because of a dispute over the requirement that he not see private patients. Apparently the town physicians felt threatened if the professor was competing with them for patients (Hercus and Bell 1964, p. 12). The university again advertised in Great Britain, and John Halliday Scott was appointed Chair of Anatomy and Physiology. In the tradition of the first Alexander Monro, the Professor of Anatomy was called on to provide the founding leadership for the school. He also had a background from the University of Edinburgh where he was Demonstrator of Anatomy. His application was strongly supported by the Professor of Anatomy at the University of Edinburgh and the Professor of Physiology at the University of Glasgow. Both were on the selection committee. Scott had an interest in the visual arts, but not humanities. He was elected an "artist" or working member of the Otago Art Society at its founding in 1875 (Jones 1945, p. 82).[4]

The Search for Medical Ethics in the Early Years

My search for medical ethics in the early years of the medical schools led to many dead ends. A look at the medical jurisprudence course, which was later established in the curriculum in 1887, was fruitless. Sometimes that is where medical ethics resided in eighteenth and nineteenth centuries. Scott began the planning of the medical faculty, coming up with seven positions, six of which were quickly filled. But Scott recommended a delay in the appointment in public health and medical jurisprudence,[5] for the hope of finding medical ethics in the jurisprudence course was a dead end.

Another possibility was to look for the use of a code or oath for graduation. If the Monro-type really prevailed, I could expect either a Hippocratic form of oath or no oath at all. At the first graduation in 1887, Coughtrey, who returned to give the commencement address, made no mention of oath or code or any other humanities perspectives. I then searched graduation programs and the New Zealand University calendar (New Zealand University 1877);[6] the graduation programs are available starting in 1889. There was no reference to any oath being taken in any of the programs through the next several decades.

Emergence of Modified Hippocratism

This pattern prevailed until the 1950s. In examining the May 1951, graduation program, I found no reference to an oath in the program, but lying next to it was another program for a December graduation that same year. It contained a "declaration" apparently taken by the graduating students. The program for this and the following December contained a list of the order of events: an address, presentation of candidates, singing of Gaudeamus, singing of national anthem, etc.[7] The same declaration appeared verbatim for the remainder of the decade. It has survived, with only minor changes, as the declaration taken by the university medical and dental students to this day.

The declaration looks very much like a variant of the Declaration of Geneva (itself a rewriting of the Hippocratic Oath). There is no indication of where it came from. Was 1951 the first year the oath was used or had it been used earlier but moved into the graduation ceremony when a separate ceremony was held for medical (and dental) students?

I checked both the Hocken (historical) Library and Registrar's office. Both had December graduation programs starting in 1951, but I was still not sure where the December 1951 declaration came from and whether it was really the first use of a graduation declaration. I decided to tackle the full minutes of the medical faculty from its beginning. Technically, the classes that started in the 1870s were in the main university. It was not until 1891 that Scott had assembled the leverage and the faculty to propose a separate medical school.

Seven thick, dusty volumes of minutes provided the history I needed. The early years were in Scott's personal handwriting, in which he provided great detail of faculty issues, making for sometimes fascinating, sometimes very boring reading.[8] For about a decade he personally recorded in the minutes in classic penmanship the grade of every student in every course in the school. The minutes contained nothing relevant to the humanities, nor did they mention anything resembling ethics, humanities, or oaths. The medical school provided a scientific education, not one dealing with the arts, literature, the humanities, or ethics.

There was also no mention of a December graduation ceremony until the meeting of November 9, 1949. In the minutes of that meeting a separate graduation for medical students was proposed by Mr. Eisdell Moore of Auckland, a medical student at the time. In his proposal he recommended the change because "few medical graduates were able to attend the annual ceremony at the University of Otago" (*Faculty of Medicine Minutes*, Vol. 6, p. 730). The announcement of December 16, 1949, meeting reported that "the Professorial Board has approved the Faculty's recommendation [for a December graduation] and extended it to include the Faculty of Dentistry" (p. 75). The minutes of that month's meeting state that the sixth-year students were to be "approached to ascertain whether they would be prepared to stay for a ceremony" (p. 87) At the meeting on June 9, 1950, "the dean stated that as directed by the faculty he had communicated with the 6th year representatives in the four centres." Generally speaking, the great majority of the sixth-year students were against holding a separate graduation ceremony in December. A number of reasons were given, including difficulty in making late travel arrangements, and uncertainty of passing, thus causing difficulties with parents' travel arrangements, and many preferred holding one graduation ceremony for the whole university (p. 108). The next mention of the December graduation appears in the minutes for September 20, 1950, where there is an entry reading, "Dr. Thomson felt that graduands would certainly wish to leave Dunedin as soon as possible and not stay over a weekend for the ceremony" (*Faculty of Medicine Minutes*, Vol. 6, June 9, 1950, p. 108). Then the minutes abruptly state, "It was agreed that an independent graduation ceremony should not be held this year but that every endeavour be made to hold it in 1951" (p. 128).

The June 9, 1950, discussion of a separate graduation actually occurred in the middle of a discussion of another proposal. The announcement of the meeting (p. 106) reads: "Mr. Jas. A. Jenkins has given notice of motion that the modified form of the Hippocratic Oath adopted by the World Medical Association and known as the Declaration of Geneva be, with suitable amendment, taken by graduands at the time of graduation." This is followed by the text of the Declaration of Geneva.[9] At first I took Mr. Jenkins for a medical student He was not a regular attendee at faculty meetings, but it turns out he was a senior lecturer in clinical surgery at the hospital. He was a graduate of the school who had received an appointment at the hospital as Assistant Lecturer and Tutor in Clinical Surgery in 1922 and was to retire in December 1951. (This is not the only school in which senior faculty nearing retirement turned to ethics or the other humanities as a symbol of their recognition of a vision of the grandeur and dignity of their profession.) The declaration referred to in the minutes was under the heading "Hippocratic Oath—modified form" or sometimes simply "Hippocratic Oath." At that meeting the following motion passed:

(a) That the modified form of the Hippocratic Oath adopted by the World Medical Association and known as the Declaration of Geneva be, with suitable amendment, taken by graduands at the time of graduation and that a sub-committee be set up to bring before the Faculty the form the Oath should take and that the sub-committee should device [sic] means whereby every graduand should attest the declaration.
(b) That the subcommittee be:—
    The Dean, Sir Charles Hercus, (Convener)
    Dr. R. S. Aitken
    Prof. F. H. Smirk
    Mr. James A. Jenkins
                                (Faculty of Medicine Minutes, Vol. 6, June 6, 1950, p. 108)

The committee then reported on September 20, 1950 the following:

(a) *Hippocratic Oath*
    The Dean presented the report of the sub-committee appointed and submitted a modified form of oath based on that of Aberdeen University Medical School.
    On motion of Dr. Thomson and second by Dr. McGeorge the modified form of oath with the deletion of the word "that" in the last line was approved.
    The oath as adopted reads:
    "I solemnly declare that, as a graduate in Medicine of the University of New Zealand, I will exercise my profession to the best of my knowledge and ability for the good of all persons whose health may be placed in my care and for the public weal. I will respect the secrets which are confided in me and maintain the utmost respect for human life. I will hold in due regard the honourable traditions and obligations of the medical profession and will do nothing inconsistent therewith and I will be loyal to the University and endeavour to promote its welfare and maintain its reputation."
                          (Faculty of Medicine Minutes, Vol. 6, September 20, 1950, p. 127)

It is now clear how the declaration was adopted at the university. It stems indirectly from the Declaration of Geneva, which, in turn, is a rewriting of the Hippocratic Oath. That activity, in turn, was an outgrowth of the horror of the medical profession when it realized that some of its members had provided leadership for and participated in the World War II Nazi atrocities. Prior to that time, the University of Otago had no notion of medical ethics or oath taking for its graduates. The oath introduced by the subcommittee actually derived from the University of Aberdeen. It was closely related to the Declaration of Geneva and perhaps the source of it.

The link between Aberdeen and the subcommittee is quite apparent. Dr. R. S. Aitken, a University of Otago Medical School graduate and one of the subcommittee members, was Vice Chancellor of the University. He was a physician who had come to Otago in 1948. Prior to that he had been Professor of Medicine at Aberdeen since 1938.

The Declaration of Geneva (and the Hippocratic Oath on which it was based) focus on the individual patient to the exclusion of the community. The Aberdeen declaration contains a more public orientation, having the student pledge, "I will exercise my profession to the best of my knowledge and ability for the good of all persons whose health may be placed in my care and for the public weal." The Aberdeen and Otago declarations also tone down the Geneva pledge to respect life from the moment of conception, simply stating that the physician will have the "utmost respect for human life," dropping the reference to "from the moment of conception." In the December 11, 1950, minutes (p. 150) the final record shows the following:

(a) *Declaration to be taken by Medical Graduates*
   It was noted that the Faculty's recommendation had been approved by the Professorial Board. Steps are being taken to implement the proposal for an independent graduation ceremony.

The April 9, 1951 minutes records graduation details:

Wed. 12th Dec. 1951–2.30 p.m. Ceremony of conferring degrees, including the taking of declaration by Graduands, to be held in Allen Hall, Sept. 24, 1951.
(a) *Medical and Dental Graduation Ceremony*
   . . . The Dean intimated that the graduands would stand to indicate their acceptance of the declaration which would be previously circulated to each graduand.

This suggests no preparation of students for receiving the text or studying its contents. It is essentially the same text used today.

The Basis of New Zealand Isolation

The reasons for the isolation of nineteenth-century New Zealand physicians are, in part, similar to those we found in Britain and the United States and, in part, unique to the New Zealand frontier. At the University of Otago, the pattern of admission to medical school at an early age with weak preparation in humanities prevailed as well. To take the admission exam in the early years of the university, the rules required that the candidate be merely 16 years of age (Jones 1945, p. 60). To make matters worse, since students went directly from secondary school to a very competitive admission process that emphasized the natural sciences, the prudent thing to do was to stress chemistry, zoology, and physics in secondary school.

At the University of Otago at its founding, one was admitted to the university by taking six examinations. Three were compulsory: arithmetic, Latin, and English.

The others could include chemistry, physics, and natural science. The closest to a humanities subject (other than languages) was history. When the fledgling medical curriculum was launched under the guidance of Millen Coughtrey in 1875, lectures were delivered on the following subjects: anatomy (general and descriptive), Anatomical Demonstrations, Practical Anatomy, and Anatomical Dissections (Professor Coughtrey); Chemistry, Theoretical and Practical (Professor Black); and Natural History (Captain Hutton) (Jones 1945, p. 57). At the first faculty meeting of the separately established medical school, on April 18, 1891, the first-year curriculum for the school was set as biology, chemistry, and physics along with Preliminary Hospital instruction and Outpatient Surgery Bandaging. The second year covered Anatomy (lectures and practical), chemistry (lectures and practical), Hospital (surgical wards), Materia Medica, and Postmortem examinations—hardly a plan to stretch the student's humanities education (*Faculty of Medicine Minutes*, Vol. 1, p. 6). Jurisprudence was available in the later years, but the focus was on practical aspects of forensic medicine. This course did not provide a vehicle for medical ethics as it had for Thomas Percival a century earlier. This was a time when medicine had been under pressure to become a real science. The successful physician was one who mastered a rapidly increasing set of medical facts. This left no time for straying into the more speculative arena of the humanities.

New Zealand has had many students entering medical school with additional university education, including some with baccalaureate degrees. However, they have not necessarily expressed special talent in the humanities. That is, in part, because many Kiwi students, like their British and American counterparts, use their extra premedical university years concentrating on chemistry, biology, and physics.

The change in social class and educational background of the physician was also relevant to the isolation of physicians in New Zealand. This was certainly true of many of the pioneering families of New Zealand in the 1870s, who had recently colonized a vast, undeveloped land only 30 years from the battles with the Maori population before and after the Treaty of Waitangi of 1840. These were families who had lived a hard frontier life in primitive housing, not in the high society of the land they had departed. Charles Hercus, the one-time dean of the medical school who was to write its history, described the school in its early years as "little more than a vocational school in which students received a sound technical training" (Hercus and Bell 1964, p. 38). Launching a medical school so few years after the founding of the colony was an ambitious plan. It was all this meager, but dedicated, faculty could do to attempt to transmit the massive scientific knowledge that was emerging so rapidly to a group of youngsters whose families had so recently settled their sheep stations and created their modest villages. Even the moral philosopher–physician brought from "home" to teach moral philosophy seemed to be oblivious to the possibility that his subject had anything relevant to offer to the medical student.

NOVA SCOTIA: ANOTHER NINETEENTH CENTURY SCOTTISH CASE

Canada's medical schools also came under the influence of the Scottish universities. Dalhousie University's medical school, which was established in 1868, provides an interesting case study to test my claim that the nineteenth-century medical community had lost touch with humanists doing medical ethics.[10] As the name implies, Nova Scotia was a target of Scottish emigration. Attempting to flee the desperate conditions that followed the Jacobite rebellion, many landless Scottish crofters took enormous risks to flee to the hope of a new life. In fact, many who eventually ended up in New Zealand came by way of Nova Scotia.

Thomas McCulloch: Nova Scotia's Liberal Intellectual Giant

Rev. Thomas McColloch (1776–1843) was one of those immigrants. He was the undisputed intellectual and academic leader who eventually became Dalhousie University's first principal and one of its three original professors. If there were a candidate in Canada for continuing the Scottish Enlightenment's conversation linking medicine and the humanities, it would be McColloch.[11]

McCulloch was born in the village of Fereneze in Renfrewshire near the textile center of Paisley west of Glasgow. The son of a textile printer, his first university studies were in medicine at the University of Glasgow, but his interests soon turned to preparation for the clergy, a pattern the reverse of Osler's. In the early nineteenth century Paisley was a center of liberal political activism and Secessionist Calvinism. The theological climate was one of Presbyterian dissent from the Church of Scotland. He studied divinity under a professor of divinity of the Secession Church (Whitelaw 1985, p. 7). McCulloch found himself in an intellectual fervor not dissimilar from the dissenting academy of Percival at Warrington a generation earlier.

McCullough served a church at Stewarton, near Glasgow, but it being a financially strapped congregation, he committed to serving a mission to Prince Edward Island. Leaving Scotland, he joined the line of Scots taking the long and perilous voyage. He arrived in November 1803 at Pictou, the center of Nova Scotian Scottish immigration, where he learned that the ice in the Northumberland Strait made passage on to Prince Edward Island too dangerous.[12] This led to acceptance of a call to a congregation in Pictou, where he stayed for the next 35 years.

McCullough was destined, however, to be more than a mere dissenting minister of another small colonial congregation. He was headed for a life of intellectual and academic leadership. To supplement his income, he opened a school in his home. This school became the Pictou Academy, the premier university-level academic institution in early nineteenth-century Nova Scotia. After a hiatus, it produced provincial premiers, lieutenant governors, judges, university presidents and professors, newspaper editors, lawyers, and physicians as well as over 300 clergy. After McCullough served as head of the school for 15 years, it fell on hard times and closed for a time. In 1838, he was tapped to become the first principal (or president) of the new Dalhousie University in Halifax, which was designed to be a nonsectarian liberal university (even though its Board of Governors eventually insisted that all its faculty other than McCulloch were to be members of the Church of Scotland) (Whitelaw 1985, p. 36). The school had been proposed by Nova Scotia's Lieutenant Governor George Ramsay, the Earl of Dalhousie, who suggested that some available funds from customs duties be applied "to the founding of a college or academy on the same plan and principle as that in Edinburgh" (cited in Murray and Murray, n.d., p. 12).

The Scottish academic influence is reflected in the books the students were to read in Pictou Academy's first term in 1818. They included Smith's *Wealth of Nations*, Hutcheson's *Philosophy*, Dugald Stewart's *Outlines of Moral Philosophy*, and Hume's *Complete Works*. McCulloch himself taught moral and natural philosophy as well as logic, Greek, Hebrew, and chemistry (Whitelaw 1985, p. 20). His thought has been described as "developed from the Scottish commonsense school and especially from Thomas Reid, the critic of Hume" (Waite 1994, p. 54). Thus, the Scottish academic originally oriented to medicine setting out to train Nova Scotia's intellectual elite had a background not unlike that of Gregory and Percival. One might expect that he would have introduced students destined to study medicine to the professional ethics of these late eighteenth-century greats. In fact, at Dalhousie McCulloch taught moral philosophy, logic, and rhetoric, but failed to make any connections to the ethics of medicine. Here was the head of a university responsible for development of professional education. He had an orientation toward both Scottish philosophy and medicine. Even though he obviously was familiar with the late eighteenth-century Scottish intellectuals—teaching Smith, Hutcheson, Stewart, and Hume—and was at a time inclined toward medicine, he never seemed to grasp a possible connection between moral philosophy and the healing arts the way Gregory, Stewart, or Percival did. His own writing was more theological and political.[13] What is missing from these writings is any evidence of interest in ethics of medicine, or, for that matter, the ethics of any of the professions. For a person with a long commitment to the preparation of students of medicine and the other professions, this is striking. For the first principal of Dalhousie, there is nothing of the agenda of Thomas Gisborne, no connection between his aborted interest in medicine and his teaching on moral philosophy to students destined to the professions.

With McCulloch's health failing, he died in 1843, and soon thereafter Dalhousie became, for a time, a moribund institution. The medical school was not created until the school's resuscitation in the 1860s. By then medical education was very much removed from what McCulloch was pursuing.

Dalhousie Medical School and the Business of Medical Science

The college reopened in November of 1863 under the leadership of Rev. James Ross, McCullough's "intellectual offspring" (Harvey 1938). He taught logic, ethics, and political economy and served as the school's second principal. Familiar Scottish names are prominent in this story. George Munro made key contributions, such as endowing the chair in metaphysics. Although students and faculty had had interests in medical education since 1843, a medical school was not established until 1868 (Waite 1994, pp. 115–17; Murray and Murray, n.d.). It was a particular interest of Ross, so there was once again an opportunity for a professor of ethics to form a bridge to medical education. An eight-person faculty (seven physicians and a lecturer on chemistry) emerged with Alexander P. Reid, another familiar surname, as dean (Harvey 1938, p. 93; Murray and Murray 1982–83). He was an Edinburgh graduate. Classes began May 4, 1868, with an inaugural address by Reid. There were 14 students. The fee was $6.00 per class.

By all accounts, Reid was the prime candidate for someone to build a bridge with the humanities—to play the Gregory role. In addition to his role as dean, he was lecturer on the Institutes of Medicine and he took on the role of senior figure in the medical school. All existing evidence fails to support any efforts to incorporate any ethics into the curriculum. Sources indicate that the curriculum was devoted to botany, chemistry, and "clinical matters" (Murray and Murray 1982–83). The Library of Congress contains a pamphlet that is his only surviving writing, an 1858 inaugural dissertation published in Canada by Alexander Peter Reid, entitled *An Inaugural Dissertation on Strychnia* (Reid 1858). Any evidence of Reid's interest in ethics or conversation with Ross and the other humanities faculty is absent. As at the University of Otago, the Edinburgh model of Gregory as a physician–humanist was superceded by one of a modern medical scientist.

The remaining research question is how and why this nineteenth-century isolation was overcome. How is it that the symbolic reconvergence of medicine and the humanities occurred in the last decades of the twentieth century? Why was the Gregory model rediscovered? To answer these questions, we turn to the establishment of the Bioethics Research Centre in the Dunedin Hospital and the Department of Bioethics at Dalhousie University's Medical School, along with the other bioethics centers teaching programs established throughout the world.

IV

THE RECONVERGENCE OF PHYSICIANS AND HUMANISTS

10

THE END OF ISOLATION: HINTS OF RECONVERGENCE

At the middle of the twentieth century, the picture was not encouraging for one who believed that any serious medical ethics required communication between those who think systematically about ethical obligations and those who think seriously about the practice of medicine. There was almost no discussion of ethics between health professionals and humanists, despite recent world events underlining the need for it. It is too bold to claim that all that was wrong in medical ethics can be attributed directly to the lack of interaction between humanists and health professionals, but the correlation is striking.

The most horrendous abuse of human research subjects ever seen occurred in World War II. The evidence is now clear that German physicians, mentally isolated from their moral roots, were not mere accomplices to the Nazi horrors. They often took the leadership in devising newer and more inhumane research projects. They shifted their more traditional ethic of promoting the health of the patient into one of promoting the health of the *Volk* (carefully limited to the Aryan race) and did whatever they could to save the race. In order to know when they could still save pilots who had bailed out into frigid ocean waters, they designed experiments placing those who were not considered part of their people into ice water and measured the time it took for death to occur. To study the effects of decompression at high altitude they placed those they considered expendable into chambers to see how radical a barometric change was needed to produce death. As

Lifton's profound and moving study, *Nazi Doctors* (1986), has suggested, the isolation of German physicians' thinking as researcher/physician from their thinking in other roles in religious and secular spheres was essential to the phenomenon. Only by mentally isolating their goal of promoting the health of the race from their roles as caring parents and spouses and parishioners could they have committed such offenses.

The Nazi physicians were not the only ones committing atrocities. Japanese physicians' involvement in research abuse is a story that is less well known, but no more defensible. The bacteriological warfare study by their medical research unit, Unit 731, which exposed Chinese citizens and even Japanese employees of their programs to lethal atmospheric release of germs, to study the dissemination, as well as other similar offenses are only recently coming to light (Harris 1994; Gold 1996). Of course, both the German and Japanese atrocities could be cited as examples of physicians connecting their medical ethics all too well with the political philosophy of the underlying culture. The medical experiments conducted in the United States around the time of the second world war, however, are harder to explain. Members of the medical profession regularly conducted medical research on inadequately informed subjects who could not be said to have consented to their roles. In Tuskegee, a southern and racially insensitive community, poor, African-American men were intentionally not treated for syphilis to study the natural course of the disease. Thousands of Americans were intentionally exposed to radiation for experimental purposes (Advisory Committee on Human Radiation Experiments 1995; Moreno 2000; Welsome 1999). While some might claim that this occurred at a time when long-term effects were not known, recently available documents make clear that serious concerns existed among the scientists, and the public, including the public being experimented on, were intentionally kept ignorant. These behaviors were sometimes supported by appeals to an ethic promoting overall public good, such as long-term public health or military victory. Such an ethic, one that assessed morality in terms of long-term overall social benefits, appealed to a principle of judging acts by consequences that had long been part of the medical community. The traditional Hippocratic ethic avoided such social implications by insisting it was only consequences for the patient that counted, but modern medicine in the nineteenth and twentieth centuries had modified that ethic so that consequences for society were considered legitimately on the physician's agenda. It was consistent with the ethic then endorsed by American organized medicine's American Medical Association. The 1847 AMA code, written during a time when social consequentialism was fashionable (but without the watchful eye of humanists who could warn against dangerous implications if safeguards were not incorporated), commited members to be "ever vigilant for the welfare of the community" (American Medical Association 1848, p. 23). This included matters in which the individual might have to be sacrificed for the good of the community, such as quarantine, public hygiene, and work in prisons. This, of course, did not mean that the AMA endorsed abuse of research subjects, but it put forward the principle upon which the mid-twentieth-century abuses could be defended and without any of the cautionary checks on this community–welfare commitment that would eventually be needed to prevent abuse. The 1957 "Principles of Medical Ethics" still included as one principle the commitment that "the honored ideals of the medical profession imply that the responsibilities of physicians extend not only to the individual, but also to society where these responsibilities deserve his interest and participation in activities which have the purpose of improving both the health and the well-being of the individual and the community" (American Medical Association 1957).

While this utilitarian view was held in check by a rigorous commitment to the rights of the individual in American society, there was no such commitment to individual rights in organized professional physician ethics of the day. In fact, as we shall see, there was not a commitment to "rights" at all until the revision of the AMA code in 1980, well after the end of the period of isolation of physicians from humanist thinkers. As early as 1947, official documents of the Atomic Energy Commission (AEC) explicitly required the written, informed consent of subjects in medical research involving radiation, but this requirement was not disseminated to all the physicians conducting this research (Wilson, 1995). In fact, there is considerable reason to believe that the physicians in the AEC and in research centers treated this requirement as a military secret that could not be shared with either investigators or the public (Moreno 2000, pp. 172ff.). A major disconnection occurred between the ethic of research physicians and the ethic of the broader public. While the American legal system and international law at Nuremberg were debating the rights of subjects in human research in the years after the war, the medical profession was not engaged in the debate and would not recognize the notion of informed consent for many years.

A similar problem existed in clinical medicine. By the mid-twentieth century the benevolent paternalism of the Hippocratic Oath, with its commitment to the duty of the physician to work only for the benefit of the patient, dominated professional physician ethics (only adjusting to include some consideration of consequences to the society). This posed a conflict between this patient-centered consequentialism and the more rights-oriented commitment of the broader culture. Hence, physicians' moral attitudes were often at odds with those of the lay public. In a 1953 survey of physicians, for example, 70 percent indicated that they did not tell their patients of a cancer diagnosis (Fitts and Ravdin 1953). In various surveys of patients and laypeople who were not patients in this period, no matter how the question was asked, the vast majority always indicated that they wanted to be told (Kelly and Friesen 1950; Branch 1956; Samp and Curreri 1957). The reasons for these dramatic differences on issues such as consent and informing dying patients of their condition are complex, but they certainly include the fact that physicians were committed to the Hippocratic standard of protecting their patients from harm. (Regardless of whether they had actually read the Oath, through their medical training they had internalized a deep commitment to the Hippocratic ideal of benevolent paternalism.) Believing that the diagnosis would be disturbing, physicians wanted to spare their patients this distress. But in general, patients not only judged differently on whether the information would be harmful, more critically, they believed that they had a right to know and to be offered a choice about their treatment, *even if the information was disturbing* (Kelly and Friesen 1950; Branch 1956; Samp and Curreri 1957). There was simply a disconnection between the moral frameworks of physicians and laypeople.

The same disconnection was apparent in decisions about forgoing life support. Mid-century physicians not only believed that it was their duty to do what they thought would benefit their patients, they were also convinced that they knew that preserving the patient's life was the highest good they could pursue. By this time, however, some patients were beginning to have doubts about this value judgment. They were beginning to wonder whether life should be preserved when the life that remained would be spent in a coma or in unbearable pain. Roman Catholic patients knew their moral tradition was committed to a doctrine of extraordinary means that accepted the wisdom of forgoing treatment that was excessively burdensome (Pope Pius XII 1958; Kelly 1958).[1] Physicians in organized medicine were no more engaged with Catholic theologians in the mid-twentieth century than they were in the nineteenth century.

Similar rifts opened up in reproductive ethics. Physicians had values related to abortion that were radically at odds with the broader culture. Similar disparities existed on contraception. In an empirical study using survey and interview methods, I documented that, as late as 1970, physicians had moral views about birth control that were very different from those of their patients (Veatch 1976c, pp. 258–59).[2] Likewise, physicians often seemed to have views about sterilization that differed from those of their patients (Scrimshaw and Pasquariella 1970). In the early and mid-twentieth-century, attitudes of lay Americans about health insurance also differed from those of organized medicine. Medicine mounted an aggressive and successful campaign to block any government-controlled universal health insurance, a policy that remained fully intact until Medicare was adopted in 1965, and that program of course only covered the elderly.

While significant disconnections between the thinking of physicians and laypeople are well documented in mid-twentieth century with regard to specific medical ethical issues, in retrospect the real misfit can be seen in normative ethical positions. As we have seen, organized professional medicine was staunchly consequentialistic. In research medicine, public health, and other more social areas, utilitarian or related social consequentialistic views had been followed since the days of Gregory and Percival. In clinical medicine the same conclusion can be drawn, except that the consequentialism is limited to promoting the good of the individual patient. In both cases, with certain qualifications, the goal was to do as much good in professional practice as possible.

By the mid-twentieth century, the ideas of the Hippocratic Oath were still in this central place in organized medicine, even if the typical physician never actually read it. The ethics of broader philosophical and theological discourse, however, had taken on a radically different character. In the Anglo-American secular world, especially in the United States, liberal political philosophy was dominant. It was a culture committed more to the philosophy of Locke, Hobbes, Rousseau, and the American Founding Fathers. It was an ethic of "rights" as well as one often reflecting more Kantian notions of duty. In the religious world, more sectarian ethical concepts—the talmudic legal tradition of Judaism, the natural law thinking of Catholicism, and the more individualistic notions of moral duty in Protestantism—took many laypeople far from the consequentialism of the medical professional ethics, whether they focused on the benefit to the individual (as in the Hippocratic tradition) or to the society (as in more recent public health and research ethics). What is critical is that the masses of laypeople and their physicians no longer relied on similar ethical traditions. Hippocratic and other professional ethics was the reserve of health professionals. Laypeople generally did not participate in the forming or evaluating of physicians' ethical documents. Moreover, physicians generally did not stray from that reservation. They cared little about liberal political philosophy or scholarship in the various religiously based medical ethics. There is not a single instance of organized medicine's use of this literature in any of its documents, or any evidence of use of its ideas.

Striking as it may be, with the exception of John Bell's comment on the AMA Code of 1847 there was apparently no use of the concept of "rights" (at least rights of patients) in any professionally written medical ethical document before the 1970s and none in the documents of physician groups before 1980. The first document endorsed by a health-professional group in English I could find that uses the word *right* is the American Nurses Association (ANA) Code of 1976 (p. 3). The first document of a physicians' group that speaks of *rights* is apparently the AMA revision reported from committee in 1979 (Todd 1979) and adopted in 1980.[3] The 1972 American Hospital Association's "Patient Bill of Rights" anticipates the ANA by four years, but it was adopted by a hospital organization that included a significant number of laypeople, not by a nursing or physician group.

The bottom line is that by mid-century, physicians writing medical ethics, particularly when they wrote officially as part of a professional organization, had been isolated from the mainstream of secular and religious medical ethical discourse— the public debates in philosophy, law, public policy, and religious ethics—for a century and a half. They relied almost exclusively on other physicians who had drafted codes or written treatises who, in turn, had relied on previous generations of physicians all the way back to the late eighteenth century. In the discourse on medical ethics, there is not a single figure in the period between 1800 and the middle of the twentieth century who was as deeply involved in the humanities as Gregory, Percival, and Rush. But that was soon to change.

It is not my purpose to write a history of the current generation in bioethics, the period from the middle of the twentieth century on. Others have done that from various perspectives (Rothman 1991; Jonsen 1998); for example, Renée Fox (1959) and Fox and Judith Swazey (1974) have written from a sociological perspective. Good historical work is also available from Robert Baker and his colleagues (Baker 1995a; Baker et al. 1999), from Chester Burns (1978), and from the contributors to the *Encyclopedia of Bioethics*. I want to tell enough of the story to see why physicians began once again to talk with humanists on medical ethical matters.

ANTICIPATING REINTEGRATION: MID-CENTURY HINTS OF SOMETHING TO COME

The trials of Nuremberg and the American radiation research mark what could be considered the beginning of the end of the era of isolation. Moral reflection was still physician dominated, still paternalistic, still largely Hippocratic (or Hippo-cratic adjusted for a more social context). Metaphorically, at mid-century we re-mained in the era of the antibiotic. Medicine addressed problems of infectious disease where the solutions were thought to be in the discovery of quick cures. The responsibility was in the hands of medical professionals. The ethical reflec-tion that grew out of the Nuremberg trials was dominated by two physicians: Leo Alexander and Andrew Ivy. Reflection on moral problems in medicine by those outside of the health professions was reserved primarily for theologians who wrote for denominational audiences. Roman Catholic moral theologians continued to produce volumes for Catholic clergy and scholars as well as for medical and nursing students (Good and Kelly 1951; O'Donnell 1955; Finney and O'Brien 1956; Healy 1956; Kelly 1958; McFadden 1967). Jewish talmudic scholarship continued, but reached an even more parochial audience (Jakobovits 1959).

Nevertheless, there were hints of an end to the separation of physician-generated medical ethics from the humanities. In medical centers a few people such as those we discuss below spoke openly to the lay public, not merely to their medical col-leagues behind closed doors. Figures such as Daniel Jenkins, Willard Sperry, and Joseph Fletcher began to cross from their humanities departments over to medi-cal campuses to see what was happening and whether they had anything to say about it. Late in the 1950s, the first modern-era interdisciplinary research center devoted to social aspects of medicine, the Boston University Law–Medicine Re-search Institute, was founded by the lawyer Irving Ladimer.[4]

Medical Scientists Stepping out of the Clinic

The opening of the community of medical scientists and clinicians to reflection on ethics in the humanities had been hinted at in Osler and Cabot. That cautious adventurism received a new, if tentative, impetus in the 1950s.

Chauncey Leake

By the middle of the twentieth century, Chauncey Leake (1896–1978), a Ph.D. pharmacologist, had become a looming presence in American medical ethics at the University of California Medical Center in San Francisco (UCSF). Paul Ramsey (1970b, p. xv) later referred to him as the "elder statesman of medical ethics." Leake was also influential in embedding the humanities and medical ethics at the University of Texas Medical Branch in Galveston, where he served from 1942 to 1955 as Executive Vice President.

I began my graduate studies in neuropharmacology in the UCSF Pharmacology Department in 1961, where Leake had been the chair. He had left by the time I arrived, but his presence was still very much alive. Planning to orient my career toward the medical humanities, it was by sheer coincidence that I chose to study pharmacology at the medical center where two of the giants of medical ethics (Leake and Guttentag) had resided.

Leake made his first significant contribution to medical ethics as a young man when he produced a 1927 edition of Percival's *Medical Ethics*.[5] Though notorious for some errors and omissions,[6] it contains a useful introduction and appendices with texts of codes from the AMA and other sources.

Leake's interpretation of Percival has fallen on hard times, but his commitments remain intriguing and on target. He was concerned about medical ethics being reduced to mere etiquette among physicians and about the absence of rigorous moral philosophy in the development of an ethic for medicine. In an attack that contemporary scholars consider an error, Leake criticized Percival for ignoring the philosophical literature on ethics (Baker 1993, pp. 180–88; Jonsen 1998, p. 9).

In writing published soon after the new edition of Percival, Leake reinforced his commitment to bridging the gulf between medicine and the humanities. He proposed an ethics course for medical students that would begin with three lectures on moral philosophy given by a member of the philosophy faculty, followed by a historical survey of ethics in medicine.[7]

Otto Guttentag

The second presence in medical ethics at UCSF was a homeopathic physician, Otto Guttentag (1900–1992). He had immigrated to the United States from Germany in 1935.[8] He returned briefly to Germany after the war. Meeting with physicians there, he was shocked at how little they were disturbed by the revelations of the medical research in the concentration camps. Returning to the United States he became the Samuel Hahneman Professor of Medicine and Medical Philosophy at UCSF.

In the early 1950s Guttentag was a lone voice speaking publicly about the ethics of human subjects research. He organized and spoke at an October 1951, symposium that introduced systematic reflection to the area and led to his paper in *Science* (Guttentag 1953) that was the first to be openly critical of the ethics of medical scientists conducting studies on humans. Three of the other speakers at the meeting were law professor Alexander. M. Kidd (1953), an authority on military law, W. H. Johnson (1953), and physician Michael B. Shimkin (1953).

Physicians were beginning to discuss such issues with non-physicians. While no philosophers or theologians were represented among the published presenters, Guttentag did acknowledge the contributions to the recent literature on the subject by Willard Sperry, dean of Harvard Divinity School. As recently as 1995, the U.S. Advisory Committee on Human Radiation Experiments (p. 141) referred to Guttentag as "among physicians . . . nearly unique in medicine in those days raising such problems in print."

Henry Beecher

In September 1964, after completing a master's degree in neuropharmacology at UCSF and a stint in the Peace Corps, I decided that I needed more formal education in medical ethics and the medical humanities to do more serious work there. I moved to Harvard for that purpose. Soon after arriving there, I received a telephone call from a critical figure in the efforts to form bridges between medicine and the study of ethics in the humanities. Henry Beecher (1904–1976), Dorr Professor of Research in Anesthesia at Harvard Medical School, had heard I was coming from Robert Featherstone, who was then the chair of the Pharmacology Department at UCSF. Dr. Beecher invited me to the first of many visits. We became friends—and sometimes adversaries—for the rest of his life.

Some of Beecher's early work was on the pharmacology of pain and the placebo effect (Beecher 1952, 1953, 1955, 1957). This was very close to work I had done in the pharmacology labs at UCSF, so I was somewhat able to keep up in the conversation in medical ethics and pharmacology. (I had long been fascinated with the use of morphine pharmacology as a model for understanding the physiological basis of how humans value things, a subject not totally dissimilar from Beecher's use of pain as a model for subjective responses [Veatch 1976a]).

Beecher's work in clinical research related to pain and placebos drove him into a direct confrontation with the ethics of clinical trials. His most famous and controversial paper was "Ethics and Clinical Research" (Beecher 1966), in which he summarized the published research methods of 22 studies involving human subjects and asked whether the sometimes horrendous research procedures could possibly be ethical. This led to a worldwide explosion of criticism about the abuses in research on human subjects. Aside from Nuremberg, Beecher's publication was the most important event in raising public consciousness about the ethics of clinical trials. Even though he published it in the prestigious *New England Journal of Medicine* and refused to make public the names of the researchers he was questioning, Beecher was attacked for washing the dirty laundry of medical research publicly. His response was to continue to speak publicly and to seek more and more interdisciplinary dialogue (Beecher 1970). To his death he continued inviting medical ethicists, philosophers, and theologians into the discussion.

These three figures in 1950s medicine hardly constitute a movement that reversed the long decades of isolation, but they signalled that something was on the horizon.

Humanists and Social Scientists Stepping into the Clinic

Throughout the 1950s there were also hints from the side of the humanities of what was to come. In November 1957, Pope Pius XII addressed the International Congress of Anesthesiologists on the subject, "The Prolongation of Life" (1958), providing the definitive Catholic statement that endorsed the forgoing of burdensome life-support for patients. This was no longer Roman Catholic theologians talking among themselves.[9] In response to the development of new technologies that could indefinitely prolong life, clinicians wanted to know what their moral options were, especially with regard to what they began to call "resuscitation." Pope Pius's endorsement of the legitimacy of forgoing life-support, based on a long and sophisticated history of Catholic moral theology, traveled well beyond that Catholic world. Because it makes clear that the Catholic church does not rigidly require life prolongation, it is cited to this day routinely in court cases, government documents, and secular medical school classrooms.

Other theologians began to communicate across disciplinary lines. As early as 1945 the American Jesuit theologian, John Ford, published in a theological journal a paper insisting on the importance of consent in human subjects' research, but it was not until 15 years later that he published on a similar topic in a pharmacological journal (Ford 1960). With a physician co-author he wrote a paper in 1953 on the legitimacy of forgoing radical surgery.

Secular non-physicians were also entering the clinic during that decade. From 1951 until 1954, medical sociologist Renée C. Fox (1959) went into the pseudonymous research ward, F-Second, at a famous teaching hospital (Boston's Peter Bent Brigham) as a participant observer in some of the critical moral decisions in medicine took place behind what had previously been closed doors.

In medical ethics, three names that deserve special attention for their contributions to medical ethics in the 1950s are Daniel Jenkins, Willard Sperry, and Joseph Fletcher.

Daniel Jenkins

Daniel Jenkins (1914–) is best known as a British Protestant theologian, but one of his earlier projects was a book entitled *The Doctor's Profession* (1949), which grew out of a series of discussions held in London between 1945 and 1948 with a group identifying themselves as "Christian doctors." This book is, in fact, a very early effort at renewal of the conversation between physicians and humanists. It is Jenkins' contribution to an ecumenical group, however, the doctors as well as the humanits identify themselves as Christians. The sponsoring group was called "Christian Frontier," a lay Christian organization. The goal of the meetings was to stimulate discussion of the future of the medical profession from this special perspective.

Jenkins wrote chapters on what would constitute a "Christian attitude" in a physician, "psychiatry and the Christian doctor," and medical missions. He also discussed some of the more traditional ethical issues in medicine: contraception, abortion, artificial insemination, and euthanasia.

Willard Sperry

Turning to Willard Sperry (1882–1954), we see a different picture. The long-term dean of Harvard Divinity School represents what I take to be a true transition figure from the era when physicians and ethicists did their medical ethics in isolation to one in which a real conversation began to cross disciplinary lines without relying on the sectarian religious identifications of the physicians as a basis for a common interest with theologians of similar commitment. Sperry produced the first volume in medical ethics of the twentieth century that is explicitly addressed to physicians while intentionally avoiding writing from a particular religious perspective.

The Ethical Basis of Medical Practice (Sperry 1950) grew out of an invitation on December 4, 1947, to Sperry from J. Howard Means, the Jackson Professor of Clinical Medicine at Harvard Medical School and Chief of Medical Services at the Massachusetts General Hospital. Sperry reproduced the original letter in his book:

> It occurred to me that perhaps you might be interested to give a talk to our staff on the moral problems of medicine, and give us some guidance on what attitude to take toward them. I have talked to parsons and theological students about medicine repeatedly, but now I would like to have the tables turned and be instructed.
>
> (Sperry 1950, p. 92)

Sperry was not unprepared for the invitation. In his preface, he recounted that as an undergraduate student he had planned on medicine, and surgery in particular, as a career, but changed direction in his senior year. A lifelong companion of his boyhood and youth had died suddenly, shifting his mind from medicine to theology. He selected his college courses with an eye toward medical education, however.

Sperry accepted Means's invitation and late one afternoon, "many of the senior members of his [Means's] staff, and most of its junior members" gathered in the historic ether dome of the old Bulfinch Building of the Massachusetts General Hospital. The editor of the *New England Journal of Medicine* later asked for the text of the talk, which found its way into the journal (Sperry 1948).

For Sperry the response to the publication was overwhelming. "Following its appearance in print a minor flood of correspondence from practicing physicians, from officials in hospitals, and from professors in medical schools all over the country poured in on my desk" (Sperry 1950, p. 9). He was subsequently asked to give similar lectures at the University of Michigan Medical School. The lectures eventually led to the book.

Sperry's book makes clear why I consider Sperry a "bridge" figure in medical ethics between the more isolated era and the decades to come when the conversation once again flowed more freely. He was a contemporary of Cabot, whose work he used. One of the chapters in *The Ethical Basis of Medical Practice* is devoted to Cabot's views on truth telling, and particularly his reliance on Joseph Conrad's *Lord Jim* as a source of a case history (Sperry 1950, pp. 56–64). My classification of Cabot as the last of the older, more isolated physicians, and Sperry (along with Leake, Guttentag, and Beecher) as the start of the new, reintegrated conversation is, admittedly, arbitrary. Someone else might have drawn the lines differently. Nevertheless, I have tried to show that Cabot, however much he was *interested* in ethics, was not skilled or knowledgeable about what was going on in the humanities disciplines and was only rather marginally engaged in real communication. I am suggesting here that, beginning with Leake, Guttentag, Beecher, Jenkins, Sperry, and (as we shall see momentarily) Fletcher, the communication became much more open and intense.

Though dean of a major American divinity school, Sperry's book was different from that of his theological and philosophical counterparts of an earlier era. He listened to his physician colleagues and learned which problems worried them in the hospital. In addition to a discussion of truth telling, the book contains chapters on euthanasia (outlining the pro's and con's), prolongation of life, and "Democratic vs. Totalitarian Medicine" (by which he meant medicine in the democratic West and Naziism).

Sperry's language is primarily secular. He incorporated occasional scriptural references as befits a divinity school dean, but this is not the literature of the Catholic moral manuals or even that of the Protestant theologian, Jenkins. It is language with which a practicing physician (or any participant in late twentieth-century bioethics discussions) would feel comfortable. Sperry is not without more abstract and theoretical interests, however. He discusses the "nature of conscience" as well as notions of the "professions in general."

In a chapter on codes of medical ethics, Sperry shows knowledge of a profession that by now had taken the Hippocratic Oath as its timeless ethic. He had access to the Jones translation of the Oath in the Loeb Classical Library (Sperry 1950, pp. 84–85). In deference to Howard Means, he also reprinted the Oath's text from the handbook of the Massachusetts Chapter of the honorary medical fraternity, Alpha Omega Alpha, which Means regarded as a better translation.

Sperry is gently critical of some problems with the Oath—its prohibition on surgery, for instance (Sperry 1950, p. 85). He lived, however, in a period when the Oath had become something almost beyond question. It was a "still classic statement," "a landmark in the ethics of medicine," with "noble rules." Moreover, it was not merely an "interesting, but probably highly idealistic bit of ancient rhetoric." The latest codes of ethics "still run true to the lead given in the historic Oath" (Sperry 1950, pp. 85–87). Here Sperry seems oblivious to the potential tensions between his own religious ethical heritage with its much more social ethic. He did not bring to bear knowledge of the history of religions or the study of Greek mystery religion. He was, after all, only starting a conversation up again.

Joseph Fletcher

Another Cambridge voice that could be heard in Boston beginning in the 1950s was Joseph Fletcher's (1905–1991). An ordained clergyman of the Episcopal Church, he was professor of pastoral theology and Christian ethics at the Episcopal Theological School (ETS) in Cambridge, Massachusetts (now Episcopal Divinity School).[10] In 1949 he was invited to give the Lowell Lectures at Harvard University.

These lectures became the basis for a pioneering book, *Morals and Medicine* (Fletcher 1954). Fletcher was aware of Jenkins' work and knew that it dealt with topics beyond medical ethics (Fletcher 1954, p. xi). He described his own book as undertaking "only a modest contribution to the *ethics* of medicine, but added, "to my knowledge, nothing of this kind has been undertaken by non-Catholics as yet" (Fletcher 1954, p. xi).

Although Fletcher's reputation as an ethical theorist became somewhat tarnished in his later years, especially from his continuing defense of his pet theory of *situation ethics* (Fletcher 1966), he was deeply committed to systematic ethics. His Anglican background oriented him toward British Anglican casuistry as well as its Roman Catholic analogues. (He served a term as a curate in a London slum parish as well as in more academic positions, such as dean of the Graduate School of Applied Religion in Cincinnati). Nevertheless, especially in his later years, his real passion was for "the case," the unique individual details that for him made ethical choices situational.

Fletcher bemoaned the lack of attention ethical theorists gave to case problems, and he saw clinical medicine as both having the greatest potential for such an approach and being the most deficient in applying it. He did not shy away from blaming physicians as well as humanists for this failure. Showing that he was already crossing the communication gulf, he bluntly attacked an official of the American

Academy of General Practice for expressing the hope that a recent episode of medical euthanasia could be kept quiet. The official was quoted as saying,

There are extremists on both sides. They will bring to the floor emotions more than anything else. The subject is emotional at present. *It is a moral question, not a scientific one. We have other fish to fry.* I shall do everything possible to keep it out of the congress of delegates.

(Fletcher 1954, p. xii, quoting an unnamed official of the Academy from a *New York Times* article, Feb. 21, 1950)

Fletcher minced no words in commenting on this attitude:

Nothing could be more subversive of medical integrity, nor more irresponsible ethically. . . . This book is a serious effort to expose the cynicism revealed in all protests that practitioners of the healing art have other fish to fry when it comes to conscience around the sick bed.

(Fletcher 1954, p. xii, xiii)

Referring to his "many friends in both medicine and morals," he provided the first indication that the communication was about to begin in earnest. His selection of the famous psychiatrist, Karl A. Menninger, as the one to write the foreword for the book is one such signal. Menninger also addressed the lack of communication between physicians and humanists at the time.

More than any other work in the field, *Morals and Medicine* was to launch a new kind of ethical analysis, one provided by moral theologians and philosophers but heavily committed to the practical ethical problems of medicine. This is illustrated by the book's chapters on human rights in life and death, the right to the truth, contraception, artificial insemination, sterilization, euthanasia, and the ethics of personality. It is, by contrast, thin on ethical theory and theology, making it accessible to physicians and other health professionals while communicating in a secular vernacular.

THE EXCITEMENT OF THE 1960s

Thus, by mid-century there were stirrings. At least in the few instances we have considered, physicians and humanists were becoming reacquainted. They were seeking one another out for some initial exchanges. These exchanges were still far from sophisticated. They were chats in which notes were compared, perspectives shared, and intuitions exchanged. In the 1960s, the social and political excitement of the civil rights movement, the antiwar movement, and the feminist movement, among others, would escalate conversations in ethics more generally. New medical technologies would pose new problems for clinicians. These included hemodialysis machines, organ transplants, new definitions of death, a movement to legalize abortion, new technologies for contraception, and the beginnings of a new genetics. New teaching efforts in medical schools emphasized the medical humanities. Each of these developments provided fertile ground for more discussions between health professionals and humanists. The public was fascinated by these developments. Jonas Salk, in developing the immunization that overcame polio, became a celebrity. The ordinary citizen was still optimistic that disease could be conquered. Medical problems were often stabilized so that there was enough time for patients and families to read about them. As the need for moral choices to be made was reported in the press and described to individual families, laypeople insisted on an increased role in those choices, just as students and other citizens demanded more of a role in national policies about race and war.

Dialysis: The God Squad

One of the earliest developments of technology that had a direct impact on the emergence of a new interdisciplinary conversation in medical ethics was the invention of the artificial kidney—the hemodialysis machine.[11] Persons in chronic kidney failure needed to have bodily wastes cleared from their blood streams. In the early 1940s Willem Kolff, a physician associated with a Dutch hospital, built the first artificial kidney and prototypes had been developed by the 1950s in the United States. They were essentially machines that could take blood from a patient's artery, cleanse it, and return it to a vein. It was a laborious, complicated process doomed to fail from complications of having to undergo surgery each time the cannulas were inserted. The breakthrough came, however, in 1960, when physician–scientist Belding Scribner and his team at the University of Washington invented a shunt that permitted access to the blood vessels without repeated surgery. Still there were moral problems. Patients had to be attached to the machines for six to eight hours a day, two to three days a week. Some, particularly a Native American patient named Ernie Crowfeather, found the mental agony or the physical effects so unpleasant that they intentionally chose to forgo the treatments (Fox and Swazey 1974, pp. 280–315).

The real moral problem, however, was that the machines were expensive. There were not nearly enough for the thousands of patients who might benefit from using them. A selection of which patients would receive treatment became inevitable—at least until sufficient machines could be built at a reasonable cost.

Both deciding whether patients could walk away from the life-saving treatment to die and deciding which patients could have access posed serious ethical problems. Dr. Scribner and other physicians were wise enough to realize that their skill in nephrology did not necessarily give them expertise in such decision making. Moreover, they would have had to face the hostility sure to result from those who were excluded. The result was the development of a committee, officially known as the "Admissions and Policy Committee," but informally referred to as the "Patient Processing Committee" or, even more informally, as the "God Squad" (Alexander 1962; Fox and Swazey 1974, pp. 215–79; Jonsen 1998, pp. 211–17).

The committee was originally made up of a lawyer, minister, housewife, labor leader, state government official, banker, and surgeon plus two physician advisors. As far as the public could tell, they never developed formal criteria for choosing, but simply decided on their priorities on an ad hoc basis. With Shana Alexander's telling of this story in *Life* magazine in 1962, everyone in America had a dramatic vision of the nature of the moral choices now being made in medicine. Almost anyone could imagine themselves as a member of the committee or as a patient subject to its choices. Moreover, this vision forced us to begin thinking about the moral criteria for such inevitable selections. The secret of the clinic was getting out.

Transplantation: Handling Scarce Resources

Even more public stir was created in December 1967, when South African surgeon Dr. Christiaan Barnard cut out the heart of Louis Washkansky to replace it with one removed from a newly dead automobile accident victim named Denise Daarvall. It was immediately apparent that such radical procedures required new public and clinical policies and that individual physicians with ongoing responsibility for the care of individual patients had neither the time nor the talent nor the neutral perspective from which to make such policy.

Almost immediately two issues of public policy making developed, both of which not only pushed medical ethical choices further into the public consciousness but forced physicians and non-physicians to work together in making choices.

Procuring Organs

The first involved development of a policy for procuring organs for transplantation. Could they be taken without formal permission from the deceased on the grounds that the organs were now useless to their former "owners"? Could they be "routinely salvaged," as one popular proposal suggested (Dukeminer and Sanders 1968)? Or did the deceased or their next-of-kin retain some legitimate interest in deciding whether they could be used for transplant?

This was simultaneously a medical, legal, and moral set of choices. The natural result was first, an increasingly public discussion of the issues and second, an interdisciplinary conversation. The team proposing "routine salvaging" involved both a physician and a lawyer. But so did the team advocating the alternative, which came to be thought of as the "gift model" (Sadler et al. 1968). The latter group wrote for the Special Committee of the National Conference of Commissioners on Uniform State Laws. While these initial legal proposals primarily involved collaborations between physicians and lawyers, almost immediately theologians and other non-physicians entered the picture as well. Princeton theologian Paul Ramsey (1970b, pp. 198–215; see also 1969) gave one of his 1969 Lyman Beecher lectures, "Giving or Taking Cadaver Organs for Transplant," on this topic. Representing a more aggressive stance in favor of procuring organs, Joseph Fletcher (1969) also weighed in on the issue before the end of the decade. It was the nature of this debate, with its drama, its need for consistent public policy, and its obviously ethical character, that opened up the discourse of medical ethics to persons well beyond the clinicians at the bedside.

The moral controversies surrounding hemodialysis and organ transplantation were the subject of one of the earliest formal interdisciplinary meetings to address these issues, the Ciba Foundation Symposium on "Ethics in Medical Progress: With Special Reference to Transplantation" (Wolstenholme 1966). The foundation, which received its funding from the Swiss pharmaceutical firm of the same name, sponsored an international meeting as part of a long series of primarily scientific gatherings to encourage scientists to meet informally to exchange facts and ideas. This was one of the most explicitly social and ethical topics the group had sponsored. Held in London, March 9–11, 1966, it provided a meeting place for transplant surgeons, hemodialysis specialists, and other physicians to exchange ideas with several of the English-speaking world's most distinguished jurists and at least a token clergyperson. In truth, it was still a gathering dominated by medical scientists, who had the inside track on confronting the moral problems generated by their technology. Philosophers were not represented, nor were other humanists with the exception of Rev. Canon G. B. Bentley from Windsor Castle. Among the lawyers, however, were some of the great minds of twentieth-century jurisprudence: David Daube, the Regius Professor of Law at Oxford; Hon. Lord Kilbrandon, Senator of College of Justice in Scotland and Lord of Session; and David Louisell, Elizabeth Josselyn Boalt Professor of Law at the University of California, Berkeley. The upshot was the beginnings of a carefully formulated consensus insisting on donation of organs rather than mere salvaging without the act of individual giving.

The Definition of Death

The second public policy issue stimulated by organ transplant was the debate over the definition of death. Here the key player was, again, Henry Beecher at Harvard. Heading up the Ad Hoc Committee of the Harvard Medical School to Examine the Definition of Brain Death (Harvard Medical School 1968), he understood that what was needed was a broad, interdisciplinary consensus to support a new, brain-oriented definition that he and others in the field had concluded was essential. He saw to it that, even though it was a medical school committee, it included a theologian (Ralph Potter), a lawyer (William Curran), and a historian of science (Everett I. Mendelsohn). The result was a report proposing a brain-based definition of death, published in the *Journal of the American Medical Association* and eventually adopted by all states in the United States and most countries throughout the world. It also produced important theoretical developments. Potter, stimulated by this involvement on the committee, went on to write one of the early contributions to the more theoretical aspects of the definition-of-death debate (Potter 1968). He warned of the dangers of changing definitions just to obtain useful organs. Talmudic scholars also entered the conversation, confronting the problem that the new definition seemed to conflict with Jewish views that associated life with breathing, a controversy that remains within Judaism to this day (Rosner 1969).

Abortion, Birth Control, and Population

A third area of health care attracted a number of theologians and philosophers with religious interests in the 1960s. For centuries the moral theologians had considered the issues of contraception, sterilization, and abortion their territory in medical ethics. In May 1960, the first oral contraceptive was approved for marketing. The availability of a relatively safe, effective, convenient contraceptive was to change the moral as well as the medical and social landscape.

It was hard to escape the thought that millennia of sexual ethics were really driven by the importance of mechanisms for limiting unplanned pregnancies, especially those outside of wedlock. Could it be that the prohibitions on sexual relations outside of marriage and the fear of failing to limit pregnancy within it were really devices for social control to escape the terrible consequences of unintentional pregnancy? If so, would the new pill provide a new set of conditions upon which the ethics of contraception would have to be reassessed?

While the centuries-long reservations in Roman Catholicism about any "unnatural" fertility control are well known, many do not realize that it was only in the twentieth century that Protestants reluctantly accepted contraception (Fagley 1960). Before the Lambeth Conference in 1930, the Anglican communion, for example, was not willing to endorse such practices. With the emergence of a simple, technical means of controlling pregnancy, major work was in store for the moral theologians as well as the clinicians who had to determine whether they would prescribe the pill.

The story was made more complicated by the simultaneous emergence of technologies such as the D&C and the abortion pill RU486 that made abortion easier and safer. These combined with the women's movement of the 1960s to require a major rethinking of this area of medical morality. Although Sperry had declared contraception to be a settled question, the increased frequency of abortions brought many humanists, especially moral theologians, urgently back to these issues. Protestant (Fagley 1960), Jewish (Feldman 1968), Roman Catholic (Callahan 1969, 1970; Noonan 1966, 1970), and secular (Lader 1966; Guttmacher 1967; Rosen 1967) scholars took it up aggressively.

At Harvard's School of Public Health, funding became available to appoint two professors with special attention to the ethics of population (the moral issues of policies related to fertility and migration). Two young professors associated with Harvard Divinity School and the Graduate School of Arts and Sciences, Arthur

Dyck and Ralph Potter, were given the original appointments. By the middle of the decade, they were largely responsible for teaching and supervising a cadre of graduate students—many oriented to biomedical ethics through a graduate seminar on the ethics of population. This helped link the graduate and divinity schools in Cambridge with the medical campuses in Boston.

The Harvard Divinity School, together with the Joseph P. Kennedy, Jr., Foundation, sponsored an important international meeting on the ethics of abortion, at the Washington Hilton, September 6–8, 1967 (Cooke 1967). It brought together hundreds of the clinical people with legal scholars and humanists who had an interest in abortion. Potter and Dyck participated along with theologian Herbert Richardson and church historian George Williams.[12] Many of the key players in the nascent medical ethics conversation were present, including theologians Charles Curran, James Gustafson, Richard McCormick, and Paul Ramsey, as well as physicians Robert Cooke, Andre Hellegers, Jerome Lejeune, Kenneth Ryan, and Christopher Tietze. Jurists David Daube, Norman Dorsen, Robert Drinan, Erwin Griswold, David Louisell, John Noonan, and Norman St. John-Stevas were also present, together with Supreme Court Justices Abe Fortas and Potter Stewart.

Daniel Callahan, who had completed his Ph.D. in philosophy at Harvard and had been a teaching assistant at the divinity school, was serving as the editor of *Commonweal* when, with grants from the Ford Foundation and the Population Council, he set out to write a book on the increasingly controversial issue of abortion (Callahan 1970). His research at the Population Council leading to the completion of the book was the step that would reorient his career toward the social and ethical aspects of medicine and the life sciences. When he discovered that his neighbor in Hastings-on-Hudson, New York, the psychiatrist Willard Gaylin, also had deep interests in the ethics of health care, they began a critical, cross-disciplinary discussion from which they would, in 1969, found the Institute of Society, Ethics and the Life Sciences, the research center that eventually changed its name to the Hastings Center (Callahan 1971; Jonsen 1998, p. 21).

In the Roman Catholic tradition, oral contraception presented a serious challenge. Some theologians thought that the estrogen/progesterone birth control pill, which worked physiologically and presented no physical barrier to conception, might not raise the same moral theological objections as previous methods of birth control. A papal birth control commission (The Commission for the Study of Population, Family, and Natality), originally established by Pope John XXIII and later increased in size with the addition of a number of lay specialists by Pope Paul VI, undertook the task of examining the issues.

A well-placed Roman Catholic layman known for imaginative theological thinking was appointed in 1964 as the Deputy Secretary General of the Commission. Andre Hellegers (1926–1979), professor of obstetrics and gynecology at Georgetown University, was a physician born in The Netherlands and educated in Great Britain. The commission he helped lead met through the years 1964–1966 and provided an extended period for moral reflection at the highest levels among theologians and physicians within the Catholic tradition.

The majority report supported the potential legitimacy of oral contraception ("Majority Papal Commission Report" 1969). Hellegers was part of the majority. A minority report endorsed the more traditional view ("Minority Papal Commission Report" 1969). Soon Pope Paul VI (1989) would side with the minority. The majority were not pleased, but continued to acknowledge the authority of the Vatican on such matters. The Commission nevertheless had brought together the leading Catholic theologians in the world with leading laypeople, including physicians, to debate a crucial issue of medical ethics. Hellegers developed contacts and friendships with theologians such as Josef Fuchs, who was one of the key authors of the majority view and among the leading, more liberal Catholic theologians in the world. Within a few years, Fuchs, along with Bernard Häring and Bruno Schüller, all became visiting scholars at the Kennedy Institute of Ethics, created by Hellegers.[13]

Another important player in the moral controversy surrounding reproductive issues was Paul Ramsey, the chair of the Religion Department at Princeton and a leading Methodist theologian and ethicist.[14] Following the work of the papal birth control commission, Hellegers invited Ramsey to spend the spring semesters of 1968 and 1969 as the Joseph P. Kennedy, Jr., Foundation Visiting Professor of Genetic Ethics at Georgetown University's Medical School. The fruitfulness of those exchanges led directly to the development of the Kennedy Institute of Ethics, which we will discuss below.

Genetics and Reproductive Technologies

A fourth area of biomedical ethics was beginning to attract some attention among the specialists in religious ethics. The discovery of the double helix promised to unlock the human genetic code and generate new opportunities both for therapy and for "engineering" an improved version of the species. While this was all quite hypothetical, hints of the future were beginning to appear. Although the specifics of gene therapy were little more than speculation, genetic counseling and screening of populations at high risk for bearing offspring with specific genetic diseases were realistic options that entailed considerations of contraception and abortion. Several moral theologians and religious ethicists took up this challenge in the 1960s and early 1970s. Stimulated by a visiting professorship at Georgetown, Paul Ramsey (1970a) published a book on genetic issues called *Fabricated Man*. At the same time, he was developing his Beecher lectures for publication. He was perceived as a more conservative alternative to Joseph Fletcher. Fletcher did not produce his own book, *The Ethics of Genetic Control*, until 1974, but was already speaking out.

In addition to hosting the Beecher lectures, Yale was beginning to orient a new generation of graduate students toward medical ethics. The most influential faculty member in this respect was James Gustafson. While he continued to work in more general areas of ethics and some of these writings would eventually be important in biomedical applications (such as his analysis of the relation between the case study and general theory, Gustafson 1961, 1966), he published from time to time specifically on medical ethics, especially genetics (Gustafson 1973). He made clear that theories and cases are reciprocally related, that one must eventually get one's case judgements and theory in harmony. Applying his work on the relation between theory and case to clinical cases, he contributed significantly to overcoming the tension between clinicians, who tended to be case oriented, and humanists, who were more inclined toward "top-down" theorizing in which one had to first work out a general ethical stance and then apply its principles to cases. He cooperated in the leadership of the genetics research group at the Hastings Center, which we will discuss below (Bergsma et al. 1974). He also helped prepare the ground for the renewal of interactions between humanists and clinicians by training graduate students who were to play key roles in the next decades.[15] The Beauchamp–Childress approach to biomedical ethics, for exmple, bears the mark of Gustafson's thinking about case–theory interactions. It is not an accident that both Beauchamp and Childress studied at Yale with Gustafson. Also on Yale's faculty were physicians Jay Katz and Robert J. Levine, who both provided leadership on issues of human subjects research. Katz later served on both the Tuskegee Syphilis Study and the Ad Hoc Advisory Panel on the Human Radiation Experiments. A law student named Alexander Capron worked with him in producing an important law anthology on human experimentation issues (Katz 1972). David C. Duncombe, the chaplain at the medical school, also had significant involvement in medical ethics teaching.

It was on genetic counseling that Union Theological Seminary's best-known bioethics graduate student eventually focused. In doing so, he became the person responsible for the National Institutes of Health's (NIH) early bioethics efforts. John Fletcher (unrelated to Joseph) worked under Roger Shinn, one of the famous seminary's ethicists. Fletcher's graduate research, which he completed in 1969, dealt with human subjects research (Fletcher 1969, 1973). In 1975 he became the staff ethicist at the NIH Clinical Center (Lipsett et al. 1979).

These developments of the 1960s have some features in common. New technologies—transplants, oral contraception, abortion, and the new genetics—posed serious problems for clinicians. New methods of making human subjects research systematic (such as double-blind trials and formally developed statistic methods that could require continued randomization after trends in results were becoming clear) did as well. These new technologies and issues all produced conspicuously moral problems. Clinicians increasingly realized that they were not equipped to resolve them. As the problems did not go away, they cried out for more formal policy guidelines as well as case-by-case help. Clinicians in academic medical centers appealed to humanists across their campuses for dialogue. At the same time, philosophers and especially religious ethicists were becoming disillusioned with the more abstract issues of metaethical theory that had dominated early twentieth-century ethics. Graduate students gravitated toward dissertation topics that were applied. Their professors moved into conversation with their medical colleagues, serving on interdisciplinary committees, giving lectures at medical schools, attending rounds, and other events. Applied work in medical ethics was becoming attractive, relevant, and doable.[16]

Physician Humanities Education

The religiously sponsored medical schools in the United States had long had faculty teaching medical ethics. These faculty members were often priests or rabbis. At Georgetown University, for example, Jesuit moral theologian Thomas O'Donnell began to serve as Professor of Medical Ethics in 1952. Texts such as O'Donnell's (1955) and Kelly's (1958) were not very different in their scope and audience from those of the nineteenth-century medico-moral literature discussed in Chapter 8.

Similarly, for many years the Catholic schools of nursing had offered courses within the framework of Catholic moral theology. Charles J. McFadden's *Medical Ethics*, first written for such schools in 1946, was, by 1967 was in its sixth edition. In the preface to that edition he claimed that the book was being used in medical and nursing schools not only in the United States but also in Canada, England, Australia, New Zealand, and Spain.

Aside from these religiously sponsored schools, almost no medical schools had faculty, either physician or humanist, with specific teaching responsibilities in medical ethics or the humanities. That began to change in the late 1960s.

Penn State Humanities Department

One critical event was the founding of the Milton S. Hershey Medical Center at Pennsylvania State University, a result of the 1960s movement in medical education away from advanced research and toward primary care and family medicine. The medical center took in its first class of medical students in 1967. Its founding dean, George Harrell, was deeply committed to incorporating humanities into medical education. This led to the creation of the first medical humanities department in a medical school. Al Vastyan, an Episcopal clergyman, was appointed its first chair. He participated in the search for people to head the more traditional medical school departments. K. Danner Clouser, who had a Ph.D. in philosophy from Harvard and a background in religious studies, joined the department in 1968. The two pioneered the development of medical humanities teaching in medical schools. The department soon offered as many as 15 elective courses in the humanities for medical students. It also hosted many pilgrimages by others seeking to learn how to develop medical humanities and medical ethics education (Vastyan 1973; Veatch and Clouser 1973; Jonsen 1998, pp. 79–80).

Stony Brook

A similar collaboration between a physician with a strong interest in the humanities and humanists willing to enter the medical center occurred at the New York State University Medical Center at Stony Brook. From 1966 to 1973, Edmund Pellegrino was the Vice President for the Health Sciences and Dean of the School of Medicine at The State University of New York, Stony Brook. A seriously committed Roman Catholic scholar, at Stony Brook he facilitated the development of teaching in the humanities that in 1973 led to the appointment of Peter Williams, a lawyer and philosopher, as a professor with responsibilities for teaching the humanities to medical students. Williams now heads the Division of Medicine in Society at Stony Brook.

By the end of the 1960s the stage was set for physicians and humanists to resume interacting on a larger scale. New medical technologies forced physicians and patients to make tough moral choices. The partial success of the ventilator, dialysis machine, organ tranplantation, genetics, and fertility control made the moral questions inescapable. Had these technologies completely solved the problems of the patients on whom they were used, the moral controversies would not have been so apparent, but half-solved problems often left patients stable enough that they did not die quickly. Their medical problems were, in fact, sufficiently treated that patients were able to think about the choices and their alternatives. By the beginning of the 1970s so many of these issues had forced themselves on physicians and the public that interdisciplinary communication had to resume on a larger scale. It is to these events that we turn in Chapter 11.

11

THE NEW ENLIGHTENMENT: THE 1970s

The civil rights, antiwar, women's, and student movements of the 1960s provided fertile ground for orienting ethicists, particularly religious ethicists, toward applied ethics. The new biomedical technologies began to call for moral reflection, but it was not until the end of the decade that social changes pressed humanists out of their academic reserves and into the clinic. As we shall see, religious ethicists, already committed to working in the real world of practical moral dilemmas, were especially receptive to responding whereas philosophical ethicists were still finding interest in and prestige from working on more abstract theoretical issues. This social milieu also made clinicians in large numbers follow Howard Means's lead and invite humanists into the clinic.

Within a five year period—30 months on either side of mid-1970—a remarkable number of events occurred that make that year a plausible candidate for the beginning of a new generation of bioethics and the reconvergence of physicians and humanists in significant numbers.[1] We have already touched on the world's first heart transplant in the closing days of 1967 and the founding of the first medical school with a humanities department. The report of Henry Beecher's Harvard Ad Hoc Committee of the Harvard Medical School to Examine the Definition of Brain Death was issued in May 1968. In July, Pope Paul VI's birth control encyclical appeared. In 1969 an ad hoc committee began to evaluate the Tuskegee syphilis study, leading to an exposé of one of the most serious abuses of human research subjects in American history. In the fall of that year, the Institute of Society, Ethics and the Life Sciences was founded and a commitment was made to form the Society for Health and Human Values. The legal case of *Berkey v. Anderson* was decided in 1969; it was the first of a critical series of court cases reforming our understanding of informed consent. In 1970 three important books on abortion appeared (Callahan 1970; Grisez 1970; Noonan 1970) as well as Ramsey's two volumes, a landmark work on the moral foundation of the patient–physician relation (Ramsey 1970b) and the volume on genetic engineering already mentioned (1970a). In December of that year, the U.S. Department of Health, Education, and Welfare (1971) published the first formal institutional guidelines on the protection of human subjects in research. Known as the "yellow book," it was the precursor to the long series of federal regulations attempting to provide formal structure for protecting human subjects. That same month the Institute of Society, Ethics and the Life Sciences organized a symposium at the American Academy of Arts and Sciences (AAAS) meetings in Chicago that brought together from diverse disciplines people dealing with the care of the terminally ill (including physicians Henry Beecher, Robert Morison, Leon Kass, and Elisabeth Kübler-Ross as well as Paul Ramsey, Daniel Callahan, and political science scholar, George Anastaplo). In the spring of 1971, The Joseph and Rose Kennedy Institute for the Study of Human Reproduction and Bioethics, which later became the Kennedy Institute of Ethics, was founded. That June the Institute of Society, Ethics and the Life Sciences held a conference on the teaching of medical ethics. In July the public learned of the Tuskegee study. A Tuskegee Syphilis Study Ad Hoc Advisory Panel was chartered August 28, 1973 (U.S. Public Health Service, 1973). That year also saw the maturing of the "reasonable person" informed-consent cases in various courts (*Canterbury v. Spence*, 464 F. 2d 772 (D.C. Cir. 1972); *Cobbs v. Grant*, 502 P.2d 1 (Cal. 1972)). Then, on January 22, 1973, the U.S. Supreme Court ruled that state prohibition of abortion was a violation of a constitutional right of privacy (*Roe v. Wade*, 410 U.S. 113, 93 S. Ct. 705, 1973). These events reflect the formalization of a movement to convert professional physician ethics into the interdisciplinary field of biomedical ethics, with institutions, teaching programs, a core set of books, a body of legal case law, and public policies.

EMERGENCE OF INTERDISCIPLINARY CENTERS AND TEACHING PROGRAMS

As important as the medical school departments were, a much more significant innovation was about to emerge. The interdisciplinary institute was a new phenomenon for medical ethics of the 1970s.

Institute of Society, Ethics and the Life Sciences

Daniel Callahan and Willard Gaylin founded the Institute of Society, Ethics and the Life Sciences in 1969. An interdisciplinary group of 70 nonresident physicians, philosophers, theologians, lawyers, biologists, and social scientists was supported by a resident professional staff in the effort to explore the issues of biomedical ethics formally and systematically (Callahan 1971).

The group at first met in hotels and operated out of an office on the second-floor porch of Callahan's home. I joined the staff on September 1, 1970, as its first professional-level employee when the formal, out-of-home office was opened. It was in a Hastings-on-Hudson office building owned by a local dentist.[2]

In the early years the Institute operated through four task forces, or research groups: death and dying, population, genetics, and behavior control (the ethics of psychiatry, electrical stimulation of the brain, and other behavior-controlling interventions). The fellows of the Institute attended research group meetings two to three days at a time, three or four times a year. Gaylin provided staff leadership for the behavior control group (Institute of Society, Ethics and the Life Sciences [1971a]). Callahan (with his Population Council experience) and I (with my population ethics work at Harvard) staffed the population group. I had initial staff responsibilities for the death and dying group, until Marc Lappé joined the staff (and again some years later). Lappé also served as the staff member for the genetics group, which was co-chaired by Massachusetts General Hospital molecular biologist Richard Roblin and ethicist James Gustafson.

In addition to the four research groups, the Institute agreed to develop a medical ethics teaching program for Columbia University's College of Physicians and Surgeons (Institute of Society, Ethics and the Life Sciences [1971d, 1971e]; Veatch 1972). Gaylin was already on the Columbia faculty and provided senior leadership for the teaching along with Associate Dean Councilman Morgan. I received a faculty appointment and took over day-to-day responsibilities for the teaching as the Program Director. Another humanist was formally present in the medical center.

The Hastings Center also contributed to the development of medical ethics teaching beyond its Columbia involvement when it began sponsoring workshops on this subject. The first one, for about 20 college and health professional school faculty (including Indiana University's David Smith and Dartmouth psychiatrist, Charles Culver) was held at Dartmouth College in 1973. Courses were held regularly in the years that followed at Manhattanville College, the University of Colorado, and other sites.

By the mid-1970s the Institute of Society, Ethics and the Life Sciences was thriving. It did not formally change its name to The Hastings Center for a number of years but almost immediately began using the shorter name informally. By the middle of the decade its list of nonresident fellows had grown to 94, including 10 honorary fellows such as Otto Guttentag, Chauncey Leake, Rene Dubos, and R. M. Hare. Its internal professional staff had expanded to nine (Institute of Society, Ethics and the Life Sciences 1976).

Kennedy Institute of Ethics

A similar humanist–clinician collaboration was evolving at Georgetown University. Pleased with the collaboration with Protestant theologian Paul Ramsey, the Catholic obstetrician Andre Hellegers set out to create a more permanent environment to facilitate interaction between physicians and humanists. The result was a research institute whose original name and structure revealed the founder's intentions. Originally called The Joseph and Rose Kennedy Institute for the Study of Human Reproduction and Bioethics[3] (reflecting Hellegers's background and the Institute's origins in the issues of fertility control and reproductive biology), it was designed to have three "centers": the Center for Bioethics, the Center for Population Research, and the Laboratories for Reproductive Biology, where bench science research would be conducted. Within its first few years, many graduate students in ethics of the previous decade were appointed to positions at the Institute, including LeRoy Walters, Tom Beauchamp, James Childress, and Roy Branson as well as Catholic ethicists such as Warren Reich and Richard McCormick. Among the ethicists who had visiting appointments were Ralph Potter, David Smith, John Fletcher, Gene Outka, Stanley Hauerwas, Albert Jonsen, and Karen Lebacqz. They joined physicians and nurses like Hellegers, the psychiatrist Seymour Perlin, geriatrician John Collins Harvey, physician Leon Kass, and nurse–bioethicist Sally Gadow as scholars of the Institute. These appointments made cross-disciplinary conversation a necessity. Gadow was one of several scholars at the Institute during the 1970s who had formal training in both the clinical sciences and the humanities. Two others with dual training who joined before the end of the decade were physician–philosopher H. Tristram Engelhardt and Jesuit geneticist Robert Baumiller. Beginning in 1975, Harvard's Arthur Dyck provided leadership in the early years for the Institute's annual "Total Immersion Course" (later called the "Intensive Bioethics Course"), which was designed to provide an intensive introduction to the discipline of ethics for physicians, nurses, and other clinicians. The course, still held annually, has had over 3000 participants to date, most of them clinicians getting their first formal exposure to ethics.

From the start, the Kennedy Institute of Ethics was committed to creating the scholarly tools of a discipline. Under the direction of faculty member LeRoy Walters and the chief librarian, Doris Goldstein, the Institute has built the largest biomedical ethics library in the world. Supported by the National Library of Medicine and receiving other government grants and contracts, the library provides a publically accessible research facility of 26,000 books, 160,000 articles, and close to 500 journals. Since 1975 it has been responsible for the production of BIOETHICSLINE, the Internet-accessible database that is associated with MEDLINE.

Early in the 1970s, Warren Reich, one of the initial appointments at the Kennedy Institute, began early in the 1970s to conceptualize an *Encyclopedia of Bioethics*. The first edition appeared in 1978 and the revised edition in 1995. The *Encyclopedia* provides further evidence of the maturing of the field and the number of people committed to scholarly interdisciplinary work. To get an idea of the expansion of the field by the late 1970s, the first edition had entries by 286 authors. Other signs of the field's rapid, early growth are the hundreds of participants in the intensive courses of the Kennedy Institute and the workshops of the Hastings Center, the 60 or so professional scholars who had been in residence at the Kennedy Institute either as permanent or visiting fellows by the end of the decade, and the hundred fellows and professional staff of the Institute of Society, Ethics and the Life Sciences. Over a thousand physicians, humanists, and other scholars were involved in these enterprises during the decade.

Georgetown, where teaching in medical ethics at the medical school had existed for many years, continually modified its courses (Baumiller 1973). Warren Reich moved his primary base from the Kennedy Institute to the medical center when he was appointed head of the new Division of Health and Humanities in 1977. That further increased the ties between the Kennedy Institute faculty and the medical center. Faculty at the Institute have taught regularly in the medical school courses since then.

By the end of the decade, the communication between physicians and humanists was more intense than it ever had been in the 1770s. New biotechnologies posed complex ethical issues that were beyond the expertise of clinicians. They had no special expertise in analyzing the social and moral dimensions of the decisions that were needed. Laypeople had learned that making such choices was not the sole domain of those with technical expertise. This led to a new willingness, indeed insistence, of laypeople to step onto the physician's turf and to countless combinations of clinicians and humanists in the movement toward a reconvergence of physician ethics with the mainstream of philosophical and religious ethics.

SECULAR MEDICAL SCHOOL TEACHING PROGRAMS

Teaching programs in medical schools evolved rapidly during the 1970s. In a study conducted by the Institute of Society, Ethics and the Life Sciences in December 1971 and reported at its June 1972 conference on the teaching of medical ethics, only 15 of 94 schools surveyed would admit to having no teaching in medical ethics (Veatch 1973). Many of the schools still had relatively little in the way of formal offerings. Some claimed that they incorporated medical ethics into their other courses. However, 33 offered elective courses and four (including two with religious affiliation) had a required course. We attempted to count faculty who devoted at least half their time to medical ethics and came up with 18.

When this survey was repeated two years later (with 107 schools responding) 47 schools offered electives in medical ethics and six had required courses. The number of faculty spending at least half their time on medical ethics was up to 31 (Veatch 1976b).

Harvard

The Harvard program in medical ethics, for example, began in July 1971. Funded by the Joseph P. Kennedy, Jr., Foundation, it offered fellowships to scholars as well as a number of courses open to medical students. The faculty included Stanley Reiser, a physician who is also a historian, lawyer William Curran, and Arthur Dyck.

Galveston

Chauncey Leake's legacy is still felt at the University of Texas Medical Branch in Galveston (UTMB), where he was Executive Vice President from 1942 to 1955. Leake initiated medical humanities efforts at the school. His interest in the history of medical ethics was furthered by Truman Blocker (1909–1984), a plastic surgeon, medical educator, and the first president of UTMB. They provided fertile ground for development of the history of medicine and the medical humanities there. Chester Burns went to UTMB in 1969 as director of the new History of Medicine Division, which evolved into the Institute for the Medical Humanities in 1973. Both a physician and a historian of medicine, having received his Ph.D. from Johns Hopkins, he has written extensively on the history of medical ethics (Burns 1977a, 1977b, 1978). Physician William Bean became the director of the Institute in 1974.

Two other faculty at UTMB played key roles during this early period. H. Tristram Engelhardt, Jr., arrived in 1972. A philosopher of medicine who also has a medical degree, he stayed in Galveston until moving to the Kennedy Institute in 1977. Harold Vanderpool, a historian and medical ethicist, joined the program in 1976 after serving as a Kennedy fellow in the Harvard medical ethics program, where he focused on ethics (with Arthur Dyck and philosopher Roderick Firth) and the history of medicine (with Stanley Reiser) and served as a teaching assistant in Dyck's and Reiser's popular course on medical ethics for Harvard undergraduates.

Tennessee

Another significant teaching program in the 1970s was the Inter-Campus Graduate Program in Medical Ethics at the University of Tennessee. Beginning in 1975, it involved a collaboration between the departments of philosophy and religious studies at the Knoxville campus, the University of Tennessee Medical Center at Knoxville, Lakeshore Mental Health Institute, and the Department of Human Values and Ethics, University of Tennessee at Memphis (UTM). The faculty included philosopher Glenn C. Graber, religious studies ethicist Charles Reynolds, and physician Alfred D. Beasley. It gained a significant early reputation for training humanists in the clinical setting.

Society for Health and Human Values

The pattern of these pairings of humanistically inclined physicians and humanists willing to enter the medical center repeated itself in a number of medical settings. In 1965 a Committee on Medical Education and Theology was formed, having its origins in the staff of the United Ministries, the organization of university chaplains (Jonsen 1998, pp. 24–25).[4] In 1968 that group sponsored a Conference on Human Values in Ministry and Medical Education at the University of Florida. Sam Banks of the University of Florida and George Harrell were among the members. By February 1969 that committee had decided to form a society for faculty and others committed to human values in medical education. The resulting Society for Health and Human Values was founded in November 1969 and held its first meeting in October 1970. For the 1970–71 year, Penn State's Al Vastyan was the President. The Council included two other humanists: Kenneth Spilman, a clergyman who was the Director of the Health and Human Values Task Force for metropolitan Philadelphia, and Ronald McNeur, the Society's executive director. Physicians included William Maloney, the Dean of Medicine at Tufts; Fritz Redlich, Dean of Yale's medical school, William Ruhe, from the AMA, as well as Edmund Pellegrino. The Society opened membership to subscription in 1972.

Closely associated with the Society was the Institute on Human Values in Medicine. It was not a research institute in the sense of the Hastings Center or the Kennedy Institute, but rather an ongoing series of meetings focusing on human values education in medical school settings. The first session was held at Arden House in Harriman, New York, April 12–14, 1971 (Institute on Human Values in Medicine [1972]). The participants list is striking in how little overlap there is with the figures we have thus far encountered. Only Danner Clouser, Al Vastyan, and Pellegrino are familiar names. Yet within the group of 28 people were many well-known physicians and humanists committed to the discussion of human value issues in the medical context. Philosophers and theologians included State University of New York professor Michael Novak, Jesuit St. Louis University professor Walter Ong, Cornell philosopher Max Black, and University of North Carolina professor Ruel Tyson. Physicians (most of whom were from the high ranks of medical school administration) included Duke's Roger Bulger, University of Florida's Leighton Cluff, University of Rochester's Louis Lasagna, Yale's

David Musto, UCLA's Bernard Tower, and the National Institute of Mental Health's E. Fuller Torrey. Ten years later the leaders of the Institute were able to provide a summary and overview of the decade of rapid growth of medical school teaching programs (Pellegrino and McElhinney [1982]).

INTERDISCIPLINARY COMMISSIONS

This interdisciplinary communication led naturally to a number of commissions and committees that helped formalize the dialogue. We have already examined the 1960s papal birth control commission. Many others, in both public and private settings, were to follow during the 1970s.

The National Commission

The most significant in this early period was certainly the National Commission for the Protection of Human Subjects of Biomedical and Behavioral Research (U.S. Government 1974), which was a direct outgrowth of the Tuskegee controversy. Troubled over reports of subject abuses, Senator Ted Kennedy introduced legislation that mandated, among other things, the formation of a national commission to study and evaluate issues of human subjects research. Public hearings were held in February through July of 1973 (U.S. Senate 1973a, 1973b, 1973c, 1973d). The subcommittee staff requested assistance from the Institute of Society, Ethics and the Life Sciences in planning the hearings, and I spent a day with Larry Horowitz and Stan Jones from Senator Kennedy's staff helping sketch out lists of witnesses. Among those who testified were Alexander Capron, Henry Beecher, Daniel Callahan, Willard Gaylin, and Jay Katz.

The National Commission was pioneering in many ways. It was the first government agency mandated to do a formal study of ethics. It produced the influential Belmont Report (National Commission for the Protection of Human Subjects of Biomedical and Behavioral Research 1978), the first formal ethical framework for public policy analysis and, to this day, the dominant public document in the field of the ethics of human subjects research. The 11-member commission included two who had been ethics graduate students of the 1960s, Karen Lebacqz and Al Jonsen; physician Robert E. Cooke, the medical advisor to the Joseph P. Kennedy, Jr., Foundation; Patricia King, a Georgetown University law professor who had regularly participated in Kennedy Institute activities; and jurisprudence scholar David Louisell, whom we met as a participant in the 1967 Harvard Divinity School/Kennedy Foundation international meeting on abortion. The commission was chaired by Harvard physician Kenneth Ryan. Both he and Cooke had also been at the 1967 meeting. Philosopher–bioethicists Tom Beauchamp and Stephen Toulmin along with Yale physician Robert Levine served on the commission staff. The commission was the first formally constituted group working in medical ethics with a legally mandated majority of medical laypeople. In effect, physicians (who had lost public confidence from the Tuskegee exposé) were forced to converse with humanists and other laypeople.

Other 1970s Commissions

Other commissions and committees also provided opportunities for interdisciplinary conversation among physicians and ethicists. For example, the Artificial Heart Technology Assessment Panel met in the early 1970s to study the issues of development of a technology that provided hope for replacing heart transplants with an entirely artificial mechanical device (Artificial Heart Assessment Panel 1973). Among the ethical controversies this proposal generated were the potentially enormous costs and the risk to third parties from nuclear-powered devices. Al Jonsen also served on this panel.

By the end of the decade the most influential government commission of all had been appointed. The President's Commission for the Study of Ethical Problems in Medicine and Biomedical and Behavioral Research was to issue a series of reports covering most of the major issues in the field and serving as the definitive consensus statements. The commission included among its members Albert Jonsen, Patricia King, talmudic scholar Seymour Siegel, and Renée C. Fox. Its executive director was Alex Capron. Among its staff who would go on to careers in bioethics were philosophers Dan Brock, Allen Buchanan, and Dan Wikler; physician Joanne Lynn; and attorneys Barbara Mishkin, Alan Meisel, and Alan Weisbard.

BRITISH RECONVERGENCE

A similar renewal of the physician–humanist interaction was on the horizon in Great Britain. The most significant early activity centered in a group called the London Medical Group and associated groups such as The Edinburgh Medical Group, the Society for the Study of Medical Ethics, and the Institute of Medical Ethics.

Society for the Study of Medical Ethics

In the early 1960s Edward Shotter was a Church-of-England priest with responsibility for medical students in London. He was not a scholar who wrote a great deal. He tended to stay in the background organizing interdisciplinary seminars and encouraging others to contribute. For example, he edited some lectures on life-and-death issues in medicine, given in 1963 under the auspices of the London Medical Group, and published them several years later (Shotter 1970). When he organized sessions in various hospitals and medical schools, they often took place under the name of the London Medical Group. Under Shotter's guidance, a Society for the Study of Medical Ethics was formed. The participants also functioned under the name Institute of Medical Ethics. Shotter developed a working relation with several scholars in Edinburgh, including Kenneth Boyd, who is currently Senior Lecturer in Medical Ethics at Edinburgh University Medical School and Research Director of the Institute of Medical Ethics, and Alastair Campbell, of the Department of Christian Ethics and Practical Theology at the University of Edinburgh. In 1975 the Society for the Study of Medical Ethics began publishing the *Journal of Medical Ethics* under Campbell's editorship. The editorial board included some of the most distinguished British health professionals and humanists of the day. Cicely Saunders, who is credited with being the founder of the modern hospice movement, was a member, as were G. R. Dunstan, a theology professor at the University of London who later co-edited the British *Dictionary of Medical Ethics*; Lord Kilbrandon, whom we met at the Ciba Foundation symposium on transplantation ethics, and Shotter. The first issue contained articles by another hospice physician, R. G. Twycross; Richard Nicholson, another physician who would spend many years working in medical ethics; and philosopher R. S. Downie, as well as two American ethicists, William W. May (of the University of Southern California) and Mark Frankel. Daniel Callahan and Vatican theologian Bernard Häring were among the editorial correspondents. From its inception, the *Journal of Medical Ethics* has been published from Tavistock House in London, the home of the British Medical Association and the *British Medical Journal*.

Dictionary of Medical Ethics

Many of these same people were involved in the first British publication of a reference work devoted to medical ethics, the *Dictionary of Medical Ethics* (Duncan et al. 1977), a shorter British alternative to the American *Encyclopedia of Bioethics*. It involved 116 entry authors, including many of the same people associated with the Society for the Study of Medical Ethics and its affiliated groups. The editors are A. S. Duncan, an emeritus professor of medical education at the University of Edinburgh; G. R. Dunstan, Professor of Moral and Social Theology at King's College, London; and R. B. Welbourn, professor of surgical endocrinology at the Royal Postgraduate Medical School, University of London.

Since the first edition of the dictionary was published in 1977, we can assume that the volume was conceptualized in the early part of the decade and that most of the entries were written in the middle years of the decade. The list of authors, then, is a good catalogue of those who were engaged in the British development of biomedical ethics during the period—at least those who were writing and recognizable on the national scene.

Of the 116 authors, many are physicians or health scientists. Judging from their backgrounds as well as their entries, they may well not have had extensive exposure to interdisciplinary bioethics. Some of them, however, were the major scientists contributing to some evolving area of medical innovation. R. G. Edwards (Steptoe and Edwards 1978), the scientist responsible with Patrick Steptoe for the development of in vitro fertilization, is an example. Another is Bryan Jennett (Jennett and Plum 1972), a key player in the British definition-of-death discussion. However, there are also many humanists among the authors, including Campbell, Dunstan, Shotter, and the American population ethicist Richard M. Fagley, whom we have previously met, and other theologians, philosophers, and non-scientists. For example, the well-known Oxford professor, philosopher Mary Warnock, is included, as is the historian of medical ethics, Vivian Nutton, who, at the time, was Fellow of Selwyn College, Cambridge, and has since moved on to the Wellcome Institute in London. That over a hundred primarily British scholars in medicine and the humanities were available and willing to write for the medical ethics dictionary is a sign that, by the middle of the 1970s, the British conversation had resumed as well.

THE IMPACT OF RENEWING THE DIALOGUE

Thus, by the mid-1970s the isolation of physician ethics was over. Health professionals were once again heavily engaged in conversation with humanists and other non-physicians. They increasingly recognized the inadequacy of their internally produced medical ethical literature. They brought theologians, ethicists, lawyers, social scientists, and eventually philosophers into the clinic to help sort out the moral issues raised by the new biomedical technologies and by the success of their therapies.[5] Patients were surviving long enough that decisions had to be made about which treatments were worth pursuing. Humanists were often appalled at what they found: anemic moral stances that physicians and other health professionals thought of as being associated with the Hippocratic Oath. Medicine had no doctrine of informed consent. It had no coherent social ethic. It had no notion of patients' rights. Once professional ethics of the nineteenth and early twentieth centuries was confronted by these more robust and sophisticated ethical systems, the old medical ethics could not survive.

In the United States, nurses were the first to move. In 1976, the American Nurses' Association revised its code of ethics, becoming the first health professional group to change from a patient-benefit approach to ethics to one acknowledging the rights of patients (American Nurses' Association 1976).

At the American Medical Association, a certain discomfort was setting in. By 1971, the AMA had been accused by the Federal Trade Commission (FTC) of conspiring to restrain free trade by using its code of ethics to prohibit advertising among its member physicians. The prohibition on advertising was perceived by many physicians as a sign that they were not mere business people, but "professionals" committed first to the welfare of patients. They considered advertising beneath the dignity of their role. It also happened that the prohibition could work to keep physician fees at high levels. Having been challenged by the FTC, Russell Roth, the Speaker of the AMA's House of Delegates, mounted a last-ditch defense of the prohibition on advertising (Roth 1971).

The AMA began to realize that its Judicial Council, the body within the organization responsible for the AMA's advertising policy and other matters classified as ethical, was ineffective. Indeed, it was perceived as irrelevant. The organization began to make changes. It invited outsiders to its Chicago offices for consultation.[6] I was the first non-physician ethicist invited to become a member of the *Journal of the American Medical Association* editorial board.

As the decade drew to a close, more effective leaders came into power, some of whom had been directly exposed to the current ethical controversies and interdisciplinary discussion of the day. James Todd had been a New Jersey physician during the Karen Quinlan debate. He was part of the interdisciplinary group that developed guidelines for implementing court rulings. He traveled to the Hastings Center to explore the issues with philosophers, lawyers, and others removed from the clinic. When the AMA decided it would have to review its old code of ethics, Todd was named chair of the committee. He single-handedly dragged the AMA into the modern world, proposing to the House of Delegates a new code that formally committed physicians for the first time to being honest with their patients. More generally, this code shifted to the language of rights, acknowledging in a physician code for the first time that patients have rights that cannot be supressed merely because physicians believe doing so would benefit patients. The new code integrated American organized medicine into the mainstream of American political philosophy and ethics. The proposed code was adopted and remains essentially unchanged to this day (American Medical Association 1981).

Todd recognized that a momentous change was taking place. Not only was the AMA shifting from its paternalistic ethics in the tradition of the ancient Hippocratic group and the nineteenth-century consequentialists to a philosophical view much more compatible with mainstream secular and religious values of the culture, it was also acknowledging that physicians would increasingly lose their exclusive place as custodians of the profession's ethic. In his report to the delegates, Todd wrote, "the profession does not exist for itself; it exists for a purpose, and increasingly that purpose will be defined by society" (Todd [1979]).

In Great Britain change was also on the horizon, but the confrontation was less dramatic. The British had not left the disciplining of wayward physicians exclusively in the hands of the medical association. Physicians charged with unethical or illegal conduct came before the General Medical Council, a body involving governmental and public members as well as representatives of the profession.

In 1970 a British physician was charged with breach of confidentiality for revealing to a 16-year-old young woman's parents that she had received birth control pills from another physician ("General Medical Council: Disciplinary

Committee" 1971). His defense was a wonderful testament to the physician's isolation. He claimed that he had acted appropriately according the Hippocratic Oath and the British and AMA codes because the codes in place at the time authorized disclosure of confidential information if the physician believed it would be for the benefit of the patient to do so. This was based on the Hippocratic Oath's confidentiality provision that limits the nondisclosure obligation to "those things that ought not be spread abroad." This was understood to restrict the duty of confidentiality to disclosures that would not benefit the patient. Since this physician was clearly acting in good faith to do what he thought would benefit the young woman, he was exonerated of any ethical violation.

The result was an international outcry and a revision of the British code so that, in the future, if a physician came to believe that a patient would benefit from disclosure of confidential information, the physician would have to seek the patient's approval to disclose it ("Central Ethical Committee" 1971). If the patient gave permission, then the disclosure could take place, but not without that approval.

Unfortunately, this re-entry of British professional medical ethics into the tradition of liberal political philosophy and patients' rights has not, as yet, been completed. In fact, the revision of the confidentiality provision of the BMA code was, in effect, repealed. The 1980 version of the code provides that there is an exception to the confidentiality rule "when it is undesirable on medical ground to seek patient's consent" to the disclosure of the confidential information (British Medical Association 1980, p. 12).

When Raanan Gillon, the physician–philosopher who edited the British *Journal of Medical Ethics* during this period, set out to produce a compendium of medical ethics he called his volume *Principles of Health Care Ethics* (Gillon 1994). This was not an accident. He knew the current debates among philosophers and other ethical theorists well enough to know that "principlism" was the dominant ethical approach in health care ethics. He put forward a set of principles—beneficence, nonmaleficence, autonomy, and justice—that were familiar to every participant in the discussion of medical ethical theory of the period. Gillon knew that principlism was not without its critics, but was convinced that the principlists had gotten it right. He recruited both the defenders of principlism and their critics to write chapters in the volume. He knew all of this because he was close to the players in the discussion. Even though he was a British physician and many of the participants in the principlism debate were American philosophers, he knew their work well. As editor of the leading British journal in medical ethics, he had read and edited their work. Gillon obviously was not isolated from the contemporary debate among humanists in philosophical and religious ethics. He was in a position far different from that of John Warren in Boston in 1808 or John Bell and Isaac Hays in Philadelphia in 1847. These nineteenth-century physician editors were essentially practicing physicians and medical scientists who were temporarily called into action to address moral problems of their time. Without background or experience in the ethics of their field, all they could do was borrow from the previous generation's physician–philosophers. Gillon was even in a position far different from the members of the AMA Judicial Council in 1970. He was more the descendent of John Gregory—a physician–philosopher engaged with other humanists in integrating medical ethics into the main philosophical and ethical debates of the day. The conversation in the Anglo-American world had resumed.

Gillon is just one example of the dramatic change that occurred during the 1970s. We began the decade with physicians essentially trying to go it alone in their medical ethics. If they needed help on an ethical issue they might turn to the AMA's Judicial Council, but it was busy with issues of an earlier era: socialized medicine, physician advertising, and protecting the orthodox practitioner's turf from alternative practitioners. Physicians quickly discovered that they were over their heads. They needed more sophisticated and experienced sources to address new problems. The time to renew the dialogue had arrived.

WHY THE RECONVERGENCE?

Whether one dates the reconvergence from Nuremberg of 1946 or Fletcher and Sperry's cautious wandering into the clinic in the 1950s; whether it began with Scribner's dialysis shunt, Henry Beecher's challenge in research ethics, or the first heart transplant in the 1960s; or whether it began with the new interdisciplinary research institutes of 1969–1971, by the early 1970s, the cross-disciplinary conversation was fully in gear. Hundreds of physicians, religious ethicists, lawyers, and social scientists (and a few deviant philosophers) had resumed a conversation interrupted two centuries earlier. Just as we asked why physicians and humanists became isolated from each other, we also need to ask why they came back together. Three elements seem critical.

The Change to Chronic Illness and Half-way Technologies

The first essential ingredient that forced physicians and humanist to resume talking was an important shift in medicine itself. Until the middle of the twentieth century, the "modal" disease—the disease that captured the public and professional consciousness—was acute illness. In the early and mid-twentieth century the modal disease could be considered poliomyelitis. It was to the early decades what cancer, heart disease, and HIV have become at the beginning of the twenty-first century. Other similar diseases were pneumonia and other acute infectious diseases. From a medical point of view they were all caused by microorganisms. More importantly, from a sociological point of view, they were acute illnesses that made people very sick, very quickly. The result was either a rapid death or, with luck, a cure.

Why is this important sociologically? First, it meant that there was no deep philosophical disagreement about whether these conditions were bad. The only expertise that was needed was someone who had a diagnosis and treatment. The physician was the relevant expert. The physician with a preventative or a cure— penicillin or polio immunizations—was the only person worth consulting.

Second, it meant that laypeople had very little reason to become involved in medical decision making. There was no disagreement that these diseases were bad and patients wanted to be rid of them. Moreover, the person with the disease was in no condition to attempt to become involved. The patient with pneumonia, delirious with a 104° temperature, was neither able to contribute any relevant knowledge nor think coherently enough to be an active participant in decision making. Other laypeople—relatives and friends—were ignorant and without useful skills. Quick decisions made by experts in an environment of complete consensus about the goals of medicine were all that was needed.

With the development of a few new technologies, all of this changed precipitously. With penicillin and other antibiotics, pneumonia was no longer a threat in any but a few special cases. With vaccines for polio and childhood infectious diseases, acute infection ceased to be the modal disease.

Just as acute disease was tamed, other new technologies brought a new type of modal disease. The dialysis machine was just one of those technologies. The invention of the ventilator was another, but there were many others in rapid succession: organ transplant, cancer chemotherapy, radiation, the birth control pill, and safe techniques for abortion.

The sociological impact cannot be overstated. Every one of these technologies leaves patients in a position in which they are relatively healthy and lucid at a time when certain key decisions must be made. Moreover, the decision-making process is generally on a much slower timetable. Thus decisions can get made over days or weeks or even years and the patient is healthy enough to study his or her condition and think about the choices, drawing on a personal framework of beliefs and values to reflect on options.

Many of those options have turned out to be controversial. Some of the technologies are only partially successful. They are "half-way technologies," to use Thomas Chalmers' phrase. They permit stabilizing of the patient in a relatively healthy condition, but do not produce a cure. Dialysis goes on two to three times a week for the life of the patient. A ventilator-dependent patient can live for years. Patients with cancer and heart disease go on for months or years facing choices about therapeutic alternatives. HIV patients on antivirals now live for years in relatively healthy condition. At least some of that time, the patient is perfectly capable of participating in the decision making. And he or she has time to become knowledgeable about the disease, the treatment options, and the potential risks and benefits. Even if the patient is not able to participate actively, the family members or surrogates are. Just when the choices become ethically problematic and controversial, the lay participants on the scene have the time and the mental capacity to become "mini-experts," experts on the small group of therapeutic choices that need to be made. Many laypeople, discovering that there are controversial choices to be made and that they can learn enough to understand the nature of those choices, insist that they have the right to make them, or at least to participate in exploring the options.

When physicians are challenged in this way, they sometimes find that their isolated physician ethics is insufficient. In fact, in some cases they have been all too eager to transfer the tough choices. Physicians such as the managers of hemodialysis programs have actively sought to transfer the decisions to some other parties. They have done so on the grounds that they are not experts in the ethical and other value choices to be made and that they have much to lose by imposing their personal moral perspective on patients. Dialysis programs have turned to allocation committees. Transplant surgeons turned to the United Network for Organ Sharing, the quasi-governmental body made up of laypeople as well as surgeons, to collectively develop allocation algorithms. Critical care medicine physicians have asked for guidance in the production of advance directives, brain-death protocols, and futile-care decisions.

In some cases patients or their surrogates have forced the issue. When Karen Quinlan's parents went to court to force Dr. Robert Morse to cease treating their daughter, they generated international publicity that educated every layperson about difficult choices they might some day have to make. When a private bed- side medical decision is taken to the courts, there are important sociological and political sequellae. The parents first talked with Father Trepasso, their priest. He brought centuries of tradition in Catholic moral theology to bear, reintegrating a major religious tradition into the bedside discussion. When they asked attorney Paul Armstrong to represent them, they brought a legal and political dimension into the discussion. When they went to court, a private debate suddenly became public. Joseph Sullivan, writing for the *New York Times*, and many of his colleagues were brought into the conversation, and they, in turn, brought millions of the public along. Soon every reasonably informed layperson knew that decisions were being made to turn off ventilators on reasonably stable, persistently vegetative patients who could not speak for themselves.

With Catholic moral theology and liberal political philosophy reintroduced into the decision making, it became harder and harder for physicians to rely on their Hippocratic Oath. This was especially true when this choice and almost all the others that were now modal were not addressed directly in the short-form ethics summary. It was even implausible for them to rely on the longer code of the AMA. Although the 1970s code was more detailed, it was often deemed by laypeople (and increasingly by physicians) as reaching implausible positions. Moreover, merely having physicians fix up the most implausible stances still left the code out of sync with the most important religious and secular moral traditions of the day and the best understandings of our common morality.

By the events of 1970 (give or take the few months discussed in this chapter) *everyone*—physician and layperson alike—realized that difficult choices were going to have to be made in medicine and that there was no rational reason to rely on physicians in isolation to make them. The new technologies and the new modal diseases were collectively one of the critical elements in the reintegration of physicians with the mainstream of religious and philosophical ethics.

The Social Rights Movement

While these new biomedical technologies were critical in this reconvergence, they were not the only element. Equally important were the social and political and moral events of the 1960s.

The 1960s were wonderful, turbulent times. As the decade opened we already had hints of what was to come. The 1954 *Brown v. Board of Education* decision escalated the ethics conversation regarding the morality of racism and civil rights. Some people were already uncomfortable with the tentative support of the Eisenhower administration for a faction in Indo-China that was not always democratic or egalitarian.

Soon after the beginning of the 1960s the civil rights and antiwar movements were launched in earnest. They taught moral perspectives that had lasting impacts on sectors of the society that were well beyond international and racial relations. They taught a language of rights and a way of using the U.S. Constitution to support minorities and other have-not, out-of-power groups. In the protest against theVietnam war, ordinary citizens learned to question the authority of military generals. In the civil rights movement ordinary citizens learned to question the authority of entrenched political powers.

With the war resistance and civil rights movements, could women's rights and student rights be far behind? These out-of-power groups adapted the rhetoric and tactics of their allies in the other movements. They adopted the moral language of rights and the moral theories of philosophical liberalism to defend freedom and equality.

The patients' rights movement was not far behind. Many of the bioethicists identified in this chapter as graduate students of the 1960s developed their moral theories and their activist inclinations in these other rights movements. They learned to challenge authority, and physician authority was soon to be the target. They learned to speak the language of rights; the benevolent paternalism of the Hippocratic ethic was soon to confront a demand for rights of patients. Ethical theories influenced by Kant, deontological ethics, and liberal political philosophy as well as Christian and Jewish religious ethics found the Hippocratic individualism and lack of respect for autonomy wanting. When ethicists were invited into the clinic, they often came with their anti-Hippocratic ethical theories in tow. Very soon thereafter their religious and secular theories also found Hippocratic ethics too individualistic for the world, as resource allocation and fair access to health care became one of the critical moral issues.

It was the combination of the new technologies of medicine with the rights movements of the 1960s that forced a reintegration of physician ethics into the mainstream of ethical discourse with humanists. Still, that reintegration probably would not have been as dramatic had it not been for a third and final factor: the dissonance between physician ethics and other ethics.

Dissonance Between Physician Ethics and Other Ethics

As we have just seen, when laypeople learned what decisions physicians were making about laypeople's health care, they were often appalled. It was not merely that the new technologies gave laypeople a chance to participate in the decisions while they were relatively healthy and gave them enough time to learn about the nature of those choices. Nor was it that the antiwar and civil rights movements gave laypeople the courage to recognize that expertise in some technology did not necessarily an expert in morals make. It was that, once laypeople had the time and knowledge to review physician choices and the fortitude to challenge the physician's authority, they discovered that physicians were very predictably making controversial moral moves, choices that at least some laypeople considered morally indefensible.

Physicians intentionally withheld grave diagnoses from patients; they did research on them without informing them; they sterilized some patients whom they thought were not worthy of being parents; they routinely kept critically and terminally ill patients alive against the wishes of those patients or their families; they intentionally broke confidences against the wishes of patients; they refused to perform sterilizations, abortions, and provide contraceptives if they thought patients shouldn't have them; they allocated scarce resources in controversial and nondemocratic ways. The more laypeople learned about the ethic that had become embedded in the medical profession, the more they protested. They began to find that the physician ethic, isolated from the mainstream of religious and secular morality, had developed such tensions with most plausible ethical positions that it was untenable and offensive. Four major tensions emerged.

Benefits vs. Rights and Duties

The first tension was between the ethic of benefits of the physicians and the more Kantian, or "rights-oriented," deontological, ethic of many other secular and religious systems. Ethical theorists at the middle of the twentieth century had been raised on a dispute in normative ethical theory between what they often called consequentialist (or utilitarian) and deontological ethics. Any theorist learns early on that ethical systems can be divided into those that strive to evaluate actions or rules on the basis of their consequences and those that rely on criteria other than consequences. An ethic that holds that it is simply wrong to lie or break a promise "regardless of the consequences" is one that evaluates actions based on certain "formal" criteria (that the action involves a lie or a broken promise). These nonconsequential ethics are often called "deontological" or "formalist."

Among the deontological ethics are those of the philosopher Immanuel Kant, those that recognize certain ethical principles beyond maximizing good consequences (such as W. D. Ross's), and those that speak of certain rights holding sway even when respecting the rights-claims does not necessarily produce the greatest amount of good.

Liberal political philosophy often incorporates two ethical principles that affirm the rightness of actions even if they do not produce the best consequences: autonomy and justice. Nineteenth-century liberalism affirms the rights of individuals to live their lives as free agents with the right of noninterference. Twentieth-century liberalism often emphasizes justice in the allocation of benefits and harms, holding that certain patterns for distribution, such as the pattern based on equality or need, take precedence over maximizing good outcomes in aggregate.

This is not the place to outline the many existing theories of ethics. What is important for our purposes is that many of these ethics recognize either autonomy or justice or some other set of principles other than good consequences as morally critical. This is true of secular liberal political philosophy. It is true of talmudic law. It is true of almost all Protestant ethics. It is true of Communism, feminism, libertarianism, and the ethics that rely on concepts of rights.

It is *not* true of secular utilitarianism often relied on by economists and social planners. One explanation for the eighteenth-century conversation between physicians and humanists going so well is that, at that time, both physician ethics and the ethics of the Scottish Enlightenment (the ethics of Hutcheson, Smith, and Hume) were consequentialist, at least to an important degree. Nevertheless, this substantial list of traditions that are to some degree deontological suggests that physician ethics, once exposed, will be in for difficult times.

The most conspicuous characteristic of the Hippocratic ethic that has emerged since physician ethics has been isolated from the humanities is that it is consequentialist. It is consequentialist with the important proviso that the only consequences that count are those affecting the patient, but it is consequentialist nonetheless. The core ethical principle is that the physician should do what is best for the patient according to the physician's ability and judgment. It is what most physicians, at least until the reawakening of the 1970s, would state as their basic moral commitment if they were cornered on a hospital floor and asked to defend their behavior. It was what the major professionally generated codes of the nineteenth and early twentieth centuries called for.

If the dominant physician ethic is consequential and so many lay ethical systems are deontological or rights oriented, it is predictable that, once the difference is recognized and made known, there will be such tension that further discourse will have to take place to resolve the disagreement. While not every ethical tradition and every ethical theorist will bristle at the Hippocratic consequentialism of traditional physician ethics, enough will that the conversation will be vigorous.

Individual vs. Social

The second tension is that, even among the ethical traditions outside of medicine that are consequentialist, there is still an important difference with the ethic that emerged in organized medicine during the period of its isolation. In its pure form, health professional ethics was individualistic. It focused on the best interests of the patient as an individual apart from society. Most of the other ethical systems that could be called consequentialist—classical utilitarianism, for example—reject this individualism. While utilitarianism considers goods and harms to be individual in the sense that they accrue to individual persons, classical utilitarianism requires consideration of the benefits and harms that accrue to all persons. It would reject the Hippocratic idea of giving consideration only to the health provider's individual patient and ignoring the benefits and harms of actions that accrue to other people.

Not all health professional ethics are individualist in this way. Both Gregory and Percival had social dimensions to their ethic. Especially Percival, who was interested in the hospital as a social institution for health care delivery, addressed the interests of those beyond the individual, isolated patient. The codes of the AMA have, from the beginning had a social dimension to them. Nevertheless, much isolated physician ethics has given priority to the welfare of the individual patient. The American Nurses' Association Code of 1976, for example, said that the "the nurse's primary commitment is to the client's care and safety" (American Nurses Association 1976, p. 8). The fact that it also said that sometimes individual rights "may temporarily be altered for the common good" (American Nurses Association 1976, p. 4) does not detract from the individualist character of its "primary commitment."

If most ethical systems outside of medicine that are consequential incorporate some social dimension to their consequentialism and many deontological ethics do as well (at least those that incorporate a principle of justice), then we can predict tension when physician ethics with its individualist tendencies comes up against these more social ethical systems outside of medicine. Thus the dissonance between Hippocratic individualism and non-physician ethics that are more social provides a second reason to expect that tensions will be recognized and that, once recognized, they will have to be addressed.

Authoritarian vs. Egalitarian

There is a third area of dissonance. Traditional physician ethics is usually paternalist. It is thus authoritarian in that it legitimates the authority of physicians to act for the welfare of their patients *even when the patients reject the proposed physician intervention*. We saw precisely this paternalism in Gregory and in many manifestations of physician ethics when they defended the legitimacy of lying to patients or withholding the truth from them to protect them from bad news. We have noticed along the way that some physicians have been more skeptical— Percival to some degree and some nineteenth- and early twentieth-century physicians, such as Hooker and Cabot—who have gotten a bit of distance from their professional peers. But even in these exceptional cases, we saw that their questioning of the paternalist position of disclosure tended to be grounded in fear of the consequences, fear that the physician who lied for benevolent motives would be found out and that, in the long run, it would do more harm than good. These reasons for opposing lying to patients are in tension with the Kantian perspective (one shared by many religious ethical traditions) that holds that lying is simply immoral regardless of the consequences.

We are left with the ethic that emerged when physicians were isolated, one with strongly paternalistic qualities, while most ethical systems outside of medicine were skeptical of that paternalism. Certainly, American liberal political philosophy with its emphasis on autonomy and informed consent is antipaternalistic. So is Protestant ethics with its affirmation of the layperson as decision-maker. When Protestant students in religious ethics, nurtured on the antiwar and civil rights movements, discover medical paternalism in decisions to hide diagnoses and force treatment on terminally ill patients against their will, there will be a dissonance that forces a confrontation.

Ethics of Rules and Ethics of Cases

The fourth and final area of difference between many physician-generated ethical stances and those of many laypeople involves a part of ethical theory that addresses how one bridges between individual case judgments and more abstract ethical principles.

Ethical theory must incorporate a method for translating abstract ethical principles down to the individual case judgment. Here professionally generated medical ethics and much of lay medical ethics are significantly different. Professionally generated ethics resist rigid rules. They take the abstract principles directly to the bedside, relying on case-by-case judgments by the clinician. Every case is so unique that no hard-and-fast rules apply. Clinicians favor making moral decisions on a case-by-case basis.

Philosophical ethics has names for various versions of theory that rely on case-by-case judgment. If the principles are utilitarian or consequentialistic, the approach is called "act-utilitarianism." If they are deontological (duty-based), the approach is called "act-deontology." The preface "act-" is meant to convey that the principles are applied directly to every instance of an action.

Some lay medical ethics also take principles directly to individual actions. As we saw in Chapter 10, in the 1960s Joseph Fletcher built a career claiming that ethics should be "situational," that is, every situation or action should be judged individually without using moral rules for anything more than summaries of past experience or guidelines. His view was called *situationalism* (Fletcher 1966). It is, in fact, act-consequentialism. It is not surprising that Fletcher became a great friend of medical professionals when he transferred his attention to matters medical. Some philosophers also accepted one of the versions of an act-based ethic, rejecting the necessity of mediating the step from principles to individual judgments through a system of moral rules. Recently, some feminist ethical theory has resuscitated a version of this view under the name *moral particularism* (Hooker and Little 2000).

Many medical laypeople, however, are skeptical about this act-based way of making individual judgments. They fear that, especially in the urgency and emotion of a medical crisis, humans are too fallible, too prone to err in judgment. In a pluralistic world, physicians will rely on their own version of ethical principles, even when the patient or the society does not accept that ethical position. Many religious ethical systems insist on placing robust moral rules between the abstract principles and the individual case judgments. Secular philosophical ethics often hold that case judgments ought to based on moral rules that are, in turn, generated by reflection on the moral principles. Depending on the principles involved, these approaches are variously called "rule-utilitarianism" or "rule-deontology." Thus, contrary to what we saw in Richard Cabot, it is possible for utilitarians to take rules very seriously and it is possible for deontologists to bring their ethical principles to individual cases without mediating judgments through a rigid system of rules.

In philosophical ethics, the philosopher John Rawls (1955) defended the rule-based approach. In theological ethics, Paul Ramsey (1967), relying to some extent on Rawls, made a similar case for religious ethical systems. Since then, most of the major medical ethical theory done by philosophers and theologians has tended toward a more rigorous application of rules (see Beauchamp and Childress 2001, for example) while much professionally generated medical ethics continues to insist that cases are unique and that codes should be taken only as guides to individual clinical decisions.

While not all health professionals favor more situational, act-based ethical systems and not all medical laypeople associate with more rule-based approaches, this is another area in which physicians and humanists need to be in communication to understand the controversies that can arise in producing medical ethics.

CONCLUSION

This complex combination of technological, sociological, and philosophical developments conspired to force a reassessment of the mutual disinterest that physicians and humanists were expressing. Humanists discovered that they wanted to work on real-world issues in ethics just at the time that physicians discovered they needed help from outside medicine. Laypeople were recognizing that the issues of controversy in medicine were not really questions of medical science so much as matters of morals. These were topics that were not the physician's domain any more than military ethics of the Vietnam war were the domain of the generals. The behavior of both humanists and physicians changed. Medical journals began appointing non-physicians to their boards and publishing articles on the ethical aspects of medicine. Medical schools added scores of humanists to their faculties. Ordinary practitioners began bringing patients into the decision-making process, asking them for living wills, informing them of treatment options, and getting their consent (at least for more major clinical choices).

Humanists were happy to reciprocate. They began offering courses in medical ethics covering all the key topics: death and dying, fertility control, human subjects research, and health insurance. They invited clinicians into their classrooms just as humanists had been asked to speak to medical students. Medicine was once again more than just a clinical science.

Afterword: The 1980s and Beyond

By the beginning of the 1980s the reconvergence was more or less complete. We have arrived at the current generation in medical ethics. All the major themes are in place. The right of competent patients to refuse treatment has been firmly established (although some loose ends pertaining to forgoing nutrition and hydration need to be tied up); the authority of lay surrogates to make medical decisions, including treatment-forgoing decisions, is established (although limits on their authority to make unexcepted or unpopular decisions are still being explored); the system for the protection of subjects of medical research is in place (although some inconsistencies in the regulations from one federal agency to another have not yet been reconciled).

By the 1980s, virtually all the other main topics of controversy in medical ethics had been identified and the main positions staked out. The fertility control issues were either settled (birth control and sterilization) or the sides in the controversy were becoming intransigent (abortion and test-tube babies). Lying to patients, even for benevolent reasons such as easing bad news, was now indisputably unacceptable for health professionals and laypeople alike (Novack et al. 1979). The informed-consent doctrine had been firmly established in law as well as in the clinic. Moreover, its foundation in the Western notion of the right to freedom of choice was clear. The legitimacy of transplanting organs from one human being to another, either from a newly dead body or from a living donor consenting to

the removal of a kidney, was beyond serious controversy. A brain-oriented definition of death was the law in every state in the United States and in almost all
other countries of the world.

Medicine was a significantly different social institution than it had been only a
decade or two earlier. The standard policy for the practice of medicine in every
one of these areas of controversy was dramatically different from what it had been
before the transition in what I have called a "new enlightenment." More importantly, those who were not health professionals were central to the new policies.
Patients or their lay surrogates were the ones who would decide whether to accept or reject life-sustaining medical treatments. The patients or healthy laypeople
who were to be subjects of medical research had, in virtually every case, to consent before they could be the targets of such research. The one whose fertility is
to be limited had the right to decide whether to use birth control, select sterilization, try in vitro fertilization, and decide whether to terminate a pregnancy.

While informed consent was totally absent from Hippocratic medical ethics
and from the modern codes for therapeutic medicine that had emerged through
the middle of the twentieth century, it had become the centerpiece of medical
decision making by the last years of the century. Lack of consent—in writing in
the case of most surgery, oral or implied in the case of other treatments—is
grounds for both legal and moral censure. In organ transplant, the social aspects
of the enterprise—the decisions to procure and allocate organs—are removed
entirely from the hands of the practicing clinician. The policy about when organs
can be procured is governed by state and federal law and the details are in the
hands of an interdisciplinary board of the United Network for Organ Transplantation (UNOS). Its ethics committee, which handles many of the most controversial issues, includes philosophers, lawyers, organ recipients, and representatives
of the families of organ donors. Interdisciplinary government committees have
addressed all of these issues and continue to set or recommend policy for issues
such as cloning.

Thus patients and other laypeople directly affected by the decisions are, by the
current generation beginning in about 1980, presumed to be the ones responsible
for making choices about their own treatment and medical laypeople, including
professionally trained humanists as well as health professionals, are routinely part
of every policy-making group.

MAJOR DEVELOPMENTS IN BIOETHICS

One of the major changes resulting from this emergence of laypeople as active
decision-makers in medical ethics is that key actions are no longer exclusively in
schools of medicine and the professional medical organizations. The federal
government–mandated National Commission for the Protection of Subjects of

Biomedical Research that shaped national policy in this area in the 1970s was just the first of a number of important government commissions since then.

The President's Commission for the Study of Ethical Problems in Medicine and Biomedical and Behavioral Research

The crowning achievement in this publicly organized interdisciplinary deliberation was the President's Commission for the Study of Ethical Problems in Medicine and Biomedical and Behavioral Research. Encouraged by the success of the National Commission, which focused exclusively on human subjects research, Congress authorized a new presidential commission with a broader mandate to study and report on ethical and legal issues in clinical medicine as well as research.

Over the course of its four years (1979–1983), it tackled virtually all the major controversies of biomedical ethics: compensation for research injuries, the decision to forego life-sustaining treatment, the definition of death, protection of human subjects and implementing human research regulations, whistle-blowing in biomedical research, genetic screening and counseling, genetic engineering, access to health care, and, under the vague heading of "making health care decisions," the controversies surrounding informed consent.

The original 11-member commission included five physicians and two medical scientists, but it also included a medical ethicist, a sociologist, and two lawyers. The sociologist, Reneé Fox, and one of the lawyers, Patricia King, as well as the medical ethicist, Al Jonsen, we have encountered before in this volume. All had extensive experience in the interdisciplinary hammering out of medical ethical controversies. Later a Jewish medical ethicist, Seymour Seigel, was added to the commission. Just as important, its interdisciplinary staff included a number of humanists in key positions as well as physicians like Joanne Lynn who were comfortable in the interdisciplinary world. The staff also provided the first significant opportunity for a number of academic philosophers to emerge as some of the best analytical minds in the field—people like Dan Brock, Allen Buchanan and Daniel Wikler.

By the end of the decade, this public interdisciplinary body had become the new authority in medical ethics, replacing organized medicine as the definitive standard for the moral conduct of physicians and patients. It is to this day routinely cited in court decisions, hospital ethics committee deliberations, and Congress as the authority on matters of American public bioethics.

Medical School Developments

The professional resources are not depleted, however. Both medical schools and medical professional organizations are about to escalate their efforts in medical ethics.

By this time, it no longer makes sense to attempt to list the examples of humanists and health professionals formally engaged in the efforts to teach medical ethics to health professional students and laypeople. There are literally thousands devoting at least part of their professional time to teaching and consultation in medical ethics. Virtually every school of medicine, nursing, dentistry, and the other health sciences has not merely a designated faculty person responsible for teaching health professional ethics; they generally have entire departments with subspecializations in medical history, medical ethics, medical law, medical literature, and social aspects of medicine.

One program, that of The State University of New York (SUNY) Upstate Medical Center at Syracuse, can be cited merely by way of illustration. It is picked not because it had any unusual role in the development of medical school humanities, but because it is typical of an institution that joined in the movement pioneered in the 1970s at places such as Galveston, Hershey, Stony Brook, Harvard, and Tennessee.

By 1975 psychiatrist Robert W. Daly had risen through the ranks from assistant to full professor of psychiatry at SUNY Upstate. He had long had an interest in the social and ethical aspects of medicine. That year he was a senior fellow of the National Endowment for the Humanities. By the end of the decade he had been appointed adjunct professor of philosophy at Syracuse University. That humanities interest continued to grow. By 1984 he launched the school's program in the medical humanities.

Meanwhile, philosopher Samuel Gorovitz had developed his interests in teaching ethics in the direction of medicine, first at Case Western Reserve University and then at Maryland. He co-edited one of the early medical ethics texts (1976), organized courses for the National Endowment of the Humanities for college humanists who wanted to develop skills in teaching medical ethics, and, for the 1979–80 academic year was the senior fellow at the federal government's National Center for Health Services Research. In 1986 he moved to Syracuse as professor of philosophy and dean of the College of Arts and Sciences. His biomedical ethics interests led him to the medical center, where he was involved in many collaborative efforts with Daly.

Here is a typical convergence of interests between two leaders in a university. Other academic health professionals and humanists from the university gathered around, and by the year 2000 a Center for Bioethics and the Humanities was formed. Under the direction of physician Kathy Faber-Langendoen, its eight faculty include Daly and Gorovitz, another physician who specializes in ethics, a lawyer with a doctorate in bioethics, a psychologist who teaches medical ethics, and two specialists in medical literature.

The program offers courses and other educational initiatives in bioethics and the medical humanities; provides a clinical ethics consultative services; and conducts research, publishing scholarly and creative writing in bioethics and the medical humanities.

The SUNY Upstate program shows that medical education is deeply penetrated by this collaborative effort across disciplines. It is in many ways typical of American and Canadian health professional education by the beginning of the twenty-first century, an effort in the spirit of Gregory, but at a level of commitment of which Gregory could only have dreamed. Today virtually every medical school can point to something analogous.

The New Face of Organized Medicine

What happened at medical schools across the country has been mirrored in organized medicine. We have seen that 1980 marked the year of the revision of the AMA Code to—for the first time in the history of organized medicine—acknowledge the rights of patients and commit to honesty in dealing with them.

That has turned out to be only the beginning of medical ethics reform at the national association for physicians. The new code was followed by an upgrading of the AMA's Judicial Council. It changed its name to the Council on Ethical and Judicial Affairs, reflecting an effort to get away from the petty, quasi-legal review functions such as punishing physicians for advertising and move in the direction of serious ethical reflection. They hired David Orentlicher, a lawyer with serious commitment to the academic study of ethics, to be senior staff person for the Council. He took the leadership in producing the first position papers and resolutions dealing with serious ethics matters in medicine including virtually every issue of the day. The anemic, platitudinous code of ethics rapidly grew to a compendium of position statements with supporting documents that now takes up a 250-page book. These are backed up with longer position papers published in *JAMA* and other journals. For the first time, academic teachers of medical ethics, courts, legislators, and administrators are taking the AMA seriously as a player in medical ethics on the national scene. When Orentlicher left the AMA to assume a position on the faculty of the Indiana University School of Law, the AMA recruited highly respected Harvard physician–ethicist Linda Emanuel to take over the work. Although she has now moved on to become the professor of medicine and director of the Interdisciplinary Program in Professionalism and Human Rights at Feinberg School of Medicine at Northwestern University, by the time she left, the AMA's ethics efforts were, for the first time since the organization's founding a century and a half earlier, on a solid footing as a respected leader in the field.

The Bioethics Program at the National Institutes of Health

Linda Emanuel is not the only dual-degreed bioethics scholar in her family. Her husband, Ezekiel Emanuel, has assumed the directorship of the new Department of Clinical Bioethics at the National Institutes of Health (NIH). The efforts originally launched by John Fletcher, the ethicist we met in Chapter 10, had evolved under the leadership of physician Alison Wichman into the NIH Clinical Center Bioethics Program during the 1980s. Ezekiel Emanuel, like his wife, has both medical and academic doctorates. His is in political philosophy. The NIH Department includes nine faculty (in philosophy, nursing, medicine) and a similar number of fellows. The philosopher along with the physician is now on the payroll of the most important biomedical research facility in the world.

The Council for International Organizations of Medical Sciences Ethics Effort

Since 1980 the expansion of the dialogue has not been limited to the United States. One of the most constructive and persistent efforts has been that of the Council for International Organizations of Medical Sciences (CIOMS). Its efforts reveal both interdisciplinary commitment an the complexity of international, interdisciplinary work. While a council of medical professional organizations, it works very closely with the World Health Organizaton and thus has the status of something approaching the official international body for medical ethics.

Led by the late Zbigniew Bankowski, a Polish physician who had a rich working list of international humanities contacts, it has now held a series of over 30 conferences in locations throughout the world. Always several philosophers have been among the conference participants. Bankowski normally relied on philosophers to plan the details of the conferences and propose the key speakers. The CIOMS conferences have been particularly important in setting the standards for international research involving human subjects, whether consent standards, for instance, of the country of the sponsor of the research or that of the subjects. There have been times when first-world drug researchers, frustrated with the rigor of the protection of subjects from their country, have attempted to avoid these inconveniences by recruiting subjects from third-world nations where regulations are more lax or even nonexistent. The CIOMS has been in the forefront of proposing policies to short-circuit these techniques.

The Intenational Association of Bioethics

In addition to the CIOMS efforts among professional organizations, a major development at the international level has been the founding of an international interdisciplinary organization that serves as an umbrella organization for scholars, clinicians, and policy-makers with serious bioethics commitments. It marks the true globalization of the interdisciplinary dialogue in bioethics. The dialogue disrupted in the English-speaking world at the end of the eighteenth century has resumed, not merely in Britain and its former colonies; it has now spread literally across the world.

CONCLUSION

The reasons why physicians and humanists quit talking at the end of the eighteenth century are complex. The social forces that had led to an intense period of rich and productive dialogue ceased to support that interaction. They stopped mutual enrichment, with only a few special exceptions like Osler and Cabot challenging that conclusion. I have claimed that, even in their cases, they really were not active participants in the ongoing philosophical and theological discussions, at least in ethics.

Likewise, something happened in a very preliminary way in the middle of the twentieth century and became manifest more vividly around 1970 with the beginning of the current generation in biomedical ethics that brought physicians and other health professionals back into communication with humanists. I suggest that it was the combination of the new technologies that made chronic disease modal, the rights revolutions that made laypeople active participants in making moral decisions in medicine, and the dissonance between more paternalistic, consequence-based morality of the professions and the ethical systems of secular and religious humanists.

Whether these or other, more subtle explanations prove to be the reasons, it seems clear that the long period of isolation of health professional ethics is over and that new systems for ethics in the professions will, in the future, be shaped by the ongoing debates in over ethics in the broader society. I suggest both the professions and laypeople will be better for it.

Notes

PREFACE

1. Here I follow a rather precise linguistic convention that seems required once one recognizes that not all ethics in the medical sphere involves norms for the behavior of physicians. I view medicine as a sphere of human social action. In this sense it is like education or labor or recreation. Medicine is the sphere of human social action concerned with the well-being of the body. No one would think of equating the sphere of education with the behavior of professional teachers. It necessarily involves students, school administrators, teacher aides, parents, school board officials, and people in many other educational roles. So, likewise, I have long insisted that medicine involves much more than the behavior of physicians. In fact, most decisions in the medical sphere are not made by physicians at all; they are made by other health professionals (nurses, pharmacists, dentists, and allied health professionals) and by medical laypeople (patients, parents, politicians, judges, and administrators). The decision to self-medicate with aspirin for a headache rather than seeking professional advice is, after all, a decision in the medical sphere. In fact, it is a decision involving medication, the sphere of medicine in a narrower, more technical sense. Likewise, decisions of pregnant women not to abort a pregnancy or of couples to use birth control I take to be decisions in the sphere of medicine. To the extent that these decisions involve ethical dimensions, they can and should be viewed as decisions involving medical ethics. In this sense, most medical decisions and most medical ethical decisions involve medical laypeople: the healthy or ill laypeople who decide about self-medication or the seeking of professional advice, their families, friends, spiritual advisors, legislators, judges, and business people who make countless decisions in the medical sphere every day.

Even within the realm of professionals in the medical sphere, only a minority of decisions are made by physicians. Here, I insist that members of other health professions refuse to cede the word *medicine* to physicians. At Georgetown University and in many other health education settings, the schools of nursing, dentistry, etc., are in the "Medical Center" along with the school for physicians. Granted, the physician school calls itself the "Medical School," reflecting the built-in systematic ambiguity in the term *medicine*. For many years I have used the word *medicine* to refer to the medical sphere in the broad sense. Among the professionals in this sphere are nurses, pharmacists, dentists, social workers, and allied health professionals.

In my usage, *medical ethics* refers to systematic ethical analysis of decisions within the medical sphere. *Professional medical ethics* refers to the ethics of decisions made by those in all the medical professions. I use the term *physician ethics* to refer to the more narrow group of ethical decisions made by physicians.

Unfortunately, the linguistic conventions must be even more complicated. It is a serious mistake to assume that only professional physician groups can reflect on and articulate ethical systems—codes, principles, oaths, etc.—for professional physician conduct. The Catholic Health Association, for example, articulates a Code for Catholic Health Facilities (United States Catholic Conference 1971). One of the central themes of this book is that religious and cultural groups should draw on their basic systems of beliefs and values to articulate a conceptualization of how medical professionals (including physician professionals) ought to act from the point of view of their system of ethics. Thus I speak of "professionally articulated ethics" as any ethics, regarding the behavior of professionals or laypeople that is put forward by members of the medical professions or their groups. This is in contrast to ethics articulated by those outside the professions, whether they are speaking of the ethics for medical professionals or ethics for medical laypeople. Thus, in this volume, I speak of both professional- and lay-articulated medical ethics. Either group may put forward ethical maxims for medical professional behavior or medical lay behavior, and among those focusing on medical professional behavior, some will deal with physician behavior while others will deal with the behavior of other medical professional roles.

2. Others have more recently suggested that this view may be too simple, but both Edelstein and others (Carrick 1985; Temkin 1991; Smith 1979) have claimed that the Hippocratic ethic was only one among many ethical stances in Greek medicine.

CHAPTER 1

1. Vivian Nutton (1995) has attempted to identify the influence of the Hippocratic Oath in modern culture. He finds some evidence for its use in sixteenth-century Germany, particularly at the University of Jena. He also finds "verbal echoes" at Giessen as well as the use of some of the language of the Oath at Wittenberg, Basel, and Freiburg during the sixteenth century. He attributes this to "the revival of classical learning in the Renaissance (p. 521)," of which the German universities stood at the very forefront. Consistent with my findings, however, Nutton stresses that the Hippocratic Oath played "a somewhat marginal role in medicine until relatively recent times (p. 519)." It is not until the nineteenth century that the Hippocratic Oath was widespread among physicians.

2. For background on the Scottish Enlightenment see Chitnis (1976), Daiches (1986), Davie (1961, 1981), Donnachie and Hewitt (1989), and Lenman (1981). For more specific histories of the development of science and medicine during the Enlighten-

ment see Christie (1974, 1975), Lawrence (1985, 1988b), and Rosner (1991). For the medical ethics of the period see Baker et al. (1993) and McCullough (1993).

3. See Donnachie and Hewitt (1989) for good, concise summaries of the roles of many of these figures.

4. Biographical information on Gregory comes from Smellie (1800), John Gregory himself (1821), Ramsay (1888), and Bettany (1890), as well as twentieth-century Gregory scholarship. The recently published critical study of Gregory by Laurence McCullough (1998) is particularly valuable.

5. A copy of each version of the lectures is in the special collections of the library of the University of Edinburgh, each part of the library of Dugald Stewart, Professor of Moral Philosophy at the University from 1785 to 1809. The collection contains a number of important medical ethics volumes, including an original edition of Thomas Percival's 1803 *Medical Ethics*, which, together with Gregory's *Lectures*, constitutes the two most important works of physicians in modern Anglo-American medical ethics. The Percival volume will be discussed at length in Chapter 2.

The 1770 *Observations* appears anonymously as "two preliminary lectures, read not long ago, in one of the universities of a neighboring kingdom, by a medical professor" ([Gregory] 1770, p. iii). Apparently, Gregory was not difficult to identify. The first lecture "treated very fully on the duties and offices of a physician: a path almost untrod till now" ([Gregory] 1770, pp. iii–iv). In the second "the author has endeavoured to ascertain the true method by which enquiries into medicine are to be prosecuted; and has likewise pointed out, with much precision, the causes which have retarded the advancement of medicine, and the inconveniences which that science in particular at present labours under" ([Gregory] 1770, p. vi). It presents what we would call philosophy of science and scientific methodology. The text contains 182 pages of approximately 160 words each. The lectures are introduced with an explanation of their purpose: "Before I proceed to the particular business of this course, I shall, agreeably to the usual custom, give some preliminary lectures. Such lectures are intended to have a relation to the proper subject of the profession, but not to be essentially connected with it ([Gregory] 1770, p. viii).

The revised manuscript, which Gregory titled *Lectures* rather than *Observations*, contains six lectures, expanding the length to 238 similar-sized pages. Each of the original lectures is divided into three parts, each termed a "lecture." Now Gregory introduces them as follows:

The following lectures have been read in the University of Edinburgh for several years past, and as many transcripts of them were, for time to time, taken by my pupils, one of them found its way to the press in the negligent dress in which they were first exhibited. The public, however, having been pleased to afford them a favourable reception even in that form, I thought it a piece of justice I owed to their candour, to give them a thorough revisal, and to make them, as far as I was able, more worthy of their acceptance. This I have now done. I hope they will be found of some use not only to students, but to the younger part of the Faculty; and that my sincere endeavours to promote the true interests of Physic, however ineffectual, will induce my Brethren to overlook any defect that, after all my care, may still be found in them.

(Gregory 1772, unnumbered pages at beginning of book)

For the most part the changes are modest and usually not substantive. It is, at this point, impossible to tell whether Gregory had a written manuscript from which the 1770 version represented good student shorthand or whether Gregory, having the benefit of one transcription in front of him, simply took that and edited it. For comparison purposes, the opening lines of the 1772 version read, "But before I enter upon the particular business of this course, I shall, agreeable to custom, give some preliminary lectures, in which I shall lay before you some considerations, which though not strictly belonging to my subject, yet deserve the attention of all those who would practice medicine" (Gregory 1772, p. 2).

While the original publications of 1770 and 1772 are available in places like the Edinburgh library, we are fortunate that the Gregory scholar, Laurence McCullough, has recently published carefully researched critical editions (Gregory 1998).

6. The St. Andrew's colleges shifted to separate professorships for each subject in 1747 (Wood 1993, pp. viii, 62, 68).

7. Whether Gregory actually completed the full three-year curriculum is questionable. An assistant was hired for him in the third year, which may imply that he did not teach the full course (Wood 1993, p. 31).

8. These included Wilkes and Charles Townshend, whom Gregory already knew, as well as George, Lord Lyttelton, and Lady Mary Wortley Montagu. Lady Montagu was involved in the publication.

9. As Smellie puts it, "he lived in habits of great intimacy with most of the Scottish Literati; such as, Doctors Robertson and Blair, David Hume, John Home, Lord Monboddo, Lord Kames, and the elder Mr. Tytler" (Smellie 1800, pp. 117–18).

10. For additional examples of Gregory's use of Bacon in the *Lectures* see Gregory (1772, pp. 120, 159, 189, 191, 209, 220); for his use of Newton see Gregory (1772, pp. 152, 153); for Boyle see Gregory (1772, p. 224).

11. Its [religion's] most dangerous enemies have ever been among the temperate and chaste Philosopher, void of passion and sensibility, who had no vicious appetites to be restrained by its influence, and who were equally unsusceptible of its terrors or pleasures. Absolute Infidelity or settled Scepticism in Religion is no proof of a bad Understanding or a bad Heart, but is certain a very strong presumption of the want of Imagination and sensibility of Heart. Many Philosophers have been Infidels, few Men of Taste and sentiment. Yet the example of Lord Bacon, Mr. Locke, and Sir Isaac Newton, among many other first names in Philosophy, is a sufficient evidence that religious belief is perfectly compatible with the clearest and most enlarged Understanding.

(Gregory 1765, pp. 165–66)

12. By 1753 Reid had emerged as a leader in the King's College curriculum revision (Wood 1993, p. 67).

13. It was not unusual for members of the Scottish school of common-sense philosophy to divide among themselves over specific issues including skepticism. Beattie attacked Locke, Berkeley, and Hume because they contradicted the maxims of common sense (Wood 1993, pp. 120, 129). Reid also was critical of Hume's skepticism and is credited with "institutionalisation of common sense philosophy in Aberdeen." On these issues Gregory is aligned with the Aberdonians Beattie and Reid, rather than Hume.

14. Adam Smith was also a member of the Edinburgh Philosophical Society, but for part of this time he lived in Glasgow. Later in life, Smith returned to the family estate in Kirkaldy, a town across the Firth of Forth about 20 miles from Edinburgh, but that would have been primarily after Gregory's death. Smith returned there in 1767; Greg-

ory died in 1773. During this period, Smith suffered from ill health and Hume complained in 1772 that he was "cutting himself off entirely from human society" (cited in Stephen 1898, p. 7). Smith reportedly also spent some of this time in London, so extensive contact with Gregory seems unlikely.

15. The detailed curriculum analysis by Wood (1993, pp. 132–3, 145) makes clear that the emergence of common-sense philosophy at Aberdeen draws widely not only on Hutcheson but also on Butler, Reid, and Turnbull.

16. The anonymous writer of the "Life of Dr. John Gregory" that accompanies the 1821 edition of his *Legacy* states, "He likewise owed much, during the whole course of his studies, to the attention of his cousin, the celebrated Dr. Reid, late Professor of Moral Philosophy in the University of Glasgow."

17. The key passage is reprinted in the "Life of Gregory," appearing with "A Father's Legacy to His Daughters" (1821, p. 150):

> Art thou, my Gregory, for ever fled!
> And Am I left to unavailing woe!
> When fortune's storms assail this weary head,
> Where cares long since have shed untimely snow,
> Ah! now for comfort whither shall I go?
> No more thy soothing voice my anguish cheers:
> Thy placid eyes with smiles no longer glow,
> My hopes to cherish, and allay my fears—
> 'Tis meet that I should mourn—flow forth afresh, my tears!

18. It appears in *Comparative View*, that is, while Gregory was still at Aberdeen (see especially the first discourse, in which the faculty psychology is first laid out, and the second, in which the faculties of reason are set out). These were read before the Philosophical Society on October 11, 1758, and August 28, 1759, respectively.

19. On "enquiries into human nature" see Gregory (1772, p. 152); on *experience* see Gregory (1772, p. 14; 1821, pp. 112, 114, 141, 201, 222); on *sympathy* see Gregory (1772, pp. 19, 20; 1821, p. 192). For appeals to *common sense* see Gregory (1772, pp. 62, 141, 185, 215, 234, 193; 1765, p. 47), for *good sense* see Gregory (1765, p. 162, 169, 170, 180). For his use of faculty psychology see Gregory (1772, p. 156; 1765, pp. 1–81; 1821, p. 156).

On the virtues, for *humanity* see Gregory (1765, p. 68; 1772, pp. 12, 19, 20, 35, 36, 68, 70, 106, 108, 217, 225, 234, 236; 1821, pp. 153, 159, 175, 184, 188); for *sensibility* see Gregory (1772, pp. 8, 9, 19; 1821, pp. 161, 171, 177); and for *steadiness* see Gregory (1772, pp. 172, 175). On his use of the concept of *improvement* see Gregory (1772, pp. 108, 196, 201, 214, 216, 221, 223, 227) See also Smellie (1800, pp. 6, 7). On *sentiments see* Gregory (1765, p. 68; 1772, pp. 196, 197; 1821, pp. 154–55, 157 [where religion is grounded in sentiment rather than reason], 169, 170, 171, 174, 177, 180, 181, 182, 183, 184, 185, 187, 188, 189, 192, 193); and for *tastes* see Gregory (1765, p. 68; 1772, p. 190). On *imagination* see Gregory (1821, pp. 62, 189), and on its link to taste see Gregory (1765, p. 72).

20. See, for example, Hume (1978, Book II, Section III).

21. Gregory says:

> Reasoning properly dignifies the exercise of that power of the mind by which it infers one thing from an other, or deduces conclusions from premises. Without

the exercise of this power, we could neither act in the common affairs of life, unless when impressed in particular cases by instinct, imagination, or passion; nor advance a step in the investigation of truth, beyond self-evident principles.
(Gregory 1772, p. 147; cf. 1765, p. 14)

22. Gregory says:

The true dignity of physic is to be maintained by the superior learning and abilities of those who profess it, by the liberal manners of gentlemen, and by that openness and candour—which disdain all artifice, which invite to a free inquiry [*sic*], and thus boldly bid defiance to all that illiberal ridicule and abuse to which medicine has been so much and so long exposed.
(Gregory 1772, pp. 237–38)

23. Gregory says:

I must observe that the same objections made against any person pretending to judge of medical subjects, who has not been regularly bred in the profession, were formerly made against the reformers from Popery. Besides the divine authority claimed by the church, it was said, that a set of men, who devoted their whole time and studies to so deep and complicated a subject as theology, were the only proper judges of whatever belonged to it; that calling their authority in question was hurting the cause of religion, and lowering the sacerdotal character. Yet experience has shewn, that since that Laity have asserted their right of enquiry into these subjects, theology, considered as a science, has been improved; the real interests of religion have been promoted; and the clergy have become more learned, a more useful, and even more respectable body of men, than they ever were in the days of their greatest power and splendor.
(Gregory 1772, pp. 236–37)

24. Gregory's sophisticated consequentialism leads him to warn against too facile a use of the appeal to consequences to avoid the unpleasant duty of the physician to disclose bad news to patients. The quotation just provided continues as follows:

It sometimes happens, on the other hand, that a man is seized with a dangerous illness, who had made no settlement of his affairs, and yet perhaps the future happiness of his family may depend on his making such a settlement. In this and other similar cases it may be proper for a physician, in the most prudent and gentle manner, to give a hint to the patient of his real danger, and even solicit him to set about this necessary duty. But, in every case, it behoves a physician never to conceal the real situation of the patient from the relations. Indeed justice demands this; as it gives them an opportunity of calling for further assistance, if they should think it necessary. To a man of compassionate and feeling heart, this is one of the most disagreeable duties of the profession: but it is indispensible [*sic*]. The manner of doing it, requires equal prudence and humanity. What should reconcile him the more easily to this painful office, is the reflection that, if the patient should recover, it will prove a joyful disappointment to his friends; and if he dies, it makes the shock more gentle."

This consequence-based pro–truth telling is consistent with the Hippocratic ethic, provided the consequences are limited to those that redound to the patient. This consequentialist-based support of a policy of disclosure is seen in a more rigorous form in Percival and in more modern dress in Joseph Fletcher.

25. The advice to students is, "It had been happy, however, for mankind, if, instead of a blind admiration of Hippocrates, justly styled the father and founder of medicine, they had imbibed some portion of his spirit for observation. Hippocrates will always be held in the highest esteem, for his accurate and faithful description of diseases, for his candour, his good sense, and the simple elegance of his style. But instead of prosecuting his plan, and building on the foundation he had laid, his successors employed their time in commenting on his works (Gregory 1772, pp. 182–83).

26. In 1826, in testimony before the Commission for Visiting the Universities and Colleges of Scotland, one of the key issues was whether medical students should continue to be tested in the classical languages, particularly Greek. A regulation had recently been adopted that dropped the testing on the translation of the Hippocratic aphorism, much to the distress of Dr. Andrew Duncan, Senior, whose tenure, dating from 1789, suggests he retained some of the eighteenth-century Enlightenment ideal. Duncan's testimony before the commission is revealing: "The new Regulations admit of examinations in English, which will lead to Edinburgh degrees being conferred upon ignorant empyrics; and they abolish entirely the examination in Greek, by relinquishing the Commentary on the Aphorism [o]f Hippocrates" (Duncan, Sr., in Commission for visiting the Universities and Colleges in Scotland 1837, p. 218).

The following exchange took place between the commissioners and the current dean, Dr. William Pulteney Alison:

"Upon the subject of the preliminary University education of medical Graduate, have you occasion to know what was the opinion of your uncle Dr. Gregory?

"I cannot say exactly; I do not at present remember having conversed with him upon that subject. He was certainly very fond of classical acquirements; I would say he was more attached to them than most men of the present day are."

(Commission 1837, p. 205)

By contrast, many of the younger faculty, including Alison, who were lobbying for elimination of the classical language requirement, were aware of Gregory's reputation for an interest in Greek medicine. At a later point in the hearings, he gives the story of Gregory's interest in the classical languages a slightly different twist:

I was asked, if I knew what Dr. Gregory's opinion was in respect to some parts of the alterations that have been talked of for the Medical Degree. I have since recommended that several times he mentioned to me, he was afraid the examinations for the Medical Degree went rather too much into collateral science, that were not clearly essential to a medical man, and from that circumstance (though I have not a recollection of his having said so to me), I think that he would not have been inclined to recommend the making imperative other studies in branches of science, not more immediately connected with medicine than those in our present Curriculum. I recollect his having stated several times, that he thought medical men were often deficient in the knowledge of general reasoning, and therefore, if he had recommended any collateral scientific studies, I think he would have recommended rather Mathematics, and a little Natural Philosophy, than Natural History. I think he would have been disposed to concur in any measure which could have been thought likely to secure a more thorough knowledge of Latin to our graduates than some of them at present have; but he never made any proposal for any plan of that kind. And in regard to the knowledge of Greek, I know, from notes on his lectures (for he used always to give a few lectures on the History of Medicine), that he thought that every physician who had a wish to be considered a scholar, ought to have a general knowledge of the writings of Hippocrates; but he did not consider it essential that he should study them in the Greek. He mentioned several works, in which those opinions could be learned, both in Latin, English, and also in French. He mentioned the same in regard to the works of Galen. Therefore I may say, as far as I can judge, that I do not think he would insist on our graduates knowing Greek.

(Commission 1837, p. 248)

27. This was still the regulation in the second decade of the nineteenth century, at least up until 1818, but had been dropped by 1823, according to the available Senate regulations for the medical degree in the Commission Report appendices (1837, pp. 137–141).
28. Essentially the same idea occurs in the approved version of 1772, in which Gregory describes these lectures as "some considerations, which though not strictly belonging to my subject, yet deserve the attention of all those who would practice medicine" (Gregory 1772, p. 2).
29. Christie goes on:

Cullen's philosophical chemistry can be described as conforming with some precision to the work of Hume and Smith. The conformity may be seen in the general feature of epistemology's cognitive priority. It is seen, too, in Hume's, Smith's, and Cullen's substantive descriptions of scepticism's relationship to theory, the psychological aspect of speculation, and speculation's analogical and conjectural status. . . .

Hume's and Smith's description of moral conduct as originating in natural feeling rather than in rational assessment, and their emphasis on its social function, could quite justifiably lead to their arguments' being seen as expressions of determinism, and this was in part the cause of the deeply disturbed reactions of some contemporaries, particularly those of the first generation of common sense philosophers: Reid, Gregory, and Beattie.

(Christie 1981, pp. 93, 95–96)

30. James Gregory says:

It is very remarkable, and not easily to be accounted for in a satisfactory manner, that long after the precepts of Bacon were generally known, and even after the example of Newton had fully explained those precepts, and had shewn how just and important they were, almost every Metaphysician would still persist in making discoveries in his science. Leibnitz [sic], though a man of uncommon talents and very extensive knowledge, and an excellent mathematician, and well versed in physical science was unluckily a great discoverer in metaphysics. . . . Berkeley and Hume followed the same plan of discovery in metaphysics with still greater diligence, and proportionable success. Dr. Priestley, and many others of less note, have followed nearly the same plan. . . .

Let it be remembered, however, for the honour of human reason, that before Dr Priestley had begun his discoveries in metaphysics, and before Dr. Reid had exposed to deserved contempt the discoveries of preceding Metaphysicians, there had been at least one author who had so much good sense, and such just notions of science, as to perceive and to explain clearly the futility of such discoveries. I mean Mons. D'Alembert. . . .

(James Gregory 1792, pp. liv–lvi)

31. Compare the following attacks on Hume and Reid as well as most of the rest of the history of philosophy:

I understand but very little of the medical system of Galen, and still less of the writings of Paracelsus; and not much more of the physics and the metaphysics of Aristotle and of Mr Hume; and I am not in the least sorry for it: nor do I wish to understand any more of them; for judging of the whole from the part which I do understand, I presume with confidence, that if it were all intelligible, it would not be worth understanding.

(James Gregory 1792, p. clxx)

It appears to me, that Dr Reid, and many philosophers who have thought and argued nearly as he hath done on this point, have gone just as far wrong on one side as Mr. Hume, Dr Priestley, and Mr Leibniz, or in general, all assertors of the doctrine of Necessity, have done on the other.

(James Gregory 1792, pp. ccxii)

32. It seems that a pamphlet came to be published apparently under a pseudonym advising students on the qualities of the various professors in the medical school. Although Gregory fared reasonably well (based on his own quotations from the infamous pamphlet [James Gregory 1793]), he considered the account of his course inadequate and the treatment of some of his colleagues even worse. Noting that all the professors except his colleague Alexander Hamilton, the professor of midwifery, were treated in a manner Gregory considered harsh, Gregory accused Hamilton and his son James, who was also a physician and eventually to be professor of midwifery, of writing the review. He demanded consideration by the academic senate, which established a committee and, as with many academic squabbles, found that there was not enough evidence to conclude that either Hamilton was the author. Unsatisfied, Gregory pursued his colleague even further, by now evoking the wrath of all eventually generating the lawsuit (James Gregory 1793).

CHAPTER 2

1. Undoubtedly, similar changes were occurring among educated women, but the impact on professional careers and the thought processes of those who pursued them is necessarily still primarily a story of males in the eighteenth and nineteenth centuries.
2. This summary of the Monros is based primarily on Alexander Monro Primus's "Life of Dr. Are. Monro Sr. in His Own Handwriting," unpublished manuscript in the collection of the Medical Library of the University of Otago, New Zealand. The manuscript copy in that library is often difficult to read. Fortunately, a published version appears in Erlam (1954), where the full text of the Monro manuscript is reprinted with great care and is accompanied by a helpful introduction. There is some question as to whether Monro, Primus, wrote the original manuscript. There is no author's name on the manuscript, only references to A.M. and P.M. (Alexander Monro and Professor Monro) throughout. Nevertheless, it is generally accepted that the biography did indeed come

from Monro's own hand. The binder carries the title "Life of Monro by himself" (although it is not clear when that was written). The handwriting appears to match that of other Monro, Primus, manuscripts in the collection (see Erlam 1954). Two other major sources are Monro, Alexander Secundus (1781) and Monro (1996). Other sources that are helpful in constructing the lives of the Monros include Moore (1894), Lawrence (1985, 1988a, 1988b), and Hamilton (1988).

3. The son, writing in the third person, described the trauma of the events: his father

> obliged him to give publick Lectures soon after he received his Commission and without his Knowledge prevailed on the President and Fellows of the College of Physicians and the Deacon of the Surgeons with his Brethren to honour the first days Demonstration with their Presence—This unexpected Company put the young Teacher into such Confusion as to make him sensible that his Memory would fail in repeting the words of the Discourse which he had mandated, and therefor beginning with the Demonstration of some Parts from the Structure of which he was to prelect [*sic*], he endeavoured to recover himself, but found still his Memory as to words fail and therefor resolved to lay aside all Attention to those which he had wrote and to express himself in such as should first occurr to express his Meaning.
>
> (Erlam 1954, pp. 82–83)

4. Norman Moore's biography of Alexander Monro, Primus, states that he studied at the University in Edinburgh and graduated from there with an M.D. degree, but this did not occur until 1756, when Primus was nearing the end of his career. Monro mentions that early in his career he had contemplated studying medicine in addition to surgery, but "He also laid aside the Design of becoming Physician by the advice of some Friends, whose Opinion he had great regard for, and who through the Business he then had as Surgeon-Apothecary was more lucrative than was to be expected by him as a Physician so young" (Erlam 1954, p. 84). In a recent publication, a descendent of Monro includes biographical information in which he states that Monro attended classes at Edinburgh in 1616 and 1617, and refers to receipt of an M.D. degree, an event not mentioned in Monro's own account of his life (Monro 1996, p. x). Although an occasional medical degree was awarded by Edinburgh before there was a medical faculty, there is no mention of awarding such a degree to any Alexander Monro in the Laureation book, which has recorded the signature of every graduate of the university since its founding in 1585 (Edinburgh, University of). Moreover, Monro, himself (assuming, as is usually done, that he is the author of the manuscript biography examined in Dunedin) never mentioned attending the university (Erlam 1954). He did mention studying for brief periods in London, Paris, and Leyden, but not at Edinburgh.

5. Only one title strays even the slightest from the science of anatomy: "Histories of successful indulgence of bad habits in patients" (Monro 1781, pp. 635–6). This is a delightful account of cases in which he had treated broken bones of patients who apparently had rather heavy drinking habits. His usual advice was illustrated by the second case, in which he reported, "I ordered him to have no drink given him, except water and milk, water-gruel, or such like." The result was that the patient reported complaints of headache, quick pulse, and thirst. A similar patient complained of fainting and sickness to the stomach. He apparently had iatrogenically produced delirium tremens commonly experienced by chronic alcoholics, which was cured when a family member prevailed on him to permit more usual doses of alcohol. This was about as far away from scientific publication as Monro strayed during an illustrious career as the leading

anatomist of his day and the single most important figure in the development of the Edinburgh medical school.

6. A newly published critical edition of the *Essay* makes access easier. See Monro (1996).

7. Monro does occasionally use the language of contemporaneous moral philosophy. For example, in his advice to his daughter he says, "Shun thus not only every thing that has a tendency to Cruelty but encourage the contrary Principle, indulge that Sympathy which Humanity prompts us to have for our Fellow Creatures in distress, enjoy frequently the glorious laudable Pleasure of relieving and assisting the afflicted" (Monro 1996, p. 40). The terminology of *sympathy* and *humanity* was so much a fabric of the society in which he lived that it is not surprising that these terms found their way into his moral language. P. A. G. Monro, the descendent of Primus who has recently published an edition of the "Essay on Female Conduct" and written an approving, detailed introduction, reflects on whether Monro was cognizant of the work of Hutcheson or other thinkers of the era: "Similarly, although the Scottish Enlightenment is now supposed to have started with Francis Hutcheson's anonymous publications from Dublin in 1725, there is nothing to suggest in *Primus's* ms. that he was aware of these, and although certainly enlightened, he borrowed nothing here. Indeed it is very difficult to identify the source of many of *Primus's* ideas; I believe that most were his own, and when similar to others', they were much better argued" (Monro 1996, p. 195; see also p. 200) P. A. G. Monro seems to be saying in a nice way that Monro was not familiar with the thought of philosophers of his time.

8. There is also a brief mention in Monro's *Life* of regular weekly dinner meetings at the home of university president Ferguson, with Dr. John Clerk, the president of the Royal College of Physicians, and Mr. Maclaurin, professor of mathematics, of whom Monro speaks fondly. They discussed "most of the sciences and parts of literature" (Erlam 1954, p. 103). Here Monro mentions that during these conversations, "Newton, Leibniz, Clerk and most of the Philosophers were attacked and defended." Once again, there are hints that Monro was close to discussions of the philosophers, but it seems unlikely that a conversation among the university president and two physicians and a mathematician really brought Monro to a sophisticated understanding of the contemporary debate in moral philosophy.

9. A question remains to be settled about whether all of the books in his library were sent to New Zealand. It appears that they were not. Monro himself says that when he returned to the family estate at retirement, one side of a particular room was formed into book cases where he put all his books except those of "Physick," that is, medicine. It appears that it was the medical portion that eventually was sent to New Zealand. The key question is what was in the nonmedical portion. We can only speculate, given Monro's expressed fields of interest. These included "subjects as could be applyed practically to the Utility and advantage of the Community" (Erlam 1954, p. 98). He particularly names interests in "uncommon machines or manufactory, Curiousities of Nature and Antiquity, handsome Houses well laid out Gardens or Grounds, or in short of anything he was unacquainted with." He expressed an interest in Mechanicks, experiments in farming, and advice on how to cultivate a field, but he never included philosophy when delineating these interests. In discussing the section of his essay for his daughter on religion, he specifically says he is "more than superficial tho' without metaphysicks" (Erlam 1954, p. 98). That the Newton volume went with the "medical collection" suggests that philosophical aspects of science were included with medicine. Although Reid would have been added to the collection later, by the time it was sent to New Zealand, there was apparently no other group of philosophical books with which Reid could be included.

10. M316 in the Taylor catalogue.
11. M153 in the Taylor catalogue.
12. M129–130 in the Taylor catalogue.
13. M131 in the Taylor catalogue.
14. M107–111 in the Taylor catalogue.
15. M139 in the Taylor catalogue.
16. When one sees the size of the volume, it is not surprising that it took 11 years to publish the full transcript.
17. Alison was "conjoint professor" with the more senior man, Dr. Andrew Duncan, Senior (Commission for visiting the Universities and Colleges in Scotland 1837, p. 218). It was the custom to appoint a junior person as conjoint professor as the senior man was reaching retirement age. In Duncan, Senior's testimony he says, "The truth is, I am an old man, and I have not attended much to the business of the Faculty of late" (Commission 1837, p. 219). His son, Andrew Duncan, Junior, following the pattern of nepotism we have seen previously, was at the time professor of materia medica. He gives much more detailed and valuable insights into the faculty of the day (Commission 1837, pp. 219–227). It was the practice that the duty of dean was given to the most junior member of the faculty, "having more trouble than any other" (Commission 1837, p. 191).
18. The testimony of four additional professors, called Regius professors because they were appointed by the king rather than the town council, were also taken. They included the professors of military surgery, clinical surgery, medical jurisprudence, and natural history. They were not technically part of the medical faculty, but were regularly involved in the students' medical education. There appeared to be considerable tension between the regular faculty and the Regius professors. For example, only the regular faculty examined students for graduation. Since the students paid a fee that was then divided among the examining professors, more was at stake than merely the prestige of faculty membership (Commission 1837, p. 234).
19. Alison summarized the justification for more practical medical training and less humanities education as follows:

> I think the fairest way of stating the result of my own observations, and also the observations of those with whom I have been able to consult upon the subject, is, that, as regards our graduates when they go into the world, a great many of them succeed very well, but they are *oftener* surpassed in practice by men who are their inferiors, than by those who are their superiors in point of general literature and science—I will say *much oftener.* . . . The leaning of the public is decidedly favourable to practical rather than literary or scientific attainments in medical men.
>
> (Commission 1837, p. 194)

20. The exchange between Alison and the commissioner went as follows:

> "Is it your opinion, and also the opinion of the Faculty of Medicine, that no literary qualification should be required before taking a degree, other than the knowledge of Latin and a little French, which you said you would suggest?"
>
> "I think I would require a knowledge of French, Latin, and Mathematics. I do not say that I would go farther than that."
>
> (Commission 1837, p. 203)

21. During the latter part of Stewart's tenure as professor of moral philosophy, Thomas Brown held the position conjointly. There is no evidence of his linking of moral philosophy with medicine. He was a physician, but may be among the nineteenth-century physicians who could gain expertise in moral philosophy simultaneously while practicing medicine without seeing any connection between the two. We will see another conspicuous example of this in Duncan Macgregor, who played a fascinating role in the founding of the University of Otago in New Zealand. That story will be told in Chapter 5.

22. This conclusion seems compatible with Christopher Lawrence's conclusion:

> By 1800 the shared and uniquely Scottish account of the body, which described the nervous system as binding the organism together by sympathy, had disappeared. . . . In place of a common model teachers and practitioners employed a variety of English and, later, French ideas. At least one of the reasons for this medical fragmentation was the expanding power of the surgeons, who in some instances aligned themselves with the local Scottish landed interest but in others identified with a wider surgical *profession*.
>
> (Lawrence 1988b, p. 262)

Lawrence goes on to say the following:

> The forty years 1790–1830 saw the draining of power and patronage from the old order of physicians, lawyers, landed gentry and literati. New social groups, or newly powerful old ones, had interests which often conflicted with those of the 'Old Thing.'. . . By the 1830s, overt reform in politics as well as medicine in Edinburgh was only the vestigial sign of a collapse of the culture that had created a Scottish Enlightenment seventy years before. 'Old Edinburgh', as Cockburn put it, 'was no more'.
>
> (Lawrence 1988b, p. 278)

23. The first three volumes (as they pertain to medical students, who were listed separately beginning in 1897), some of which are now in very fragile condition, are entitled *Record University of Edinburgh Laureations and Degrees 1585 to 1809, Record University of Edinburgh Laureations and Degrees 1810 to 1896,* and *University of Edinburgh: Record of Degrees in Medicine, 1897–1953.* The final volume, which is still currently used, entitled *University of Edinburgh: Record of Degrees in Medicine 1954–; Degrees in Dental Surgery, 1954–; Degrees in Veterinary Medicine and Surgery, 1957–1964; Degrees in Medical Sciences, 1966–. Registry Office, University of Edinburgh,* is in the Registry Office. I am grateful to the staff of the special collections of the library and the Registry Office for helpful assistance in gaining access to these volumes.

24. The full text appears in the first volume of the Laureation book (Edinburgh, University of, Vol. 1) above Cockburn's name and is reprinted in an 1846 compendium of all medical school graduates up to that time. See "Nomina Eorum . . ." (1846, p. v).

25. At several places in the books, the sponsio is not redrafted for each signature, but signatures are appended, apparently still conveying affirmation of the sponsio above their names. In later years this pattern becomes routine with the sponsio being written once for each class.

26. The text appears written in Latin in long-hand for each class and is reprinted in "Nomina Eorum . . . ," 1846, p. v.

27. This translation is from the current Laureation book used by the university, which first included an English translation in the book in 1962. Since the included translation is from a copy pasted in the book, signed by a graduate who graduated in absentia, it is possible that the English translation existed on separate sheets prior to this time, but there is no record of the translation in the book until this year.

28. The only change from 1762 until 1995 is that at some point along the way, what was referred to as the Edinburgh Academy (Academiam Edinburgeanam) became the University of Edinburgh (Universitatem). Starting in 1968, only the English version is used.

29. The commission elaborated:

> There are considerable numbers almost every season of a more advanced age than the general body of the class; there are young men from the country in narrow circumstances who have not been able to get a regular early education, and they do not come up to town until 16 . . . and most frequently they are not so far advanced, and not so accurately taught with regard to the elements of the languages [as] those younger boys who have been at preparatory academies.
>
> (Commission 1837, p. 80)

30. Dr. James Hamilton, Junior, Professor of the Theory and Practice of Midwifery, also expressed concern that medical students were too young, testifying, "those who are inhabitants of the city attend a great deal too soon. . . . [T]here were so many young men applying for degrees, under twenty-one, that a regulation was made, some years ago, that no man should have a degree until he was twenty-one, which is a perfect evidence of the youth of the nature students; but we have them of all ages here" (Commission 1837, p. 311). In London at the College of Surgeons the minimum age was 22 (Commission 1837, p. 206).

31. Alison gave the following testimony on preparation for the medical profession:

> It has been said by some that the medical profession ought to have a more aristocratic form than it has at present in this country, and that this might be given by the degree in the University being made to require a greater outlay of time and expense than it does just now, and by the graduate in the University acquiring in return a higher rank in society. But we conceive the idea that that could be done by University education, is attributing more to education in the University than experience entitles us to suppose it can do for medical men. In former times regular instruction in the fundamental branches of the Medical science was rare and not easily obtained; and those men who had a regular instruction in Anatomy and the other fundamental branches of Medicine were few in number, and they formed a kind of aristocracy; but from the education being now more generally and easily obtained, we conceive it as merely a visionary speculation to suppose that it is in the power of the University but any education it can give, to confer this distinction at once upon medical men.
>
> (Commission 1837, p. 193)

32. The exchange between the commission and Dunbar continued:

> "In the examinations for Medical Degrees, is there any inquiry as to their literary qualifications, apart from their medical knowledge?"

"I fancy not further than their knowledge of the Latin language, and such literary knowledge as many come under their consideration in connection with the various branches of the study, such as Chemistry and Botany, &c.,; there is no specific examinations as to literary qualification."

(Commission 1837, pp. 83–84)

33. As the dean put so bluntly, he would have liked very much

to make the qualifications for the medical degree higher, and likewise to make the examination such that no man should ever become Doctor of Medicine in this University without much greater attainments in literature and science than they at present possess. But if we could not at the same time secure that these men, with this degree and this increase in learning, should be practitioners of Medicine, neither the University, nor the medical profession, more the public at large, would benefit by the change. . . . [T]he only rule we can go by is to adjust the supply to the demand among the public. . . .

[I]f it were found that our graduates, after a more expensive education than they have now, and after the acquisition of a good deal more literature and science, were continually passed in practice by men whose education had been cheaper, and who did not pretend to any attainments, but those which were merely professional, the consequence would be, that our degree would become unpopular; we should lose, and the public would not gain by the change. . . . The leaning of the public is decidedly favourable to practical rather than literary or scientific attainments in medical men.

(Commission 1837, pp. 193–94)

CHAPTER 3

1. Biographical information on Wesley comes from Abelove (1990), Armstrong (1973), Ayling (1979), Baker (1970), Brantley (1984) Edwards (1933), Eli (1993), Hill (1958), Holifield (1986), Rogal (1983), Shepherd (1966), Vanderpool (1986) and Wilder (1978), as well as Wesley's journals and other primary sources. Ayling and Baker are authoritative and relied upon when there is disagreement among sources. For Wesley's primary works I had access to both the Jackson (1958) and Oxford (1975ff.) editions.
2. The most recent edition, begun in 1975 as the Oxford edition, is not yet complete, but is projected to be 34 volumes.
3. An account of the full 50 volumes as well as the definitive bibliography of works by Wesley is still Green (1896). For a more recent and thorough bibliography of the secondary literature see Jarboe (1987).
4. I made use of the first edition (Wesley 1747) at the Wellcome Institute library, as well as the twenty-first edition (Wesley 1785), a copy of which I possess. Many other editions were also consulted. (The Welcome Institute library holds 24 different editions, all but one from the eighteenth or nineteenth centuries.) However, for our purposes, the key text is the preface, which appeared in the first edition and has been reprinted in all editions since.
5. Arminianism is a doctrine attributed to Jakob Arminius (1559–1609), a Dutch theologian who held that, once God gave humans initial grace, they were capable of doing good works. It is a major competitor to the Calvinist doctrine of predestination.
6. As Wesley put it:

Physicians now began to be had in admiration, as persons who were something more than Human. And Profit attended their employ as well as Honour; so that they had now two weighty reasons, for keeping the bulk of Mankind at a distance, that they might not pry into the Mysteries of the Profession. To this end they increased those Difficulties by Design, which began in a manner of Accident. They fill'd their writings with abundance of Technical Terms, utterly unintelligible to plain Men. They affected to deliver their Rules, and to reason upon them, in an abstruse, and philosophical manner.

(Wesley 1747, pp. x–xi)

7. Showing nuance, Wesley equivocated somewhat on mercury (quicksilver):

It is because they are not safe, but extremely dangerous, that I have omitted (together with Antimony) the four *Herculean* medicines, Opium, the Bark, Steel, and most of the preparations of Quicksilver. *Herculean* indeed! Far too strong for common men to grapple with. How many fatal effects have these produced, even in the hands of no ordinary Physicians! With regard to four of these, the influences are glaring and undeniable. and whereas Quicksilver, the fifth, is in its native form as innocent as bread or water: has not the art been discovered, so to *prepare* it, as to make it the most deadly of all poisons?

(Wesley 1785, pp. xvii–xviii)

Again, showing his subtlety, he added an asterisk to his condemnation of opium, bark, and steel, saying, "except in a very few cases."

8. Somewhat later in his life, Wesley had an admiring relation with the Swiss physician S. A. A. D. Tissot, whose practical advocacy of simple, healthful practices was written as advice to people when no physician was available. Wesley arranged to have the English translation of the second edition of Tissot's volume printed together with his *Primitive Physick* (Tissot 1769). This version of Wesley's volume also went through many editions, both before and after his death. Several, including the eighth edition of 1810, are available in the Wellcome Institute library in London. Even when reprinting an ally, Wesley was not above criticism, as, for example, when Tissot advocated bleeding. Wesley observed, "some would esteem as such, his violent fondness for *bleeding*; his recommending it on the most trifling occasions; and prescribing very frequent repetitions of it, as indispensibly [*sic*] necessary in several diseases, which may be perfectly cured, without ever bleeding at all" (Tissot 1769, p. iv). Wesley also condemned his use of "glyfers" (i.e., enemas), Peruvian bark, and "that uncleanly, stinking ointment, which he prescribes for the cure of the itch" (Tissot 1769, pp. iv–v).

9. Hawes registered the following complaint of Wesley:

This representation of the gentlemen of the faculty may possibly not be thought very candid, nor very equitable: and if Mr. Wesley's character and conduct, as a divine, a politician, and a practitioner in physic, were to be examined with the same degree of candour that he hath exercised towards others, he would certainly not appear in the most advantageous light. At least it would be manifest, that he was far enough from *perfection*, though that is a doctrine for which he is well known to be a very zealous advocate. . . . But however uncandid, unfair, or unjust, Mr. Wesley's representation of the gentlemen of the faculty may be, it seemed necessary to promote the sale of his *Primitive Physic*.

(Hawes 1776, pp. iii–iv).

10. The original edition is dated 1761. The edition I consulted at the Wellcome Institute was published in 1771, bound together with an edition of his *Primitive Physick*.

11. Wesley reflected on the possible mechanism of electricity in treatment:

> But still one may upon the whole pronounce it the *desideratum*, the general and rarely failing remedy, in nervous Cases of every kind (Palsies excepted); as well as in many others. Perhaps if the nerves are really perforated (as is now generally supposed) the electric ether is the only fluid in the universe, which is fine enough to move through them. And what if the *nervous juice* itself, be a fluid of this kind? if so, it is no wonder that it has always eluded the search of the most accurate naturalists.
>
> (Wesley 1771, p. vi)

12. The editor of the nineteenth-century edition of Wesley's *Works* added footnotes translating the Latin, something not needed and not appearing in the original. For *quanta de spe decidel!* he translated "From how great expectations am I fallen!" For *ad Græas calendas* he supplied "At no future time" (Wesley 1958, Vol. 14, p. 243).

13. The endorsement of electricity immediately following his exposure to it in the late 1750s is also seen in his 1760 addendum to the "Preface" of his *Primitive Physick*, which covers the period of five years since his previous additions to his prefatory comments:

> In this course of time I have likewise had occasion to collect several other Remedies, tried either by myself or others, which are inserted under their proper heads. Some of these I have found to be of uncommon virtue, equal to any of these which were before published; and one, I must aver, from personal knowledge, grounded on a thousand experiments, to be far superior to all the other medicines I have known; I mean *Electricity*. I cannot but intreat all those who are well-wishers to mankind, to make full proof of this. Certainly it comes the nearest an universal medicine, of any yet known in the world.
>
> (Wesley 1785, p. xix)

14. Gisborne's biographical information is taken from Leslie (1886) and Porter (1993).

15. It should be noted that Gisborne used the title that approximates the unauthorized 1770 edition of Gregory, not the more polished 1772 version that speaks not of "duties and offices" but of "duties and qualifications." Even though Gisborne refers to Gregory's "Lectures," thus using the 1772 appellation rather than the 1770 term "Observations," it is clear that Gisborne was actually using the 1770 text. In a section to be discussed below, he quotes Gregory's "Lectures," giving the wording from the 1770 edition (that is, from the "Observations") and citing the page number that is appropriate for it. He cites page 45, while the comparable passage in the 1772 *Lectures* is on pages 47–48.

16. It is this quotation that provides definitive evidence that Gisborne was using Gregory's 1770 *Observations*, not his endorsed and more polished 1772 *Lectures*. Not only does the page reference match the 1770 edition, the wording does as well. In the 1772 version, several words are edited. For example, in the 1772 text, "pain and indignation" is changed to read simply "indignation." None of the word changes makes a significant difference, however. The only change in the text that Gisborne makes is in punctuation and capitalization.

17. The biographical details of Percival's life are based primarily on the "Memoirs" by Edward Percival (1807). More recent sources base their accounts, either directly or indirectly, on this biography (see Nicholson 1937–38; Pellegrino 1986, Baker 1993,

Pickstone 1993, and Haakonssen 1997). The Haakonssen study is a particularly useful examination of the sociocultural context of the environment surrounding the writings of Gregory, Percival, and Benjamin Rush.

18. John Wesley was known to have visited Warrington in 1768 and 1772, among other
times (McLachlan 1943, p. 83).

19. This paragraph is based on the historical research of McLachlan (1943, pp. 39–45)
and Haakonssen (1997, pp. 96–107). Bright (1859), upon which McLachlan draws,
was also consulted.

20. In 1760, just the time when Percival would have been studying with Taylor, Taylor published two pamphlets as guides to his students: "An Examination of Dr. Hutcheson's
Scheme of Morality" and "A Sketch of Moral Philosophy" (McLachlan 1943,
p. 45). Taylor was influenced by William Wollaston's *Religion of Nature Delin-
eated* (1724).

21. The exact length of Percival's stay in Leyden is not known, but he did not turn 25
until September 29 of that year. If he was 25 when he went to Leyden, as his son
states, he actually received his degree at least two months before he arrived.

22. These public health essays reveal the societal orientation common to many eighteenth-
and nineteenth-century utilitarians. The subjects are revealed through the following
titles: *Observations on the State of Population in Manchester, and Other Adjacent
Places* (Percival 1773b); *Further Observations on the State of Population in Manchester, etc.* (Percival 1774a); *On the Disadvantages Which Attend the Inoculation of Children in Early Infancy* (Percival 1768b); *Experiments and Observations on Water;
Particularly on the Hard Pump Water of Manchester* (Percival 1769); *Observations
and Experiments on the Poison of Lead* (Percival 1774b); *Thoughts on Hospitals/ with
a letter to the author* (Percival 1771); and *Experiments on the Peruvian Bark* (Percival
1768a). At least three of these public health–oriented essays have commanded recent
interest, as seen by the reprinting of "Observations on the State of Population in
Manchester" and "Essay on the Small-pox and Measles" in *Population and Disease
in Early Industrial England* (1973). These are, in fact, photographic reproductions
from a 1789 reprinting of the two population essays, to which a "concluding section"
was appended by Percival together with the small pox essay (Percival 1789). For a
recent secondary review of Percival's role in public health efforts see Howard (1975).

23. Like many others discussed in this chapter (including Wesley and Gisborne), Percival
was a zealous supporter of the antislavery movement, having participated in the presentation of the Manchester "Petition to Parliament for the Abolition of the Slave-
Trade." He based his position on the natural-law arguments he learned from reformers
in Scottish universities and the dissenting academies (E. Percival [1807], pp. lxxxiv–
lxxxv; see also Haakonssen [1807], p. 110). He corresponded with both Beattie and
Robertson on the issue.

24. I had access to several editions, but have cited the 1807 edition throughout.

25. The key text reads

> Mr. Hume seems to ascribe *belief* entirely to our *experience* of the truth of the tes-
> timony. But belief is a fundamental principle in human nature, of the most extensive
> importance, and manifests itself in the earliest periods of life, being the necessary
> antecedent to knowledge, which may serve either to confirm or reject it.
>
> (T. Percival 1807, p. 340)

26. Percival embeds his critique of Paley in a continued criticism of Hume:

I dwelt long on Mr. Hume's essay concerning Miracles, because I well know the impression which it makes on the minds of young persons; and recollect that at an early period of my own life, it staggered for a while my faith in Christianity. Indeed the influence which this pleasing and ingenious writer has had over the opinions of mankind, not only on subjects of religion, but of ethics and politics, has been extensive in a very remarkable degree. His principle of *utility*, which he makes the rule of moral duty, has obtained almost universal currency first as a force by himself; then as sanctioned, though on different grounds, by Dr. Paley, under the denomination of *expediency*; and afterwards as enlarged, and carried to all its extravagant and injurious consequences by Mr. Godwin, in his Enquiry into *Justice*. The History of England by Mr. Hume is so interesting, philosophical, and instructive, that it has nearly superseded every other; and has effected a considerable change in the public mind, with respect to various constitutional points of great importance. Yet this work has been shewn to abound in prejudiced and partial representations. . . . It systematically exaggerates the oppressive government of the Tudors, to extenuate the arbitrary conduct of the Stuarts. And such is the attachment of the author to his political hypothesis, that in the Memoirs of his own Life, he thus expresses himself: 'I was so little inclined to yield to the senseless clamour of the Whigs, that in above a hundred alterations which farther study, reading, or reflection engaged me to make in the reigns of the two first Stuarts, I have made *all of them invariably to the Tory side*.' This fact marks a pertinacious adherence to his prepossessions: for it is almost morally impossible, actuated as he was by the spirit of party, that all his mistakes should have been confined to one side of a disputed question; or have proved uniformly unjust to the cause he so warmly espoused.

(T. Percival 1807, pp. 346–47)

27. Edward Percival made the following comment on this section: "The Discourse forms the first part of a plan which he has long had in contemplating, of teaching his elder children the most important branches of Ethics, viz. *veracity, faithfulness, justice, and benevolence*, in systematic and experimental manner, by examples" (E. Percival 1807, p. lxiii)

28. Among the members of the Literary and Philosophical Society was Thomas Barnes, Percival's friend from the Warrington Academy days, who was to become the Academy's professor of divinity.

29. For a sample of this active correspondence see Edward Percival (1807): *From James Beattie, LL.D. to Dr. Percival Aberdeen. Dec. 24, 1786* (p. cxix); *From Dr. Franklin to Dr. Percival Passy, near Paris. July 17, 1784* (p. cxiv); *From Dr. Beattie to Dr. Percival Aberdeen. Jan. 29, 1788* (p. xxviii); *From Dr. Percival to Dr. Beattie, Manchester. Feb. 1788* (p. cxxxii); *From the Same [Percival], to the Rev. Archdeacon Paley. Manchester, June 20, 1788* (p. cxlvi); *From the Rev. Archdeacon Paley to Dr. Percival. Carlisle, June 25, 1788* (p. cxlvi); *From Dr. Percival to Dr. Priestley. Manchester, Sept. 27, 1788* (p. clii).

30. Edward was the second of Thomas's sons to carry that name. The first, Edward Bayley Percival, died before age two of hooping cough and acute asthma on May 25, 1780. The date of the second Edward's birth is uncertain, but some sources suggest 1783. *Bayley* is probably taken from Thomas Butterworth Bayley, Percival's closest friend at Edinburgh and a student of Adam Smith's philosophy.

31. I used the copy that once belonged to Edinburgh philosopher Dugald Stewart, whom we met in Chapter 1. It is presently in the rare book collection of the University of Edinburgh. It is inscribed, "For Professor Dugald Stewar . . . , With Dr. Percival's very frien . . . respects." (The ellipses indicate the edge of trimmed pages. The volume is rebound and appears to have been trimmed at rebinding, as has occurred in other volumes in the Stewart library.) Several later editions were also consulted, including the 1827 version and the 1849 version, both of which were used at the library of the Wellcome Institute in London. The 1827 edition has been edited by an unidentified editor who observes in the preface that "this work, *so much wanted at the present time*, in a separate form, has long since been out of print, and a continued demand for it, could not be supplied. The Publisher, desirous to comply with the wishes of the profession, has brought out the present edition, which the writer of this article was chosen to edite [*sic*]" (Percival 1827, p. xvii). The editor goes on to point out that the appendices have been omitted, including "supplementary notes and illustrations, of a miscellaneous kind, by the Rev. T. Gisborne, M.A. &c. and author of an enquiry into the Duties of Man" (Percival 1827, p. xic). The editor observes that "much is familiar to the public, or no longer consonant to public taste" (Percival 1827, p. xx).

  In the 1849 edition, which is labeled the "third edition," the editor observes aggressively, "a new edition was published in 1827, but the editor's notes are of such a nature as to render the book absolutely mischievous" (Percival 1849, p. 1, note b). The editor of the 1849 edition, by contrast, conveys in his preface his attempt to be faithful to the original:

  As the late Dr. Percival's Code of Medical ethics is commonly quoted as a work of authority, not only in this country, but also in America[a] and the original edition[b] has now become somewhat scarce, it was thought that it might be usefully republished.

  The present edition is reprinted from that published by Dr. Percival himself, (8vo. Manchester, [2]1803,) corrected occasionally by his unfinished and unpublished edition,[c] and also by the posthumous reprint contained in vol. ii of his collected 'Works,' (94 vols. 8v0. Bath 1807.) The references have been verified, and in several instances the quotations have been corrected, but no other alteration has been made in the *text* of the work; as, even when the statements contained in it were positively erroneous, the Editor preferred correcting them (where necessary,) in a note. Of the Notes and Illustrations added by Dr. Percival several have been omitted, as being no longer wanted, as also has the 'Discourse on Hospital Duties' by his son.

                                                                                                          (Percival 1849, pp. 1–3)

The editor of the 1849 English edition, in another footnote, makes clear he is aware of the influence of Percival's *Medical Ethics* in America (Percival 1849, p. 1, note a).

  In the United States an edition called *Extracts from the Medical Ethics of Thomas Percival* was printed in 1821 in Lexington, Kentucky, and again in 1823 in Philadelphia (Percival 1823). (The 1823 edition exists in the College of Physicians library in Philadelphia. I have not personally examined the 1821 Kentucky edition. It is reported by Baker 1993, p. 209.) The next edition did not appear until 1927 when Chauncey Leake produced an edition. That version also contains significant omissions and textual errors. It was reprinted in 1975 without any changes. In 1985, Edmund Pellegrino produced a photographic reproduction of the original 1803 edition together with a

substantial introduction. I used that edition for checking certain citations after returning to the United States from Edinburgh. Finally, an edition described as containing
excerpts was reprinted in 1987 (Percival 1987). For a history of the various editions
see Baker (1993, p. 209).

32. A copy is in the library of the College of Physicians and Surgeons in Philadelphia.
The editor of the 1849 edition had access to a copy. He notes the following:

> Of this rare volume the only copy that the editor has seen or heard of is in the
> library of the Manchester Royal Infirmary, and was given by Dr. Percival him-
> self. In the beginning there is a following Note in his own handwriting:—'The
> completion of the Medical Jurisprudence has been long suspended; and it is un-
> certain when the undertaking will be resumed.' A title-page; and introduction; a
> fifth and sixth section; and an appendix, containing Notes and Illustrations, are
> wanting to finish *Manchester, March* 17, 1794. It ends abruptly on p. 96, which
> terminates chap. iv. The text for the most part agrees with that which was after-
> wards published, except that this latter contains about twenty paragraphs that are
> not to be found in the original sketch, and that great part of what forms Note XIV.
> in the present edition is there found in the *text*. At the end of the treatise there is
> the following Note, also in Dr. Percival's own hand-writing:—'Two sections
> wanting. Sect. V. On the Powers, Privileges, Honours, and Emoluments of the
> faculty. Sect. VI. On the Moral, Religious, and Political Character of Physicians.
> (Percival 1849, p. 2, note c)

33. In the passage quoted, Aiken reflects the current consensus that the purpose of the hospital was to cure the working population quickly so they could return to work. He also
makes clear that he is concerned about what we would call iatrogenic illness: "Inbred
disease of hospitals will almost inevitably creep, in some degree, upon one who continue a long time in them, but will rarely attack one, whose stay is short"
(Dr. [John] Aiken [Jr]'s Thoughts on Hospitals, p. 21, quoted in Percival 1803, p. 17).

34. In addition, the volume contains two dedications. The first (p. v) is to Sir George Baker,
Bart. "physician to their majesties; fellow of the Royal Society, and Late President of
the College of Physicians." Percival notes that the book has been "honoured with his
sanction, and improved by his communications, is gratefully and respectfully inscribed,
by his obliged and affectionate friend." The second is to E. C. Percival, i.e., his son
Edward, who was studying medicine at Edinburgh. In the spirit of the eighteenth-
century writings of fathers to their children, he says of the writings that he will "claim
the privilege of consecrating them to you, as a paternal legacy" (Percival 1803, p. x).

35. For Gregory's influence on Percival see Baker (1993, pp. 193–98), Haakonssen (1997,
pp. 134–36), and McCullough (1998, pp. 274–76).

36. For references to Bacon see Percival (1803, pp. 3, 87, 88, 97, 111, 172, 200, 201,
205, 221). There are but two mentions of Locke, one where Locke's views on justifiable homicide against an aggressor are quoted (p. 72), and the previously mentioned
note on physicians as sceptics and infidels where Percival notes that before his death
Locke received the sacrament according to the rites of the Church of England. It is
also here that Thomas Brown is referenced (Percival 1803, pp. 182, 183, 186).

37. Montesquieu is quoted on the importance of punishment being appropriate to the of-
fense and again in the dueling note (Percival 1803, pp. 85, 216–17). Franklin makes
an important appearance in Percival's *Medical Ethics* in the dueling note as well where
Percival inserts a 1784 letter he received from Franklin in which Franklin acknowl-

edges Percival's recent letter and "the most agreeable present of your new book." Franklin goes on to speak of dueling, "which you so justly condemn" (Percival 1803, p. 226).

38. However, a contemporary of Percival and one of the most famous utilitarians of all time, Jeremy Bentham, does not seem to have been in Percival's conversation. Bentham's "An Introduction to the Principles of Morals and Legislation" appeared in 1789.

39. In fact, Pickstone (1993, p. 166) just straight-out labels him a nonutilitarian. I think that is conceding far too much to the anti-utilitarian influences. As we shall see in the discussion of truth-telling to patients, in the end the utilitarians carry the day for Percival.

40. There is a debate in the recent literature over the interpretation of Percival's contractarianism that suggests that further research would be helpful. Lisbeth Haakonssen claims that some commentators (she cites Robert Baker [1993, p. 200] and Carleton Chapman [1984, p. 80]) have seen Percival operating "without any recognizable contact between doctor and patient, and that the interests of the patient were simply determined through the duties of the physician to each other and to their profession" (Haakonssen 1997, p. 126). She counters with the claim that "this ignores the contemporary notion of the unformulated and implied contract inherent in any office, a notion that is crucial to understanding the development of the modern idea of a profession" (Haakonssen 1997, p. 126). In the accompanying endnote she states that Percival drew on the "Protestant Natural Law tradition" and wryly points out that neither Percival nor Gisborne was an "original philosopher" (Haakonssen 1997, n. 114, p. 180). No doubt Percival drew on Blackstone, Bacon, and presumably Calvinists who were sympathetic to the natural-law tradition for their contractarianism. But the real issue seems to be not so much whether Percival was exposed to this philosophical tradition but whether he corrupted it by mutating the compact from one among all the members of the broader society to one among professionals in which those outside the profession were reduced to mere passive recipients of professionally agreed-upon conceptions of their duties. When Percival says that the "tacit compact" is entered into when the physician enters the "fraternity" of physicians and its content is to submit to its laws and promote its honor and interest, he appears to have a compact in mind that is radically different from the more fundamental social contract that formulates the basic moral principles for the broader population. The critical issue is how this more fundamental, broader social contract relates to Percival's intraprofessional compact. When he restricts the compact among professionals to behaviors "so far as they are consistent with morality, and the general good of mankind" (Percival 1803, p. 46), is his reference to the more traditional social contract? I don't see any direct evidence in Percival that this is the case.

41. This does not imply that Percival advocated what twenty-first–century medical scientists would call experimental method with randomized trials, formal research design, and the like. Rather, Percival was advocating the trial of new remedies, but what is critical is that he explicitly did so in the name of the "public good."

CHAPTER 4

1. For a more detailed account of these editions see note 31 of Chapter 3.

2. Nutton (1995) claims that the pattern was similar in Germany. Citing Nolte, he notes, "from the 1750s onward in Germany, there developed specifically medical oaths, combining loyalty to state and university with more generalised moral affirmations

about what a doctor should do or think; but of the Hippocratic Oath itself there are at best a few verbal echoes" (p. 522).

3. Biographical information on Ryan comes from Norgate (1937). The card catalogue of the Wellcome Institute Library in London contains a note claiming that the *Dictionary of National Biography* has the wrong death date, that his actual death date is Dec. 11, 1840.

4. It is this second edition to which all references are made in this volume.

5. Another piece of evidence is a listing inside the back cover of the 1849 edition of Percival's *Medical Ethics* of related publications from John Churchill, the publisher. The list includes Harvard professor John Ware's *Duties and Qualifications of Physicians*, which Churchill had published the same year. (I have been unable to locate any copies of the English publication. It is not available at the libraries of The Wellcome Institute or the university libraries at Edinburgh, Oxford, Cambridge, or University College, London. Copies of Ware's original 1833 lecture as well as the 1847 American edition of *Discourses on Medical Education, and on the Medical Profession* in which it was reprinted, are available at The Wellcome in London and at various American libraries.) The advertisement continued with a Churchill publication of the American Medical Association's new Code of Ethics as well as a reprinting of Gisborne's *Duties of Physicians: Resulting from Their Profession*. Clearly, there was a modest resurgence of interest in medical ethics by mid-century in England. What is striking, however, is that what we see is not original English scholarship but a reproducing of either 50-year-old English material (Percival and Gisborne) or American literature, which, as we shall see in the next chapter, is itself a reproducing of the older British literature.

6. Ryan complains:

> It is not easy to conceive the reason why the cultivation of ethics, a matter of primary importance to the success of medical practitioners, in the commencement of their career, should be almost totally neglected in the medical schools of an age so enlightened as the present. The fact is so, however incomprehensive it may appear. It is now the custom to initiate men into the mysteries of medicine, without the slightest allusion to the duties they owe each other or the public; or the difficulties to be encountered on the commencement of their practice.
>
> (Ryan 1836a, p. 44)

7. A typical title is *A Treatise on the Most Celebrated Mineral Waters of Ireland Containing an Account of the Waters of Ballyspellan, Castleconnel, Ballynahinch, Mallow, Lucan, Swadlinbar, Goldenbridge, Kilmainham, &C. &C.: and of the Spa Lately Discovered at Brownstown, near Kilkenny, with Plain Directions During the Use of Mineral Waters and an Account of Some of Those Diseases in Which They Are Most Useful* (1824). Other titles include *A Manual on Midwifery; or a Summary of the Science and Art of Obstetric Medicine, Including the Anatomy, Physiology, Pathology, and Therapeutics, Peculiar to Females; Treatment of Parturition, Puerperal, and Infantile Diseases; and an Exposition of Obstetrico-legal Medicine* (1828a, 4th ed. 1841); *A New Practical Formulary of Hospitals of England, Scotland, Ireland, France, Germany, Italy, Spain, Portugal, Sweden, Russia, and America; of Mm. Magendie, Lugol, Etc. or a Conspectus of Prescriptions in Medicine, Surgery, and Obstetrics. With the Doses of All New and Ordinary Medicines / Translated from the new French ed. of Milne Edwards and P. Vavasseur, and considerably augmented* (1835, 2nd ed. 1836b); *The Obstetrician's Vademecum; or Aphorisms on Natural and Difficult Parturition;*

the Application and Use of Instruments in Preternatural Labours; on Labours Complicated with Hemorrhage, Convulsions, Etc / Considerably Augmented and Arranged According to the Present State of Obstetricy (9th ed. 1836c); *Remarks on the Supply of Water to the Metropolis: with an Account of the Natural History of Water in its Simple and Combined States, and of the Chemical Composition and Medical Uses of All the Known Mineral Waters Being a Guide to Foreign and British Watering Places* (1828b).

8. It carries the quaint title, *The Philosophy of Marriage, in its Social, Moral, and Physical Relations; with an Account of the Diseases of the Genito-urinary Organs . . . with the Physiology of Generation in the Vegetable and Animal Kingdoms; Being Part of a Course of Obstetric Lectures Delivered at the North London School of Medicine* (4th ed., 1843).

9. Biographical information on Taylor comes from Webb (1921–22). See also Crowther (1995).

10. Taylor's medical degree was honorary, from St. Andrews in 1852, and there is no evidence of any training in law. He was elected a fellow of the College of Physicians and made a member of the Royal Society in 1845.

11. In the *Elements* (1843, p. 66) Taylor refers to the accuracy of Hippocrates's description of a dying man. Hence, he uses Hippocrates as Gregory and Percival do, as an exemplar of a careful empirical scientist, not as the prototypical ethicist–physician. Also in the *Elements* (1843, p. 106) Taylor mentions someone named Percival in connection with a volume on the history of Ceylon. Presumably, this is a reference to Robert Percival's *An Account of the Island of Ceylon, Containing Its History, Geography, Natural History, with the Manner and Customs of its Various Inhabitants; to Which Is Added, the Journal of an Embassy to the Court of Candy. Illustrated by a Map and Charts*, 1803. Robert Percival is identified in the book as "esq. of His Majesty's 19th Regiment of Foot." I know of no relation to Thomas Percival.

12. "Poisons in Relation to Medical Jurisprudence," "On Poisoning by Strychnia, with Comments on the Medical Evidence at the Trial of W. Palmer for the Murder of J. Cook," and "A Thermocentric Table on the Scales of Fahrenheit, Centigrade, and Reaumur, Compressing the Most Remarkable Phenomena Connected with Temperature" are examples.

13. Almost everything known to recent scholarship about Jukes Styrap comes from the research of Bartrip. His work (1995) is the source of the biographical and ethical code information presented here. The 1878 text of Styrap's code is published in full along with Bartrip's analysis (Styrap 1995). Styrap is one of the few British figures in this study who did not make the *Dictionary of National Biography*. He is a minor player, but nevertheless worthy of attention as the only contributor to English medical ethics during this period.

14. I had access to the second (1886), third (1890a), and fourth (1895) editions at the Wellcome Institute, as well as the reprint of the first edition (Styrap 1995). All quotations are from the first edition.

15. In the second paragraph the AMA begins, "Every case committed to the charge of a physician should be treated with attention, steadiness, and humanity." Styrap's edit reads, "Every case (rich and poor alike) entrusted to the care of a practitioner should be treated with attention, kindness, and humanity" (Styrap 1995, p. 150). The "physician" becomes a "practitioner," "steadiness" becomes "kindness," and a parenthetical "rich and poor alike" is inserted. Yet Percival's second paragraph, which deals explicitly with the status of hospital patients, contains a second sentence that also addresses the equal treatment of rich and poor patients. Percival, after acknowledg-

ing that hospital patients cannot be permitted a choice of physician or surgeon, adds, "Yet personal confidence is not less important to the comfort and relief of the sick-poor, than of the rich under similar circumstances" (Percival 1803, p. 10). The para-phrasing continues for several paragraphs, sometimes with Styrap cleaning up less felicitous phrasing of the Americans. For example, in a paragraph in which the AMA had rather pejoratively commented, "A patient should never weary his physician with a tedious detail of events or matters not appertaining to his disease" (Chapter I, Art. II, paragraph 5), Styrap more gracefully says, "A patient, when narrating the symp-toms and progress of his malady, should avoid unnecessary prolixity and detail which would weary the attention and waste the time of his doctor" (Styrap 1995, p. 153). Aside from copyedits of this character, Chapter 1 of Styrap matches that of the AMA. In Chapter 2 Styrap is a bit more free in supplementing the text, but all seven sections parallel the AMA's second chapter and many of the sentences are identical. Likewise, the first two sections of Chapter 3 match. Wheras the AMA document ends here, Styrap adds a final, one-paragraph section and a single-paragraph fourth chapter. The added section addresses ownership of the prescription formula. Styrap challenges the "com-mon assumption" that the "right of property" transfers to the pharmacist or chemist, claiming that it must remain the property of the physician. In the added fourth chap-ter, entitled "'Medical' Etiquette, or the Rule of the Profession on Commencing Prac-tice, Etc.," Styrap stipulates that it is the duty of every practitioner who moves into a community to call upon "every duly qualified, legitimate medical practitioner resi-dent within a reasonable distance of his own selected place of abode" to "courteously announce his intention to practise in the locality." The copyedits and this modest addition, which, incidentally provides additional evidence that the remainder of the code cannot be taken as "medical etiquette," is all that separates Styrap's text from the 1847 AMA document.

16. Personal communication, July 16, 1979, from Audrey J. Porter, Executive Secretary, Central Ethical Committee.

17. This was true even though, at least in 1970, the "Medical Ethics" chapter had been reprinted as a separate pamphlet so that its dissemination would not require disclos-ing the official secrets of the members' handbook (see British Medical Association 1970).

CHAPTER 5

1. The historical summary of this and the following paragraph is based on Girdwood (1988) and Rosner (1991).

2. This account is based on Beall and Shryock (1954) and Murdock (1957).

3. The manuscript was never published during his lifetime and hence lacked the impact of Wesley's medical writing. Significant portions of the manuscript were finally pub-lished in 1954 (Beall and Shryock 1954, pp. 127–234).

4. This section also draws on Sudds (1957), Goodman (1934), Hawke (1971), and Binger (1966).

5. In addition to Rush's biography, the detailed intellectual history of Rush by D'Elia (1974, pp. 20–35) provides a comprehensive account of Rush's Edinburgh years. D'Elia concludes that "Gregory served prominently in introducing Rush to the Scot-tish Philosophy of Common Sense in its classical age" (p. 29).

6. These are not a series of six lectures given each year to beginning students in the manner of Gregory, but single lectures given in various years (with the exception of two given on November 2 and 3 of 1801). The titles include the following: "On the Necessary

Connection Between Observation and Reasoning in Medicine," delivered November 7, 1791; "On the Character of Doctor Sydenham," delivered December 9, 1793; "On the Causes of Death in Diseases That Are Not Incurable," delivered November 26, 1798; On the Influence of Physical Causes in Promoting an Increase of the Strength and Activity of the Intellectual Faculties of Man," delivered November 18, 1799; "On the Vices and Virtues of Physicians," delivered November 2, 1801; and "Upon the Causes Which Have Retarded the Progress of Medicine, and the Means of Promoting Its Certainty and Greater Usefulness," delivered November 3, 1801.

7. Much of Rush's family arrived in the New World as Quakers (Rush 1948, p. 24), but Rush was educated as a Presbyterian.

8. Correspondence of Benjamin Rush with Granville Sharp, especially Sharp's letter of Oct. 31, 1774, cited in Carlson and Simpson (1965, p. 23).

9. The lectures are taken from Rush's manuscript of lectures for his medical school course on the institutes of medicine, a course that he began teaching in 1791 (Rush 1981, p. 14).

10. Gregory shows up elsewhere as well, such as in an attack on deism in which Rush cites Gregory: "Dr. *Gregory* has observed, that a cold heart is the most frequent cause of deism. Where this occurs in a physician, it affords a presumption that he is deficient in humanity" (Rush 1789, p. 5). In his introductory lecture of 1791, "On the Necessary Connection Between Observation and Reasoning in Medicine," Rush, describing his course organization in dealing with pathology, says, "I shall depart from the order of Dr. Gregory, in his Conspectus Medicine Theoreticæ, by separating this part of our course from the physiology" (Rush 1801, p. 21). The implication is that he thinks of himself as generally following Gregory's organization.

11. Also, in his *Scottish Journal* Rush writes, "Dʳ: *Cullen* in particular will always be dear to me. I have experienced not a little of his private friendship. I never asked a Favour from him but wt: I obtained it. In a word I loved him like A Father, & if at present I entertain any Hopes of being eminent in my Profession I owe them entirely to this great man" (cited in Binger 1966, pp. 35–36).

12. There are no direct references to Hutcheson or Adam Smith, two other Scottish figures that one might have expected to appear. Rush does refer to them, as well as Adam Ferguson, elsewhere, however (Carlson 1965, p. 23).

13. Other examples include the use of Newton (Rush 1789, p. 4), Locke and Rousseau (for example, Rush 1772), and even Pascal (Rush 1947, p. 226). Again, in all of the *Selected Writings* there is only one reference to Hume, and that was merely to his history of England (Rush 1947, p. 331). Rush also corresponded with Beattie (Carlson 1965, p. 23).

14. Included in this volume, for example, are the 1772 *Sermons to the Rich and Studious upon Temperance and Exercise*, with its distinctly Wesleyan tone (Rush 1772; cf. 1947, pp. 358–72); the 1773 "On Slave-keeping" (Rush 1947, pp. 3–18); "On Punishing Murder by Death" (Rush 1947, pp. 35–53); and the 1791 "The Bible as a School Book" (Rush 1947, pp. 117–30). It also includes essays directed to physicians, such as "Vices and Virtues of Physicians" (1801; reprinted in Rush 1947, pp. 293–307), and "Observations on the Duties of a Physician" (1789; reprinted in somewhat different form as "Duties of a Physician" in Rush 1947, pp. 308–321). There also are found more abstract pieces, such as his annual oration to the American Philosophical Society, "The Influence of Physical Causes Upon the Moral Faculty" (1786, reprinted in Rush 1947, pp. 181–211), which spells out the beginnings of his theory of the moral faculty.

15. These introductory lectures were not as systematic and comprehensive as Gregory's but included "On the Application of Metaphysics to Medicine" (1794), "On the Du-

ties of Patients to Their Physicians" (1808, reprinted in Rush 1811, pp. 318–349), "On the Study of Medical Jurisprudence" (1810, reprinted in Rush 1811, pp. 363–396), "Upon the Duties of Physicians to Each Other" (1812), and the above-mentioned lecture "On Vices and Virtues of Physicians."

16. Hawke mentions Hippocrates twice. The first occasion is merely a reference by Hawke to Sydenham, whom he refers to as the "English Hippocrates" (1971, p. 30). The second is in a long quotation, not from Rush but from Samuel Bard, who we shall encounter later in this chapter. Bard describes his Edinburgh education as including examinations that consisted of "writing commentaries on up two aphorisms of Hippocrates and defending them against old Dr. Munro and Dr. Cullen" [from a letter of Samuel Bard to John Bard, 15 May, 1768, cited in Hawke 1971, p. 60]. Thus neither reference is associated with Rush.

17. In "Medicine Among the Indians of North America" (1774) Rush makes the following comment on Hippocrates:

> I honour the name HIPPOCRATES: But forgive me ye votaries of antiquity, if I attempt to pluck a few grey hairs from his venerable head. I was once an idolater at his altar, nor did I turn apostate from his worship, till I was taught, that not a tenth part of his prognostic corresponded with modern experience, or observation.
>
> (Rush 1947, p. 277)

I have looked in vain for any written evidence of Rush's worship of Hippocrates. This essay was written when he was still a young man (28 years old), having graduated from Edinburgh only six years previously. If he worshiped the Greek father of medicine, it must have been very early in his life. One passing reference to Hippocrates that is moderately supportive of his observational and reasoning skills appears in one of Rush's early introductory lectures, "On the Necessary Connection Between Observation and Reasoning in Medicine" (Rush 1801, pp. 7–22). Even here, however, he adds (referring to both Hippocrates and Sydenham), "their theories, it is true, are in many instances erroneous, but they were restrained from perverting their judgments, and impairing the success of their practice, by their great experience, and singular talents for extensive and accurate observation."

18. In this essay Rush offers two Hippocratic quotations, (*1*) the well-worn "Ars longa, and vita brevis" and (*2*) "In a physician there should be a contempt of money, a sense of shame, modesty and cleanliness in dress, judgment, gentleness, urbanity, promptness of speech, freedom from superstition, and great integrity."

19. This account is based on Burrage (1957, pp. 598–99) and McVicker (1822).

CHAPTER 6

1. The biographical information on Chapman is based on Richman (1967) and Lanza (1957).

2. The Wistar group included bankers (Langdon Cheves), lawyers (Horace Binney, Thomas Cadwalader, Peter Duponceau, John Sergeant, Thomas I. Wharton, and Nicholas Biddle and William Meredith, both of whom were also bankers), engineers (Samuel Vaughan Merrick), judges (Joseph Hopkinson, John Kane, and William Tilghman), army officers (Clement C. Biddle), businessmen (Henry Carey, John Vaughan, Roberts Vaux, John Price Wetherill, and William McIlvaine), a mayor of Philadelphia (Benjamin W. Richards), architects (William Strickland and Thomas Walter), and publishers (Mathew Carey, who was Chapman's publisher, and Isaac Lea, Carey's son-

in-law) as well as many physicians (Alexander Dallas Bache, William Dewees, Joshua Francis Fisher, William Gibson, Robert Hare, Thomas Harris, Hugh L. Hodge, William Horner, Thomas C. James, Rene LaRoche, Charles D. Meigs, John K. Mitchell, Robert M. Patterson, Jacob Randolph, George B. Wood, and Robley Dunglison).

3. This membership list of the Wistar Association comes from the Wistar archives at the American Philosophical Society in Philadelphia. The identification of the professions of the members comes from Stephen W. Williams, *American Medical Biography*, 1845; Hampton L. Carson, "The Centenary of the Wistar Party: An Historical Address;" *Dictionary of the American Medical Biography*, 1928; Henry Simpson, *Lives of Eminent Philadelphians*, Philadelphia: W. Brotherland, 1859; Digby Baltzell, *Philadelphia Gentlemen*, Glencoe, IL: Free Press, 1958; and the *Proceedings of the American Philosophical Society*. I am grateful to Nicholas Crosson, who conducted the research identifying the professional interests of each of these members of the Wistar Association. He also made every effort, but in vain, to refute the claim that humanists–philosophers, theologians, clergy, and other humanists were absent from this group.

Crosson's notes are worth repeating:

> The American Philosophical Society (all of those in the Wistar Party members were members, as it was one of the few requirements for membership in the Wistar Party) clearly proclaimed during the mid 19th Century that it was dedicated to the "promotion of useful knowledge." *The Proceedings of the American Philosophical Society* of that era were filled with papers on current scientific and technical advances of the day—new methods of engineering, descriptions of biological studies and investigations, etc. Many of these men were amateur scientists (and quite a few were professionals, of course) and they also supported the founding, funding, and operations of The Franklin Institute and The Academy of Natural Sciences in Philadelphia—both dedicated to scientific research and the latter being a center for the research and study of the natural world and a pioneering institution for fossil research and dinosaur bone exhibitions in the latter parts of the 19th Century. Many of these men saw "science" as an important ideal.
>
> Many of these folks were utilitarians, not in a Millian sense but in the American Pragmatist tradition as it descended from Franklin (whom they obviously were familiar with and honored). Useful knowledge was to be found and promulgated, science was the method of doing this.
>
> Thus, the Wistar Party may be seen as the premier social gathering place for these men. It wasn't simply a snobbish, exclusive gathering of rich folks with society connections to one another. It may have been that—obviously the majority of these folks were well off and from established families—and it was criticized as such during its time. But to one degree or another, in some ways conscious and in other ways not, many of these men shared this ideology. (I.e., it may have been a social club for snobbish society folks, but they were snobbish society folks many of whom were dedicated to the support of scientific investigation.)

4. Officers included judges Joseph Hopkinson (who was the president), Joseph R. Ingersoll (one of the vice presidents), and John K. Kane (one of the corresponding secretaries) as well as Chapman and John Bell, both of whom were vice presidents. All were members of the Wistar Party. Others with joint membership included physicians Mitchell, Patterson, and Dunglison, architects Strickland and Walter, and Thomas Dunlap, whom I have not been able to otherwise identify. At least three clergy were also members

(George W. Bethune, W. H. Furness, and S. W. Fuller), but that does not seem to have oriented the group to particularly weighty matters of theology or philosophy.

5. The information regarding the Athenian Institute is derived from Richman (1967) and Jackson (1931, pp. 188–89). I am grateful to Nicholas Crosson and his wife, Erika, for locating it.

6. "[T]he seminal liquor is . . . applied to the ovaries . . . by a law of the animal system called Sympathy or the consent of parts" (cited in Richman 1967, p. 96).

7. The text is in the University of Pennsylvania archive.

8. There is a potentially significant problem for historical research here. At the time in Boston there were two John Warrens, father and son, both distinguished physicians. It was only with considerable difficulty that I could confirm what I had expected— that it was the father who was the senior member of the committee that wrote the *Boston Medical Police*. The point is confirmed in the biography of John Collins Warren, the son, written by his brother Edward Warren (1860, p. 87). The point made here (that the committee members were not in conversation with contemporary humanists) holds for either man. The son was usually referred to as John Collins Warren (or simply John C. Warren, to be distinguished from another John Collins Warren [1842–1927], who was his grandson and also a surgeon). He was born in 1778, attended Harvard, studied medicine under his father, spent three years at hospitals in Europe, and then assisted his father in his practice. He eventually was made adjunct professor of anatomy at Harvard (under his father), and participated in the founding of the *New England Journal of Medicine* and the Massachusetts General Hospital. He, like the Monros, was a surgeon (indeed was the first to use ether and the first in the United States to operate on a strangulated hernia), but was not an eclectic scholar of the humanities in the tradition of Gregory or Rush. He received his medical degree from Edinburgh, but just after the turn of the century. He would thus have been there contemporaneously with James Gregory, but three decades after the height of the Enlightenment in medical ethics. His nonmedical interests are reflected in his participation in the Bunker Hill Monument Association and the Massachusetts Temperance Society. His publications were medical and scientific. For example, he wrote "Surgical Observations on Tumors" (Boston 1837, cited in Mumford 1928). He was a nineteenth-century scientific practitioner of medicine, not a physician–philosopher in the tradition of the previous century (Warren 1860, Mumford 1928.)

9. This account is based on Cash (1984), Viets (1964b), J. Collins Warren (1928), and Edward Warren (1874, 1860).

10. Lemuel's biography is based on "Hayward, Lemuel" (1930) and Thacher (1828, pp. 287–88).

11. A biography notes that "in his later years he preferred reading history, theology, and works of fancy" (Thacher 1828, p. 288), but he is also described as "wholly unambitious of literary and professional honors, and never could be brought to overcome the reluctance he felt to publishing" (Thacher 1828, pp. 287–88).

12. Fleet published his 11-page Harvard Medical School dissertation in 1795 (Fleet 1795). It dealt with surgery and was dedicated to John Warren. Then two years later he published the 25-page *A Discourse Relative to the Subject of Animation* (Fleet 1797).

13. Biographical information about Ware comes from Viets (1964a).

14. The full text is reprinted in Walsh (1907, pp. 140–150), which is the text used here and cited below.

15. "It is enjoined in the sacred obligations which Hippocrates imposed upon the pupils of the noble science of medicine and surgery, which is also the model of the like en-

gagement offered to the candidates for graduation in this and other countries, that they
shall respect and assist their preceptors and masters, their seniors by experience or
age, and shall contribute as far as in their power, to the honor, improvement and utility of their professions" (Walsh 1907, p. 148).

16. The generally recognized date of Pascalis's death is 1833, but one source says 1840.
The difference is not significant to his contribution to the *System of Medical Ethics* in
1823 or his philosophical exposure up to that time.

17. Pascalis published *Medico-Chymical Dissertations on the Causes of the Epidemic
Called Yellow Fever, and on the Best Antimonial Preparations for the Use of Medicine, by a Physician, Practitioner in Philadelphia* in 1796 and followed this two years
later with *An Account of the Contagious Epidemic Yellow Fever, Which Prevailed in
Philadelphia in the Summer and Autumn of 1797*. He was an editor the *Medical Re-
pository* from 1813 to 1820.

18. I am grateful to the extensive research done for this section by Nicholas Crosson. It
incorporates much material from his research notes. He had access to published and
unpublished records of the Philadelphia chapter housed at the library of the College
of Physicians of Philadelphia.

19. The text continues:

> The state of the profession in this country so imperiously calls for reformation that
> we have thought a Society modelled on similar principles might do much to raise
> it to its legitimate standard. Knowing that we have not that rank and influence in
> the community which as members of a liberal profession, we are entitled, and
> believing that our present humble condition has principally resulted from the sin-
> ister conduct of some of our unworthy brethren we have determined under a sol-
> emn oath of duty to associate on just principles for the purpose of elevating the
> character of our vocation.
>
> (Kappa Lambda [1824–26])

20. Similar observations can be made about the New York branch of the society. Its oath is
committed to promoting "professional respectability and welfare of the members of this
association." It contains a Hippocratic-style commitment to instruct fellow society
members gratuitously, but has lost all of the Hippocratic commitment to benefit patients.
The New York Society's oath reads, "I ____ do solemnly promise, that by all proper
means, I will *promote* the *professional respectability* and *welfare* of the *members* of
this association, and *vindicate their character*s when unjustly assailed, and that I will
not demand any pecuniary acknowledgement for such instruction as it may be convenient for me to afford to the *son* of any indigent *member*, as may be in the opinion of the
society qualified by his previous education, and talents, and moral character, to become
a respectable and useful member of the profession, but that *I will afford such instruction gratuitously, in conjunction with the members of the society*" ("Report of the Committee of the Medical Society, of the City and County of New York" 1831, p. 4).

21. The cross-hatched box is a symbol for the Kappa Lambda Society often used as a shorthand for "society."

22. Bache also wrote:

> The Philadelphia Society has [illegible] their attention to an important point of
> regulation, [fruitful?] to professional respectability, that of adopting by common
> [cause?] [illegible], some scale of charges for professional services. A committee
> on this subject has been for some time appointed, but owing to the difficulties of

this subject, no report has yet been made. Without doubt, the New York Society considers this subject as [illegible] for professional regulation.

While the chief object of the KΛ Institution is the cultivation of medical ethics, a secondary and [illegible] important one is the improvement of medical science itself.

23. Nicholas Crosson, who did extensive review of the Kappa Lambda records in Philadelphia for this book, searched for but could not locate any evidence of Chapman's participation, even though it appears that all the other physicians of the Wistar Party at that time were members of Kappa Lambda.

24. The history of the founding of the AMA is based on Mumford (1903, pp. 427–45), Konold (1962), Rothstein (1972, pp. 114–21), Burns (1978), King (1984, pp. 37–41; 1991, pp. 210–14), Chapman (1984, pp. 103–24), Reiser (1995), and Baker (1995a), as well as American Medical Association (1848) and the full-text reprint that includes the introductory material in Baker (1995b, pp. 65–87). A promising secondary work is N. S. Davis's *History of the American Medical Association from its Organization up to January 1855* (Davis 1855), but it turns out to provide little about the development of the code of ethics that is not available from primary sources.

25. This concern about the protection of the reputation of the profession is seen in Nathaniel Chapman's opening address at the 1848 meeting:

The profession to which we belong, once venerated on account of its antiquity— its varied and profound science—its elegant literature—its polite accomplishments—its virtues—*has become corrupt* and *degenerate to the forfeiture* of *its social position* and with it, of the homage it formerly received spontaneously and universally.

(Davis 1855, p. 56)

26. Some of the key players in the AMA's founding were also key members of the various local medical societies and of Kappa Lambda chapters. Alexander H. Stevens, who was to be elected the second president of the AMA in 1948 (Davis 1855, p. 49), was a member (and likely an officer) in the New York Kappa Lambda. A physician named Yardley, who was on committees during the formation of the AMA, was a member of the Philadelphia chapter.

27. Aside from Hays and John Bell, the committee was made up of Gouvernor Emerson (of Philadelphia), W. W. Morris (of Delaware), T. C. Dunn (of Rhode Island), A. Darious Clark (of New York), and Richard D. Arnold (of Georgia). None of them appears in any history of nineteenth-century medicine I have consulted. See Kelly (1928) and "Arnold, Richard Dennis" (1928) for the only information on these figures that could be located. Gouvernor Emerson, another surgeon, was actively involved in the smallpox epidemic in Philadelphia and worked extensively in agriculture, editing the *Farmer's and Planter's Encyclopedia of Rural Life*. The College of Physicians of Philadelphia has a manuscript book that Emerson wrote, entitled *Case histories, notes on medical topics . . .* , which is really a sort of medical commonplace book that he used from 1821 to 1827. Most of it consists of notes he made concerning specific cases, notes on particular diseases, or medical events in the city, such as hepatitis, spina bifida, cataracts, sea scurvy, smallpox epidemic (1823–4), syphilis, and yellow fever epidemic (1820). There are also some entries and newspaper clippings on medically related oddities, such as Siamese twins and trained rattlesnakes. Along with Bell and Hays, he was a member of Kappa Lambda, thus making at least three of

the seven committee members associates in that society. I have been unable to determine whether Clark was involved in the New York chapter of Kappa Lambda. Arnold was one of the physicians at the Savannah Poor-House for over 30 years. He was active in the Georgia State Medical Association and was its president in 1851. His presidential address carried the familiar title, "Reciprocal Duties of Physicians and the Public to Each Other." He funded the Savannah Medical College, becoming its professor of the theory and practice of medicine. He also served as president of the Board of Water Commissioners and in the legislature of Georgia. He eventually became mayor of Savannah. Aside from his presidential address, however, he never did anything in ethics other than serve on the AMA committee.

28. Short biographies of Hays appear in Burrage (1928), McCrae (1957) and "Hays" (1968, 1967–71). A more detailed biography appears in Stillé (1881).

29. The literature on the "internal morality of medicine" is emerging as a basis for criticizing managed care, as a way for physicians to claim they are not beholden to any external authorities. See Brody (1994, p. 877), Brody and Miller (1998), and Pellegrino and Thomasma (1988, p. 115). For a critique see Veatch (2000).

30. Titles of Bell's works on mineral baths include *Dietetical and Medical Hydrology. A Treatise on Baths: Including Cold, Sea, Warm,. Hot, Vapour, Gas, and Mud Baths: Also on the Watery Regimen, Hydropathy, and Pulmonary Inhalation; with a Description of Bathing in Ancient and Modern Times* (Bell 1850), *The Mineral and Thermal Springs of the United States and Canada* (Bell 1855), and *On Baths and Mineral Waters* (Bell 1831).

31. This is illustrated by his *Report on the Importance and Economy of Sanitary Measures* (Bell 1859).

32. The John Bell (1796–1872) we are discussing should not be confused with a British surgeon of the same name (whose dates are 1763–1820) who was widely published. This John Bell once published "Letters on Professional Character and Manners: on the education of a Surgeon, and the Duties and Qualifications of a Physician: Addressed to James Gregory, M.D." (Bell 1810). The two are not related.

CHAPTER 7

1. Biographical information on Hooker is available in Thoms (1957, pp. 201–02) and Beauchamp (1995, pp. 105–19).

2. In 1851, Hooker wrote a monograph on homeopathy (Hooker 1851).

3. The reference is to Percival's note VII for Chapter II, Section III (Percival 1803, p. 162).

4. After these writings in the years between 1844 and 1851, Hooker turned his attention again to medical science, writing a text in human physiology (1854) and eventually producing texts for younger students, including *A First Book in Physiology, For the Use of Schools* [1883].

5. Flint's books include *Clinical Medicine: A Systematic Treatise on the Diagnosis and Treatment of Diseases: Designed for the Use of Students and Practitioners of Medicine* (1879); *A Manual of Percussion and Auscultation: of the Physical Diagnosis of Diseases of the Lungs and Heart, and of Thoracic Aneurism* (1876); *Phthisis: its Morbid Anatomy, Etiology, Symptomatic Events and Complications, Fatality and Prognosis, Treatment and Physical Diagnosis: in a Series of Clinical Studies* (1875); and *A Practical Treatise on the Diagnosis, Pathology, and Treatment of Diseases of the Heart* (1859). All of these were important works in clinical and scientific medicine, but hardly excursions into the humanities.

6. Some of Pilcher's publications on surgery include *Clinical Studies of the Surgical Diseases of the Female Generative Organs; from Observations Made During Ten Years' Work in the Methodist Episcopal Hospital in Brooklyn* (1898); *Fractures of the Lower Extremity or Base of the Radius* (1917); and *The Treatment of Wounds; its Principles and Practice, General and Special* (1883).

7. For example, see Pilcher's essay, "An Account of the Yellow Fever Which Appeared on Board the United States Ship Saratoga in June, 1869" (Gihon 1872).

8. For reference to Percival see Osler's speech upon the presentation of the Warrington collection, a library he arranged to purchase for the Johns Hopkins Medical School (Osler 1940c). For a reference to Rush see Osler (1896; 1905b, pp. 175, 184; 1905g, p. 324). Osler arranged for the purchase of Benjamin Rush's Edinburgh thesis, apparently as part of a collection from the library University of Edinburgh's professor Hope. He presented these to the library of the Medical & Chirurgical Faculty of Maryland (Cushing 1940, p. 606). He once wrote a review of a sketch of Rush's work on psychiatry and was instrumental in promoting the funding for a monument to Rush that now stands in Washington, D.C. For reference to Bard see Osler (1905b, p. 175). For reference to Warren see Osler (1905b, pp. 175, 185). Osler's movement to Philadelphia was occasioned by the retirement of Alfred Stillé. That chair was filled by William Pepper, making his chair available for Osler. Osler had always held Stillé in high regard, leading to Osler's biographical tribute to him in an address at a meeting of the College of Physicians of Philadelphia in 1902 (Osler 1908a). On Chapman see Osler's letters to Joseph Leidy, Jr. (Cushing 1940, p. 245). On Cotton Mather (referring to Mather's reference to "the angelic conjunction of medicine with divinity" see Osler (1905c, p. 370).

9. The *Bibliotheca Osleriana* (1929) is the full catalogue of Osler's library divided into eight sections. It consisted of 7787 works, including a copy of the 1803 edition of Percival; 8 volumes of Rush; 1 of Bard; 1 of John Warren; 4 of John Gregory (including both the 1770 and 1772 versions of his lectures on the duties of physicians [the latter being a 1788 reprint], *A Comparative View of the State and Faculties of Man with Those of the Animal World* [a 1798 reprint], and *A Father's Legacy to his Daughters* [a 1798 edition] plus two manuscript editions of notes from Gregory's lectures mysteriously dated June 19, 1773, and 1775—both being after Gregory's death); some correspondence of Chapman; 5 works of Wesley (including the first, ninth, and twenty-sixth editions of *Primitive Physick*; *The Desideratum: or Electricity Made Plain and Useful*; and an additional 1915 edition of *Primitive Physick*); and 5 works of Mather. It is impossible to tell the extent to which Osler read these volumes. Some were acquired late in life and in one case (with memories of Monro's copy of Thomas Reid), the volume of Gregory's unauthorized lectures of 1770 was uncut. By contrast, the library contains 174 separate Hippocratic writings, including 11 editions of the collected works. Osler loved to collect libraries.

10. Osler makes one reference that I am aware of to Cullen, and that is to Cullen's views on the humoral theory of disease (Osler 1905e, p. 230).

11. Ample biographical information is available on Osler, who is a much better-known figure than many who were involved in nineteenth-century medical ethics. This account is based on Cushing (1940), Reid (1934), Barker (1957), and many of the essays in Abbott (1926). The Cushing biography is massive (originally appearing in two volumes). I used the 1940 reprint, which is over 1400 pages long. It contains full texts or long excerpts of many of Osler's more obscure speeches and letters, many of which I have relied on for this discussion.

12. The book literally went to the grave with him. It was placed on his coffin at his death. The other of the first two books he owned was a gift from his older brother, entitled, "Varia: Readings from Rare Books" by J. Hain Friswell (London, 1866). It contained an essay on Thomas Browne, which may have led him to *Religio Medici*.

13. Although Harvey Cushing, his biographer, notes that this was the chair held by Gregory, Osler made no mention of him.

14. Thucydides was cited in Osler's *Science and War* (1915, excerpt reprinted in Cushing 1940, p. 1179); and Marcus Aurelius and Epictetus were cited in Osler's "Sir Thomas Browne" (1905, reprinted in Osler 1908e, p. 276). Cushing (1940, p. 899) documents Osler's reference to Lucretius and the fact that Osler had chosen Lucretius's "De Rerum Natura" from a colleague's library after the colleague's death. Lucian is cited in a 1915 letter to a Mrs. Brewster, in which he refers to his copy of Lucian and recommends it to her (Cushing 1940, p. 534, 1142) and in Osler's "Nerve and 'Nerves'" (1915a, excerpt reprinted in Cushing 1940 p. 1178). Pythagorus is cited in "The Lessons of Greek Medicine" (1910, excerpt published in Cushing 1940, p. 906); Seneca is cited in "After Twenty-five Years" (1905a, p. 214); and Protagorus is cited in Osler's "The School World" (1916, excerpt reprinted in Cushing 1940, p. 34) and in *Thomas Linacre* (1908f, excerpt reprinted in Cushing 1940, p. 810).

15. It is clear that Osler was a great admirer of Plato. Osler gave a lecture to the Johns Hopkins Hospital Historical Club on December 14, 1892, entitled "Physic and Physicians as Depicted in Plato." It was later published in the *Boston Medical and Surgical Journal* (Osler 1893) and is reprinted in Osler's *Aequanimitas, with Other Addresses to Medical Students, Nurses and Practitioners of Medicine* (1905, pp. 47–76). Osler relied on the third edition of Jowett's translation (Cushing 1940, p. 370). Cushing, referring to Osler's interest in Plato at this time, claims that Osler had come to mention Plato almost as often as Sir Thomas Browne, Osler's earliest and most prominent model for combining humanities and medicine. In this lecture he reviews Plato's dialogues, speaking first of his physiological and pathological speculations, then his allusions to medicine and physicians, and, finally, the social standing of the Greek doctor (see Osler 1905f, p. 50). It is a remarkable tour de force. As another piece of evidence of Osler's knowledge of Plato, Osler caught a mistake in his copy of Thomas Browne's *Religio Medici*. Where Browne says, "Plato's historian of the other world lies twelve days uncorrupted. . . ," Osler has changed "twelve" to "ten" with a marginal reference to the *Republic*, Book X. This suggests a rather thorough knowledge of Plato's text.

Osler left much more evidence of his intimate knowledge of Plato. One of Osler's patients was Walt Whitman, which led him to seek out and read some of "Leaves of Grass," about which he admitted to having "never read a line of his points." Osler commented that "'twas not for my pampered palate, accustomed to Plato and Shakespeare and Shelley and Keats" (the quotation is included in a long excerpt reprinted in Cushing 1940, p. 265, which apparently is taken from "Walt Whitman's Message. The Glory of the Day's Work," a letter that appeared in *The Times* of London, June 4, 1919.) On May 6, 1892, Osler married Grace Gross, the widow of Philadelphia physician Samuel Gross. It is reported that Osler read Jowett's Plato during his honeymoon (Cushing 1940, 367n). Also see Osler's "Teacher and Student," which was a lecture given at the University of Minnesota, October 4, 1892. In it he used a quotation from Jowett's translation of Book IV of the *Republic* as its text (Osler 1905h, p. 22). Similarly, a quotation from Jowett's introduction was the text for his lecture a decade later, "On the Educational Value of the Medical Society" (Osler 1905d, p. 344) and then again several months later in "The Master-Word in Medicine" (Osler, 1905c, p. 364). Additional examples include Osler's "After Twenty-five Years" (excerpt in Cushing 1940, p. 504). He even quoted Plato in his letters; in one of them he referred to Plato as "my old master" (text excerpted in Cushing 1940, p. 672). In another, he indicated he would send a copy of Jowett's introduction to the recipient, Mrs. Mabel Brewster, a patient and long-term friend (text in Cushing 1940, p. 783). In still another he referred to Plato's "two mother forms of the state"—monarchy and democracy (text in Cushing 1940, p. 940). In 1913, in another letter to Mabel Brewster, he indicates, "I have sent you a nice little edition of the *Phaedo* for your bedside library. The translation is not so good as Jowett" (text in Cushing 1940, p. 990). Osler knew his editions of Plato's dialogues. In a 1912 letter to Dr. Raymond Crawford, who served as secretary of the history of medicine section at an international congress, he indicated that he had acquired another edition of Plato, which he referred to as the "Ed. princ" and "Ed. princ. . . . Aldine 1513" apparently, first edition (text in Cushing 1940, p. 1010). He mentioned this acquisition on at least two other occasions, once as one of "my latest treasures" (Cushing 1940, p. 1303, cf. p. 1293).

16. Osler served a term as president of the Classical Association. This was at the end of his life. He commanded attention, no doubt, as much for his enormous efforts as a bibliophile, acquiring rare books and whole libraries, often donating them to scholarly institutions.

17. Cousin is Victor Cousin (1792–1867), whose works included *Cours De L'histoire De La Philosophie Moderne* (1847) and *Du Vrai, Du Beau Et Du Bien* (1883). Jouffroy is Théodore Jouffroy (1796–1842), who wrote an *Introduction to Ethics* (1848). No works by either of these men are in the *Bibliotheca Osleriana*.

18. Another mention of Descartes occurs in a letter three years later (text in Cushing 1940, p. 854).

19. The Osler bibliography is enormous, occupying over 130 pages of citations of his writings alone, so it is possible that these figures get mentioned some place, but in a thorough search for them I failed to find a single instance. In *Master-Word in Medicine* (Osler 1905c, pp. 370–71), Osler provides another list of the modern philosophers that Bovell liked to read: "Kant, Hamilton, Reed [*sic*], and Mill." In the Cushing excerpt, "Reed" is corrected to "Reid," presumably Thomas Reid. There is no evidence, however, that Osler himself read, much less endorsed, these authors. Some are included in the *Bibliotheca Osleriana*, however, if in very modest proportions. Hume is limited to his essays on "Suicide and the Immortality of the Soul" and text in a collection sampling modern philosophers. Adam Smith is represented by a biography, but no primary sources. Beattie, Reid, and Hutcheson are not accounted for at all.

20. While in Groningen, he sought out an edition of the Bible that had belonged to Martin Luther and then Erasmus. Later he called Erasmus "the greatest scholar of the age." In 1911, he was thrilled to be able to buy a translation of Erasmus at a bibliographical auction and then, at another occasion, 25 of his letters (Cushing 1940, pp. 558, 811, 969, 1013).

21. The Servetus was a 1790 copy of *Restitutio Christianismi*, which Osler described as "now almost impossible to get" (in a letter to H. B. Jacobs, excerpted in Cushing 1940, p. 944). In the same letter he indicated that he owned "the Calvin," not indicating which book he meant. He writes, "Many thanks for the book—I like C. so much." The context seems to imply he was referring to Calvin, suggesting a somewhat different opinion of the man than the one seen when Osler defended Servetus. The only primary work of Calvin in his *Bibliotheca Osleriana* is *Defensio orthodoxae fidei de*

sacra Trinitate, contra prodigiosos errors Michaelis Serueti Hispani. Presumably, this is the source to which he referred. Calvin was placed in the library under the heading of Servetus, who qualified for the *prima* section.

22. Osler's reference to Paracelsus is in "The Past Century: Its Progress in Great Subjects: Medicine" (Osler 1905e, p. 273). Cushing (1940) documents Osler's reference to Confucius (p. 624), to Averroes (pp. 866, 1217, 1272, 1275, 1281 [letters], and to Avicenna (pp. 856, 612, 951 [letters]. Averroes is also mentioned in "Treatment of Disease" (excerpt reprinted in Cushing 1940, p. 866). Osler spent time on a 1911 trip to Cairo searching for an early Avicenna manuscript (Cushing 1940, p. 954). By the next year he had acquired such a manuscript (Cushing 1940, p. 992). In 1913 he pursued a volume of Avicenna's poems and became concerned about the disrepair of Avicenna's tomb, hoping to raise funds for its needed repair (Cushing 1940, pp. 1054, 1063, 1079). By 1914 he had cost estimates for the repair and attempted to provide an income for a caretaker (Cushing 1940, p. 1091). In late 1914 the beginnings of the war led him to conclude that the effort would have to be postponed (Cushing 1940, p. 1122). In a letter of July 1919, just a few months before his death, he was still concerned that the project was not complete. It is noteworthy that, in all of this effort, Osler never made mention of any of Avicenna's thought.

23. They all qualify for the *bibliotheca prima* section, the part reserved for Osler's group of 67 authors whom Osler considered first-rank to the advancement of science. The section also included Aristotle, Hippocrates, and Galen and the moderns, Bacon, Galileo, and Sydenham as well as Berkeley and Priestley, but not the Scottish philosophers, even those such as Hume who made substantial contributions to science. The library contains 40 works by Paracelsus, 32 by Avicenna, and 5 by Averroes.

24. For another reference to Mather see Osler, "Books and Men" (1958a, p. 39).

25. Almost all the other works also have more literary and historical than philosophical merit. They include the Bible, Montaigne, Plutarch's *Lives*, Marcus Aurelius, *Don Quixote*, Emerson, and Oliver Wendell Holmes's Breakfast-Table series.

26. The early twentieth century scholar Charles Whibley assessed Browne's abilities as follows:

> Sir Thomas Browne's *Religio Medici* is less a theological treatise than a work of art. Those who look to its pages for guidance in religion will be disappointed. . . . Its ostensible theme, indeed, is of less interest than the style in which it is composed, or than the ingenious epigrams which give a luster to its pages. Though the Doctor sets out to tell us of his religion, he very soon wanders by the way and discourses at hazard of all things that touch his curiosity, and most especially of himself. The book is various and wayward. No secure thread of thought holds the argument together.
>
> (Whibley 1913, pp. 288–89) See also Huntley (1962, pp. 104–105)

27. Osler's essay was "Locke as a Physician" (1908a, pp. 68–107).

28. See Osler's, "Vienna After Thirty-four Years" (1908g). In 1912 he wrote to H. B. Jacobs that he had visited the University of Edinburgh library and was pleased to see a third copy of the *Restitutio Christianismi*, which was missing the first 16 pages (excerpt of letter reprinted in Cushing 1940, p. 1017).

29. See Osler's, *Michael Servetus* (1909).

30. Others who combined medical and humanist interests that interested Osler included Maimonides (see Osler, "Men and Books: XXIV. Israel and Medicine," 1914, excerpt reprinted in Cushing 1940, p. 1090) and Elisha Bartlett, whom Osler described as

Rhode Island's "one great philosopher" (Osler 1908b, p. 108). Bartlett wrote on topics in philosophy of medicine, which no doubt interested Osler. It is noteworthy that, with the possible exception of Maimonides, these physician–philosophers and other humanists who combined interests in medicine and humanities were not particularly noted as contributors to ethics. None are remembered for their contribution to medical ethics, either within the medical profession or within the various philosophical and theological traditions. Thus it is really not surprising that Osler showed almost no interest in Gregory or Percival (but see Cushing 1940, p. 761, where it is clear that Osler was at least aware of Percival's existence). Osler did not discuss the American Medical Association's efforts at code writing. He also paid no attention to Worthington Hooker.

31. See note 19 for evidence that Osler was aware of Mill. He also referred to Sidgwick (see Osler 1958c, p. 208) but not to discuss utilitarianism.

32. He made reference to the Hippocratic writings and the knowledge we have of the state of medicine from those documents (Osler 1905f, pp. 47–49).

33. See Osler (1908b, pp. 147–58). It is not clear from Osler's publication whether the 12-page reprinting is the entire essay of Bartlett's.

34. There are numerous other references to Hippocrates in Osler's work (Osler 1905c, p. 373; 1940a, p. 940). In a 1916 address at the opening of the Bodley Shakespeare Exhibition at the Oxford Divinity School, he included references to both Aristotle and Hippocrates: "What naturalist is uninfluenced by Aristotle, what physician worthy of the name, whether he knows it or not, is without the spirit of Hippocrates?" Cushing 1940b, p. 1195). On another occasion, again attacking Bacon, Osler saw all of modern science as being saved by two English physicians, William Gilbert and William Harvey, who led a return to Aristotle and Hippocrates. According to Osler,

> Greek philosophy, lost in the wandering mazes of restless speculation, was saved by a steady methodical research into nature by Hippocrates and Aristotle. While Bacon was philosophizing like a Lord Chancellor, two English physicians had gone back to the Greeks. 'Searching out nature by way of experiment' ('tis Harvey's phrase), William Gilbert laid the foundation of modern physical science, and William Harvey made the greatest advance in physiology since Aristotle.
>
> (Osler 1958b, p. 4)

35. A portion of the previously unpublished lecture is included in Cushing (1940, p. 907). The reference to Gomperz refers to Theodor Gomperz, who wrote *Greek Thinkers: A History of Ancient Philosophy* (London: J. Murray 1929–39, Vol. 1, p. 281).

36. In this lecture Osler states that "the highwater mark of professional morality is reached in the famous Hippocratic oath, which Gomperz calls 'a monument of the highest rank in the history of civilization. . . .' For twenty-five centuries it has been the 'credo' of the profession, and in many universities it is still the formula with which men are admitted to the doctorate" (Osler 1921, p. 63). Osler did not document the quotation from Gomperz (it is from p. 280) and did not provide any documentation for the grandiose claim that the Hippocratic Oath had been the credo of the profession for 25 centuries or that it was "still" the formula with which men were admitted to the doctorate.

37. Biographical information on Cabot is taken from Cabot (1977), Carvalho (1984), and Williams (1977).

38. The book began as *Physical Diagnosis of Diseases of the Chest*, published in 1901. It was expanded in 1905 to include other diagnoses and went through 12 editions by the time of Cabot's death and more afterwards under the editorship of F. Dennette Adams.

39. Osler also had an interest in developing the social work dimensions of health care, an interest for which he is often not given adequate credit. Osler was 20 years older than Cabot and knew him, at least to some degree. He referred to Cabot in letters (once calling him "Dick Cabot"), took part in at least one meeting with him, and hosted him when Cabot visited England (Cushing 1940, pp. 653, 747, 775, 816).

40. The references for these books are Cabot, Ella Lyman. *Everyday Ethics.* New York: Henry Holt & Co. 1906, and *Ethics for Children.* New York: Houghton Mifflin Co. [n.d.].

41. Cabot's recollection of his first philosophy class reveals much about Cabot's interest in ethics:

> Most high-minded and conscientious ethical teachers are talking today, so far as I know. They are too modest and unassuming to teach ethics. They confine themselves to teaching *about* ethics. Nor have their students any idea of being changed in character. I have never got over the shock of discovering that the men with whom I took Philosophy 4 under Professor George Herbert Palmer as a Harvard undergraduate had no idea of bettering themselves, of changing their habit or building up their own plan of life. They took ethics "as a part of general culture"—to find out what it was about, not with any practical aim concerned with their own characters.
>
> This I abhorred and still abhor. When I accepted the chair of Social Ethics I pledged myself to the adventure of trying to make men better themselves, the most unfashionable attempt, I suppose, in all the modern educational world. I hoped and still hope to do in ethics what any competent music teaching does in music, namely, to stimulate men to grasp for themselves something which includes the best that I know.
>
> (Cabot 1926, p. 99)

42. When Cabot did offer reference to intellectuals in the humanities it was, as we saw in Osler, far more likely to be to literary figures than to philosophers or theologians. In the pious platitudes of *What Men Live By: Work, Play, Love Worship* (parts of which were originally written for *Atlantic Monthly*), Cabot mentions Hans Christian Andersen, Robert Browning, Thomas Carlyle, G. K. Chesterton, Emily Dickenson, Ralph Waldo Emerson, Goethe, Charles Lamb, Robert Lewis Stevenson, and Leo Tolstoy. He also mentions Christ as well as Francis of Assisi and Martin Luther (once each), but no philosopher except G. H. Palmer (his Harvard teacher) and Josiah Royce. To Palmer he attributed the quotation, "A man of average capacity never feels so small as when people tell him that he is great" (Cabot 1914, p. 289). To Royce he attributed a quotation condemning formalistic worship full of "vain repetitions such as the heathens use" (Cabot 1914, p. 328). Neither quote suggests that Cabot was engaged with the philosophical or theological problems of his day, at least as seen by the great minds that were potentially available to him. Cabot is reported to have attended a course taught by Royce at "Harvard Seminary" (one supposes the Divinity School), where he gave lectures in 1903 and 1904 (Williams 1977, p. 317).

43. The publisher is Free Press Printing Co., Burlington, Vt., cited in Cabot (1926, pp. 75–77). No date is given, but it was apparently published in 1924.

44. The other principles were related to "cooperation." Two expressed the idea: "all to the end that our chosen business may be known as a genteel business as well as a fairly-prosperous one" (two codes) and "Anglo-Saxon ideals and historic Americanism" (one code).

45. In addition to the moral interests suggested here, it is also known that Cabot got into trouble with the Massachusetts Medical Society for being scrupulously honest in criticizing the errors in diagnosis of his colleagues, based on a series of 3000 autopsies he

conducted (Burns 1977a, p. 359). Being so attacked could incline one to praise the virtues of honesty.

46. This essay was reprinted at least twice, as recently as the late 1970s (Cabot 1977, pp. 223–63; 1978). I have used the 1978 reprint, which is more complete than the 1977 version.

47. See Kant, Immanuel. "On the Supposed Right to Tell Lies from Benevolent Motives." 1797. Translated by Thomas Kingsmill Abbott and reprinted in Kant's *Critique of Practical Reason and Other Works on the Theory of Ethics*. London: Longmans 1909, pp. 361–365. Williams (1977) speculates that it was Cabot's training in philosophy "in the days when the teaching of Immanuel Kant were in much favor [that] helped to foster his absolutism" regarding truth telling, but there is no evidence whatsoever for this suggestion. Certainly, Cabot's argument is very un-Kantian. If he was stimulated by Kant, he got Kant all wrong.

48. This discussion of Cabot, especially the more mature Cabot, was greatly strengthened by the thorough research assistance of Nicholas Crosson.

49. I have in mind, for example, the theory informed by Catholic moral theology of Edmund Pellegrino (1973) and of Edmund Pellegrino, and David Thomasma (1988); the Talmudic wisdom of Fred Rosner (1972); the rich blend of Orthodox Christian thought and philosophical libertarianism in Tristram Engelhardt (1996); the secular liberalism of Troyen Brennan (1991); the liberal communitarianism of Zeke Emanuel (1991); and the Islamic scholarship of Hassan Hathout (1992).

50. I have never been able to locate a copy of the 1947 edition. For the AMA's claim that a major revision took place that year, see American Medical Association (1971, p. iv).

51. Throughout the nineteenth century, scholarly editions of the Hippocratic corpus appeared, providing physicians with a substantial stimulus to focus on this particular medical ethical literature. Among the editions are the following:

> 1821–30. Karl Gottlob Kühn's (1754–1840, professor at Leipzig) edition of the Greek medical writers, 26 vols., including a Latin translation, with critical and exegetical commentary and indices. Galen 20 vols., the rest devoted to Hippocrates, Arataeus, and Dioscorides.
>
> 1834. Friedrich Reinhold Dietz (1804–1830, professor at Königsburg). *Scholia in Hippocratem et Galenum*. 2 vols.
>
> 1839–1861. Maxmilian Paul Emile Littré's (1801–1881, trained as a physician but never practiced) edition and translation of Hippocrates, 10 volumes. Sandys (1967) states that Littré "laid the foundation for the modern criticism of this author" (Vol. 3, p. 252).
>
> 1846. John Redman Coxe, M.D. *The Writings of Hippocrates and Galen. Epitomised from the Original Latin*. Philadelphia: Lindsay and Blakiston.

In the section "To the Reader," dated September 16, 1846, Coxe offers the following commentary:

> With the exception of a few of the Hippocratic treatises, an *English* translation has never appeared. Of the writings of Galen, not one has received that form, for the benefit of the English reader. And yet the names of both of these great men are familiar to our ears, as though they were the daily companions of our medical researches. Our teachers refer to them ex cathedra; our books continually quote them; and yet, not one in a hundred of the Profession, at least in America, have ever seen them, and if interrogated, could not inform us of what they treat.
>
> (Coxe 1846, pp. iii–iv)

For "the Oath of Hippocrates" he gives a description of the Oath and a summary, but not a translation of the Oath itself (pp. 41–3). He notes that "this book of aphorisms [is] the most extensively known perhaps, and that which has probably been more frequently given to the world in an isolated form than any of the other writings that have reached us under the imposing title of Hippocrates." He notes the C. J. Sprengel edition of London 1708 and the de Gorter edition of Amsterdam 1742 (p. 451).

> 1846. "Hippocrates" by W. A. Greenhill in Smith's *Dictionary of Greek and Roman Biography and Mythology*.
> 1849. Francis Adams (surgeon). *The genuine works of Hippocrates translated from the Greek with a preliminary Discourse and Annotations*. 2 vols. London.

The work was commissioned by the Sydenham Society and published in their series of books, which, with few exceptions, were quite technical books of weighty medical matters. He explains that he has included rather detailed annotations because

> It is well-known that many parts of my author's works are very obscure, owing to the conciseness of the language and the difficulty which now exists of properly apprehending the views entertained on certain abstracts and questions at so very distant a period; and, consequently, it will be readily understood, that a simple version, without either comment or illustration, would have been nearly as unintelligible to most of my readers as the original itself.
>
> (Adams 1849, pp. v–vi).

Adams goes on to note,

> I have consulted all the best authorities to which I could obtain access . . . especially Dr. Ermerins of Holland and MM. Littré and Malgaigne, of France. . . . It is proper, however, to acknowledge that I have derived great assistance from M. Littré's excellent edition, of which the parts already published embrace all the treatises here given, with the exception of the last four [the last four are "On Ulcers," "On Fistulae," "On Hemorrhoids," "On the Sacred Disease"]. (Adams 1849, pp. vi, vii)

> 1859–64. F. Z. Ermerins. 3 vols. in Latin.
> 1864–1866. Reinhold. 2 vols. in Greek.
> 1877, 78. J. E. Petrequin. Chirgurie d'Hippocrate. 2 vols.
> 1886. An American edition of the Adams work was published by William Wood and Company, New York.
> 1894, 1902. Kuhlewein. 2 vols. in Latin.

CHAPTER 8

1. During this period there were a total of 11 references in seven different authors to Hippocrates or Hippocratic writings, but the remainder have nothing to do with ethics. Hippocrates' eloquence in Greek, for example, is cited by Cassiodorus (Veatch and Mason 1987, pp. 88–89).
2. See, for example, Finney (1962) and Bushnell (1962; original edition 1861). For the links among Protestant Christianity, the Great Revival, the voluntary benevolent societies, and abolitionism see Barnes (1964) and Fuller (1960, pp. 28–47). For a short, general history see Walker (1959).

3. I find no nineteenth-century evidence that Catholic commentators used the language the way they did for this reason. The term *moral theology* had been in use for years. Perhaps they were simply accustomed to this language.
4. Much of this account relies on work by Kelly (1979).
5. For examples see Kendrick (1860–61), Gury (1869), Scavini (1860), Konings (1880) and Sabetti (1889).

CHAPTER 9

1. I am grateful to Barbara Brookes, who was at the University of Otago during my research there, for the provocative suggestion that medical school might not have been the nineteenth-century locus of medical ethics in New Zealand. Perhaps the medical association, which was a branch of the British Medical Association, handled medical ethical disputes and was the custodian of the code of ethics. While this is plausible, it turns out that, as we have seen, the British Medical Association resisted adoption of a code during the nineteenth century (see also Baker 1995b). While the Americans were busy adopting professional association codes at the local, state, and national levels, the British did not accept this idea. In spite of strong encouragement by Jukes de Styrap and the increasing acceptance of his codification by some physicians, the association rejected all efforts to formally adopt it or any other code.
2. According to C. E. Wright-St. Clair (1974), John Halliday Scott, the first dean of the medical school, "with Scottish thoroughness . . . set quietly about establishing a school on the model that he knew from Edinburgh."
3. In later years Macgregor had something of a falling out with the Presbyterians who still controlled the funds for his chair (Thompson 1920, p. 124). They accused him of having a "materialistic and rationalistic spirit" (p. 124). They attempted to separate the mental from the moral philosophy and create a new chair in moral philosophy, leaving the less controversial mental philosophy (what we would call psychology) to him.
4. The closest I was able to find to an interest among the faculty in the humanities was a report that Lecturer in Medicine, Daniel Colquhoun, conducted a correspondence with "Rev. W. H. Hewitson, Master of Knox College, dealing with Colquhoun's suggestions that medical students in residence might devote some time to the reading of poetry. The admirable proposal fell on stony ground."
5. Scott wrote the chancellor on March 11, 1884, saying, "I believe it is the desire of some of the members of the Council to make the appointment of the lectureship of Public Health and Medical Jurisprudence at an early date. I don't think this course, if followed, will prove to be for the good of the Medical school. I therefore take the liberty of asking you to defer the appointment" (Jones 1945, p. 81).
6. For many years the University of Otago was technically part of the University of New Zealand. The graduates were designated graduates of the University of New Zealand and the calendar (what today in the United States would be called the "catalog") was published for the whole national institution.
7. The declaration reads:

> Declaration to be made by graduands in the degrees of M.B., Ch. B., and B.D.S.
> "I solemnly declare that as a graduate in Medicine [Dentistry] of the University of New Zealand, I will exercise my profession to the best of my knowledge and ability for the good of all persons whose health may be placed in my care and for the public weal. I will respect the secrets which are confided in me and maintain the utmost respect for human life. I will hold in due regard the honourable tradi-

tions and obligations of the medical (dental) profession and will do nothing inconsistent therewith and I will be loyal to the University and endeavour to promote its welfare and maintain its reputation."

The one dramatic departure from the Declaration of Geneva (and from the Hippocratic Oath) is the conspicuous pledge to work "for the public weal."

8. For example, in August 1906, the minutes report that the "annual sum of £50 for the
purchase of periodicals and books for the Medical section of the University Library
had been granted." The November 1906 minutes show a list of 27 periodicals and
5 books the faculty considered desirable. There is no record of how many they were
able to buy for their 50 pounds.

9. The declaration included the controversial sentence, "I will maintain the utmost respect for human life, from the time of conception," which was later edited out.

10. Three other medical schools existed in Canada by that time—Ontario's Queen's University, Kingston (1854), and two schools in Quebec: McGill (1829) and Université
Laval (1853).

11. Information about McColloch is available from the Public Archives of Nova Scotia,
M.G. I vols. 550–558 (Halifax) and a privately printed biography written by his son,
William McCulloch (1920). The most accessible source is a biographical volume pub-
lished by the Nova Scotia museum (Whitelaw 1985). Information also comes from
Waite (1994, pp. 12–14) and Harvey (1938).

12. The immigration to Nova Scotia was stimulated by aggressive marketing by recipients of land grants that carried with them the condition that the land be settled in order
for the land companies to retain possession of their grants. One of the leaders of the
Philadelphia Company, one of the most prominent of these companies, was none other
than Dr. John Witherspoon, the Presbyterian minister and graduate of the University
of Edinburgh, whom Benjamin Rush helped persuade to become the principal of the
College of New Jersey.

13. McCulloch sometimes, psudonyminously, wrote scathing editorials. Under the name
of Mephibosheth Stepsure, he published satirical comments on provincial life in the
Acadian Recorder that were of such lasting importance that they were finally collected
and published in 1960 as *The Stepsure Letters* (McCulloch 1960). His unpublished
essays include "Popery Condemned" and "Popery Again Condemned," which dealt
more with legitimate theological issues than with anti-Catholic prejudice, and the
never-completed *Auld Eppie's Tales*, which treated in a humorous manner the ideals
of Scottish life, focusing on an unscrupulous "Abbott of Paisley."

CHAPTER 10

1. Some readers will be confused about the fact that some treatments at stake were statistically quite common and therefore apparently not "extraordinary." But the Catholic doctrine of extraordinary means never judged the treatment by whether it was
statistically ordinary, only by whether it was excessively burdensome.

2. The existence of differences on birth control among different professional and social
groups was also found in the work of the study of the Institute of Society, Ethics and
the Life Sciences (1971) prepared for the Commission on Population Growth and the
American Future.

3. A noteworthy qualification to this sweeping absence of the use of "rights-talk" appears in John Bell's introduction to the AMA Code of 1847. Here he speaks explicitly of the "rights of a physician" (Bell 1995, p. 65). Nevertheless, he never extended

the term to patients. More significantly, the generalization that no medical ethical document of a *professional physician group* referred to rights is not contradicted by the fact that one individual adopted rights language, at least as applied to physicians.

4. The Institute would in a few years produce the first compendium of reflection on matters in biomedical ethics, especially human subjects research (Ladimer and Newman 1963).

5. Jonsen (1998, pp. 9–10) provides a helpful summary.

6. Some of the crucial notes are omitted and errors have crept into the text. Nevertheless, it contains a useful, long introductory essay that shows that Leake is quite familiar with the history of American and British professional medical ethics.

7. See Jonsen (1998, p. 9), citing Chauncey D. Leake, "How Is Medical Ethics to be Taught?" *Bulletin of the Association of American Medical Colleges* 3 (1928): 341–43.

8. The account here is based on Jonsen (1998, pp. 137–38).

9. Five years earlier, in 1952, Pope Pius XII had also addressed the International Conference on the Histopathology of the Nervous System on "The Moral Limits of Medical Method of Research and Treatment," but that address never received the attention of the "Prolongation of Life" document (Pope Pius XII, *Linacre Quarterly: Official Journal of the Federation of Catholic Physicians' Guilds* 19 (Nov. 1952): 98–107, as cited in Advisory Committee on Human Radiation Experiments 1995, p. 169, note 75).

10. Fletcher was the instructor of the first graduate-level ethics course I ever took. (James Luther Adams, the professor at Harvard responsible for the course at the time, was on leave that semester and Professor Fletcher was invited to come across campus to teach in his absence.)

11. The account of the hemodialysis machine is based on Fox and Swazey (1974), Jonsen (1998), and Alexander (1962).

12. I had the privilege of attending as a graduate student, my first introduction to high-level international, cross-disciplinary medical ethics conversation.

13. Fuchs was present on a number of occasions for extended stays. Häring was present in 1974 and 1975. Schüller was present in 1977. Among the other leading Catholic theologians residing at the Institute (in addition to Richard McCormick and Warren Reich, who had permanent appointments) were Charles Curran (1972) and John Connery (1972–73, 1975–76). Hellegers' interests were eclectic. He thought that ethics flourished in an ecumenical context. Protestant theologians in the early years of the Institute, in addition to Ramsey and those of the younger generation already mentioned, included Frederick S. Carney (1973–74), Jack Padgett (1979), and Robert Nelson (1979–80). Jewish scholars included Seymour Siegel (1976–77) and Isaac Franck (for several years beginning in 1979). Hellegers even managed to have a Muslim scholar in residence—Mehdi Y. Hairi (1978–80). John Ford, who was a key author of the Papal Commission minority report, was not part of the Kennedy Institute fellowship.

14. As with Potter and Dyck at Harvard, Ramsey was also supervising graduate students during the 1960s at Princeton. His best-known students who have worked in biomedical ethics are David Smith (Director of the Poynter Center at Indiana University); Robert Weir (Director of the Program in Biomedical Ethics and Medical Humanities); and Gil Maelaender (professor at Valparaiso College).

15. Among those with training at Yale, either as divinity school or graduate students, were Tom L. Beauchamp (Professor of Philosophy at Georgetown University, Senior Research Scholar at the Kennedy Institute of Ethics, and co-author of *The Principles of Biomedical Ethics*); James F. Childress (the former Joseph P. Kennedy,

Sr., Professor of Christian Ethics at the Kennedy Institute and currently the Edwin B. Kyle Professor in the Department of Religious Studies at the University of Virginia), who is the co-author of *The Principles of Biomedical Ethics*); Margaret Farley (Gilbert L. Stark Professor of Christian Ethics at Yale University Divinity School); Stanley Hauerwas (Professor at Duke Divinity School and author of several volumes resuscitating virtue theory in biomedical ethics); Albert Jonsen (former Professor of Bioethics at the University of California, San Francisco, and the University of Washington Medical Center, as well as member of the National Commission for the Protection of Human Subjects of Biomedical and Behavioral Research and of The President's Commission for the Study of Ethical Problems in Medicine and Biomedical and Behavioral Research); and LeRoy Walters (one of the early Senior Research Scholars at the Kennedy Institute and its eventual Director). The Yale Philosophy Department also contributed Robert Neville during this period. He became one of the early professional associates at the Institute of Society, Ethics and the Life Sciences.

16. For example, as a Harvard graduate student my professors included theological ethicists Ralph Potter and Arthur Dyck, sociologist of medicine Renée Fox, and Henry Beecher, as well as sociologist Talcott Parsons and philosopher John Rawls. My interest in the definition-of-death debate traces directly to the stimulus from Beecher and Potter's participation in the Harvard Ad Hoc Committee.

CHAPTER 11

1. Picking the date for the beginning of an era is an inexact science, no doubt influenced by the particular interests and parochial perspective of the one doing the dating. Two historians of bioethics have offered other proposals. David Rothman (1991), whose interests have focused on the ethics human subjects research, emphasizes the importance of the issues of research, which led him to identify the critical transition in the 1960s. Meanwhile, Albert Jonsen, whose base at the University of Washington with its hemodialysis program, has suggested 1962, the time when the Admissions and Policy Committee's selection activity received public awareness from Shana Alexander's *Life* article, as a critical date. My case for the later date rests on the importance of the institutionalization of the new bioethics and the development of more formal codes, institutes, teaching programs, and government activities. It is these more formal interdisciplinary activities that makes the 1970s significantly different from the more individualized scholarly activities and occasional cross-disciplinary conversations that had occurred in the 1950s and 1960s.

2. I am proud to claim that I opened the offices of the center, showing up for the first day the Institute was to occupy the offices. On my first day on the job, I obtained the key from the dentist and unlocked the door.

3. Whether Hellegers or the Kennedy Foundation's Sargent Shriver had a hand in coining the term *bioethics* remains controversial (Reich 1994, 1995b). We know that Wisconsin biologist Van Rensselaer Potter used the term in the title of his 1971 book, *Bioethics Bridge to the Future*. Reich, in his study of the emergence of the term, determined that the book appeared in January of that year. Moreover, Potter had used the term in two 1970 articles (Potter 1970a, 1970b). Reich cannot rule out the possibility that Hellegers or Shriver used the term independently. In any case, they gave the term a meaning quite different from that of Potter, one much closer to the meaning that the term eventually acquired.

4. The publication of the first Institute on Human Values in Medicine (1972, p. 3) contains a brief history of the Society. According to Edmund Pellegrino, who is the author, the origins of the Society are a bit different. He traced the organization to a group of humanists and medical educators who had formed the Committee on Health and Human Values in March 1963. I simply report both the Jonsen and the Pellegrino versions.

5. In addition to the many humanists who have already appeared in this chapter, many more could be mentioned. By the end of the 1970s there were easily 20 or 30 from each of these disciplines actively engaged in the interdisciplinary dialogue at the national level in the United States.

   Among the lawyers, in addition to William Curran, Alex Capron, Patricia King, and Blair Sadler, who have already been mentioned, George Annas (Boston University), John Robertson (University of Wisconsin and now the University of Texas), Harold Edgar (Columbia University), Robert Burt (Michigan and now Yale), Judith Areen (Georgetown University), and Alan Weisbard (The New Jersey Commission and the University of Wisconsin) have all been engaged with colleagues in other disciplines for many years.

   Among physicians, in addition to Otto Guttentag, Robert Morison, Leon Kass, Elisabeth Kübler-Ross, Willard Gaylin, Andre Hellegers, Edmund Pellegrino, John Collins Harvey, Jay Katz, Chester Burns, James Todd, and Tristram Engelhardt, many others have played the crucial role of either inviting humanists into the clinic or stepping outside to engage in public discourse. In the early years of the reconvergence, they included Harvard's Gerald Klerman, UCLA's Jolly West, Michigan State's Howard Brody, and Wisconsin's Norman Fost.

   By contrast, mainstream philosophers were relatively late to arrive at the conversation. Throughout most of the twentieth century most British and American philosophers were looking elsewhere, primarily to abstract questions of metaethics. It was, and in some places still is, considered professionally risky to take up practical questions or applied ethics. Nevertheless, even in the early years some philosophers were what, with tongue only partly in cheek, we could call "deviant." We have seen that while their colleagues were debating the subtleties of the natural fallacy, some philosophers had the courage to communicate across disciplines. In addition to Daniel Callahan, Tom Beauchamp, Danner Clouser, and others we have encountered in this chapter, all had serious interests in matters of religion at some point in their careers and thus may not be as far removed from the religious ethicists who moved quickly into the dialogue with physicians. Other philosophers who were relatively early include British philosopher R. M. Hare; President's Commission staff members Dan Brock, Allen Buchanan, and Dan Wikler; The New School's Hans Jonas, Brown's John Ladd, Tufts' Norman Daniels, Union College's Robert Baker, Kentucky's Dallas High, MIT's Judith Thomson and Baruch Brody (now at Rice), Vanderbilt's John Lachs and Richard Zaner, and Texas A&M's Laurence McCullough (now at Baylor).

6. In the early 1970s (about 1972), Willard Gaylin and I were among a group of consultants attending sessions in the AMA's board room in which we were asked to identify ethical issues the AMA should be addressing.

Bibliography

Abbott, Maude E., ed. *Sir William Osler; Memorial Number, Appreciations and Reminiscences.* [Toronto: Murray Printing Co., Limited,] 1926.

Abelove, Henry. *The Evangelist of Desire: John Wesley and the Methodists.* Stanford, CA: Stanford University Press, 1990.

Advisory Committee on Human Radiation Experiments. *Final Report.* Washington, DC: U.S. Government Printing Office, 1995.

Alexander, Shana. "They Decide Who Lives, Who Dies." *Life* 53 (1962): 102–25.

American Medical Association. *Code of Medical Ethics: Adopted by the American Medical Association at Philadelphia, May, 1847, and by the New York Academy of Medicine in October, 1847.* New York: H. Ludwig and Company, 1848.

———. *Code of Medical Ethics: Adopted by the American Medical Association.* New York: William Wood & Company, 1871.

———. *Code of Medical Ethics: Adopted by the American Medical Association,* 3rd ed. New York: William Wood & Company, 1879.

———. *Current Opinion of the Judicial Council of the American Medical Association.* Chicago: American Medical Association, 1981.

———. "Principles of Medical Ethics of the American Medical Association." *Journal of the American Medical Association* 164 (1957): 1119–20.

———. "Principles of Medical Ethics of the American Medical Association [1903]." In *Percival's Medical Ethics, 1803.* By Thomas Percival, reprint edited by Chauncey D. Leake. Baltimore: Williams and Wilkins, 1975a, pp. 239–56.

———. "Principles of Medical Ethics of the American Medical Association [1912]." In *Percival's Medical Ethics, 1803.* By Thomas Percival, reprint edited by Chauncey D. Leake. Baltimore: Williams and Wilkins, 1975b, pp. 257–71.

———. Judicial Council. *Judicial Council Opinions and Reports*. Chicago: American Medical Association, 1971.

American Nurses' Association. "Code for Nurses with Interpretive Statements." Kansas City: American Nurses' Association, 1976.

Armstrong, Anthony. *The Church of England, the Methodists and Society*. London: University of London Press, 1973.

"Arnold, Richard Dennis." In *Dictionary of American Medical Biography*. Edited by Howard A. Kelly and Walter L. Burrage. New York: D. Appleton & Co., 1928, p. 37.

Artificial Heart Assessment Panel. "The Totally Implantable Artificial Heart." In Report by Artificial Heart Assessment Panel, National Heart and Lung Institute. June, 1973. Reprinted September 1973. Available from the National Heart and Lung Institute, National Institutes of Health, Bethesda, MD.

Ayling, Stanley. *John Wesley*. London: Collins, 1979.

Baker, Frank. *John Wesley and the Church of England*. London: Epworth Press, 1970.

Baker, Robert. "Deciphering Percival's Code." In *The Codification of Medical Morality: Historical and Philosophical Studies of the Formalization of Western Medical Morality in the Eighteenth and Nineteenth Centuries*. Vol. 1, *Medical Ethics and Etiquette in the Eighteenth Century*. Edited by Robert Baker, Dorothy Parker, and Roy Porter. Dordrecht, The Netherlands: Kluwer, 1993, pp. 179–211.

———, ed. "The Historical Context of the American Medical Association's 1847 *Code of Ethics*." In *The Codification of Medical Morality: Historical and Philosophical Studies of the Formalization of Western Medical Morality in the Eighteenth and Nineteenth Centuries*. Vol. 2, *Anglo-American Medical Ethics and Medical Jurisprudence in the Nineteenth Century*. Edited by Robert Baker. Dordrecht, The Netherlands: Kluwer, 1995a, pp. 47–63.

———. *The Codification of Medical Morality: Historical and Philosophical Studies of the Formalization of Western Medical Morality in the Eighteenth and Nineteenth Centuries*. Vol. 2, *Anglo-American Medical Ethics and Medical Jurisprudence in the Nineteenth Century*. Dordrecht, The Netherlands: Kluwer Academic Publishers, 1995b.

Baker, Robert B., Arthur L. Caplan, Linda L. Emanuel, and Stephen R. Latham. *The American Medical Ethics Revolution: How the AMA's Code of Ethics Has Transformed Physicians' Relations to Patients, Professionals, and Society*. Baltimore: The Johns Hopkins University Press, 1999.

Baker, Robert, Dorothy Parker, and Roy Porter, eds. *The Codification of Medical Morality: Historical and Philosophical Studies of the Formalization of Western Medical Morality in the Eighteenth and Nineteenth Centuries*. Vol. 1, *Medical Ethics and Etiquette in the Eighteenth Century*. Dordrecht: Kluwer, 1993.

Bard, Samuel. *An attempt to explain and justify the use of cold in uterine hemorrhages: with a view to remove the prejudices which prevail among the women of this city, against the use of this safe and necessary remedy*. New York: Printed by H. Gaine, at the Bible, in Hanover-Square, 1788.

———. *A Compendium of the theory and practice of midwifery: containing practical instructions for the Management of women, during pregnancy, in labour, and in childbed . . .* New York: Printed and sold by Collins and Perkins, 1807.

———. "A Discourse upon the Duties of a Physician: with some Sentiments on the Usefulness and Necessity of a Public Hospital." Delivered before the president and governors of King's College, at the commencement, held on the 15th of May, 1769. As advice to those gentlemen who then received the first medical degrees conferred by that university. New York: Printed by A. & J. Robertson, at the corner of Beaver-Street, 1769.

———. *An enquiry into the nature, cause and cure, of the angina suffocativa, or, sore throat distemper, as it is commonly called by the inhabitants of this city and colony.* New York: Printed by S. Inslee and A. Car, at the new printing-office in Beaver-Street, 1771.

———. *Tentamen medicum inaugurale, de viribus opii . . . Eruditorum examini subjicit Samuel Bard, Americanus.* Edinburgh: Apud A. Donaldson and J. Reid, 1765.

Barker, Lewellys F. "Osler, William." In *Dictionary of American Biography,* Vol. 7. Edited by Dumas Malone. New York: Scribners, 1957, pp. 83–87.

Barnes, Gilbert Hobbs. *The Anti-Slavery Impulse: 1830–1844.* 1933. New York: Harcourt, Brace & World, 1964.

Bartrip, Peter. "An Introduction to Jukes Styrap's *A Code of Medical Ethics.*" In *The Codification of Medical Morality: Historical and Philosophical Studies of the Formalization of Western Medical Morality in the Eighteenth and Nineteenth Centuries.* Vol. 2, *Anglo-American Medical Ethics and Medical Jurisprudence in the Nineteenth Century.* Edited by Robert Baker. Dordrecht: Kluwer, 1995, pp. 145–48.

Baumiller, Robert C. "Medical Ethics at Georgetown." In *The Teaching of Medical Ethics.* Edited by Robert M. Veatch, Willard Gaylin, and Councilman Morgan. Hastings-on-Hudson, New York: The Hastings Center, 1973, pp. 93–96.

Beall, Otho T., and Richard H. Shryock. *Cotton Mather: First Significant Figure in American Medicine.* Baltimore: Johns Hopkins University Press, 1954.

Beattie, James. *Elements of Moral Science.* 2 vols. Edinburgh and London: Printed for T. Cadell, William Creech 1790, 1793.

Beauchamp, Tom. "Worthington Hooker on Ethics in Clinical Medicine." In *The Codification of Medical Morality: Historical and Philosophical Studies of the Formalization of Western Medical Morality in the Eighteenth and Nineteenth Centuries.* Vol. 2, *Anglo-American Medical Ethics and Medical Jurisprudence in the Nineteenth Century.* Edited by Robert Baker. Dordrecht: Kluwer, 1995, pp. 105–19.

Beauchamp, Tom L., and James F. Childress, eds. *Principles of Biomedical Ethics,* 5th ed. New York: Oxford University Press, 2001.

Beecher, Henry K. "Clinical Impression and Clinical Investigation." *Journal of the American Medical Association* 151 (1953): 44–45.

———. "Ethics and Clinical Research." *New England Journal of Medicine* 274 (1966): 1354–60.

———. "Experimental Pharmacology and Measurement of Subjective Response." *Science* 115 (1952): 157–62.

———. "The Measurement of Pain—Prototype for the Quantitative Study of Subjective Responses." *Pharmacological Review* 9 (1957): 59–209.

———. "The Powerful Placebo." *Journal of the American Medical Association* 159 (1955): 1602–06.

———. *Research and the Individual: Human Studies.* Boston: Little, Brown and Company, 1970.

Bell, John (1763–1820). *Letters on Professional Character and Manners: on the education of a Surgeon, and the Duties and Qualifications of a Physician: Addressed to James Gregory, M.D.* Edinburgh: Printed by John Moir . . . and sold at all the booksellers in London and Edinburgh, 1810, xxiii.

Bell, John (1796–1872). *Dietetical and Medical Hydrology. A Treatise on Baths: Including Cold, Sea, Warm, Hot, Vapour, Gas, and Mud Baths: Also on the Watery Regimen,*

Hydropathy, and Pulmonary Inhalation; with a Description of Bathing in Ancient and Modern Times. Philadelphia: Barringtron and Haswell, 1850.

———. *An Inaugural Dissertation on the Liver: Its Influence Over the Animal Economy in Health and Disease.* Philadelphia: Printed by William Fry, 1817.

———. "Introduction to the Code of Medical Ethics" 1847. In *The Codification of Medical Morality: Historical and Philosophical Studies of the Formalization of Western Medical Morality in the Eighteenth and Nineteenth Centuries.* Vol. 2, *Anglo-American Medical Ethics and Medical Jurisprudence in the Nineteenth Century.* Edited by R. Baker. Dordrecht: Kluwer, 1995, pp. 65–72.

———. *The Mineral and Thermal Springs of the United States and Canada.* Philadelphia: Parry and McMillan, 1855.

———. *On Baths and Mineral Waters. Part I: a History . . . Of the Chief Mineral Springs of the United States and Europe.* Philadelphia: H.H. Porter, 1831.

———. *Report on the Importance and Economy of Sanitary Measures.* New York: Jones, 1859.

———. *A Treatise on Physiology Applied to Pathology.* Philadelphia: H. C. Carey and I. Lea, 1826.

———, ed. *The Eclectic Journal of Medicine.* Began with Vol. 1 (1836) and ceased with Vol. 4 (1840). Philadelphia: Barrington and Haswell, 1836–1840.

Bell, John, Isaac Hays, G. Emerson, W. W. Morris, T. C. Dunn, A. Clark, and R. D. Arnold. "Note to Convention" [1847] *The Codification of Medical Morality: Historical and Philosophical Studies of the Formalization of Western Medical Morality in the Eighteenth and Nineteenth Centuries. Volume Two: Anglo-American Medical Ethics and Medical Jurisprudence in the Nineteenth Century.* Edited by R. Baker. Dordrecht, The Netherlands: Kluwer Academic Publishers, 1995, pp. 73-74.

Bergsma, Daniel, Marc Lappe, Richard O. Roblin, and James M. Gustafson, eds. *Ethical, Social and Legal Dimensions of Screening for Human Genetic Disease.* New York: Stratton Intercontinental Medical Book Corporation, 1974.

Bettany, G. T. "John Gregory." In *Dictionary of National Biography*, Vol. 23. Edited by Leslie Stephen and Sidney Lee. London: Smith, Elder & Co., 1890, p. 102.

———. "William Cullen." In *Dictionary of National Biography*, Vol. 13. Edited by Leslie Stephen. London: Smith, Elder & Co., 1888, pp. 279–82.

Binger, Carl. *Revolutionary Doctor: Benjamin Rush, 1746–1813.* New York: Norton, 1966.

Boston Medical Police. Boston: Snelling and Simons, 1808.

Branch, C. H. "Psychiatric Aspects of Malignant Disease." *CA: Bulletin of Cancer Progress* 6 (1956): 102–04.

Brantley, Richard E. *Locke, Wesley, and the Method of English Romanticism.* Gainesville; FL: University Presses of Florida, 1984.

Brennan, Troyen A. *Just Doctoring: Medical Ethics in the Liberal State.* Berkeley: University of California Press, 1991.

Bright, Henry A. *A Historical Sketch of Warrington Academy.* Transactions of the Historic Society of Lancashire and Cheshire, Vol. 11, read November 11, 1858. Liverpool: T. Brakell, 1859.

British Medical Association. *Handbook of Medical Ethics.* London: British Medical Association, 1981.

———. *Medical Ethics.* London: British Medical Association, 1970.

———. *Members Handbook.* London: British Medical Association, 1963.

———. *Rights and Responsibilities of Doctors.* London: British Medical Association, 1988.

Brody, Howard. "The Physician's Role in Determining Futility." *Journal of the American Geriatrics Society* 42, no. 8 (1994): 875–877.

———. *The Healer's Power*. New Haven: Yale University Press, 1992.

———, and Franklin G. Miller. "The Internal Morality of Medicine; Explication and Application to Managed Care." *Journal of Medicine and Philosophy* 23 (1998): 384–410.

Burns, Chester R. "Medical Ethics, History of: North America—Seventeenth to Nineteenth Century. In *The Encyclopedia of Bioethics*. New York: The Free Press, 1978, pp. 963–68.

———. "Richard Clarke Cabot (1868–1939) and Reformation in American Medical Ethics." *Bulletin of the History of Medicine* 51 (no. 3) (1977a): 353–68.

Burns, C. R., ed. *Legacies in Ethics and Medicine*. New York: Science History Publications, 1977b.

Burrage, Walter L. "Bard, Samuel." In *Dictionary of American Biography*. Vol. 1. Edited by Allen Johnson. New York: Scribner's Sons, 1957, pp. 598–99.

———. "Hays, Isaac." In *Dictionary of American Medical Biography*. Edited by Howard A. Kelly and Walter L. Burrage. New York: D. Appleton & Co., 1928, pp. 545–46.

Bushnell, Horace. *Christian Nurture*. 1861. New Haven: Yale University Press, 1962.

Cabot, Richard C. *Adventures on the Borderlands of Ethics*. New York: Harper & Brothers, 1926.

———. *Christianity and Sex*. New York: Macmillan, 1937.

———. *Differential Diagnosis*. Philadelphia: W. B. Saunders Company, 1911–14.

———. *Honesty*. New York: Macmillan, 1938.

———. *The Meaning of Right and Wrong*, rev. ed. New York: Macmillan, 1936.

———. *Physical Diagnosis*. New York: W. Wood and Company, 1905.

———. *Richard Cabot on Practice, Training and the Doctor–Patient Relationship*. Edited with introductions by John Stoeckle and Lawrence A. May. Oceanside, NY: Distributed by Dabor Science Publications, 1977.

———. *Social Service and the Art of Healing*. New York: Moffat, Yard and Co., 1909.

———. "The Use of Truth and Falsehood in Medicine." *Connecticut Medicine* 42 (1978): 189–94.

———. *What Men Live By; Work, Play, Love, Worship*. Boston, New York: Houghton Mifflin Company, 1914.

Callahan, Daniel. *Abortion: Law, Choice and Morality*. New York: Macmillan, 1970.

———. "Profile: Institute of Society, Ethics and the Life Sciences." *BioScience* 21 (1971): 735–37.

———, ed. *The Catholic Case for Contraception*. New York: Macmillan, 1969.

Canterbury v. Spence, 464 F. 2d 772 (D.C. Cir. 1972).

Capellmann, Carl. *Pastoral Medicine*. Translated by William Dassel. New York: Pustet, 1879.

Carlson, Eric T., and Meribeth M. Simpson. "Benjamin Rush's Medical Use of the Moral Faculty." *Bulletin of the History of Medicine* 39 (1965): 22–33.

Carrick, Paul. *Medical Ethics in Antiquity: Philosophical Perspectives on Abortion and Euthanasia*. Dordrecht: D. Reidel Publishing Company, 1985.

Carvalho, Joseph. "Cabot, Richard Clarke." In *Dictionary of American Medical Biography*. Edited by Martin Kaufman, Stuart Galishoff, and Todd L. Savitt. Westport, CT: Greenwood Press, 1984, pp. 112–13.

Cash, P. "Warren, John." In *Dictionary of American Medical Biography*. Edited by Martin Kaufman, Stuart Galishoff, and Todd L. Savitt. Westport, CT: Greenwood Press, 1984, pp. 778–79.

Cassell, Eric J. *The Healer's Art.* Cambridge, MA: MIT Press, 1985.

"Central Ethical Committee." *British Medical Journal Supplement* (May 1, 1971): 30.

Chapman, Carleton B. *Physicians, Law, and Ethics.* New York: New York University Press, 1984.

Chapman, N. *Discourses on the Elements of Therapeutics and Materia Medica.* Philadelphia: James Webster, 1817–1819.

———. *Discourses on the Elements of Therapeutics and Materia Medica*, 3rd ed. Philadelphia: Mathew Carey, 1823–1824.

———. *An Essay on the Canine State of Fever.* Philadelphia: Hugh Maxwell, 1801.

———. *Lectures on the More Important Eruptive Fevers, Haemorrhages and Dropsies: and on Gout and Rheumatism. Delivered in the University of Pennsylvania.* Philadelphia: Lea and Blanchard, 1844.

———, ed. *Select Speeches Forensick and Parliamentary.* 5 vols. Philadelphia: Hopkins, 1807–1808.

———, et al. *Essays on Practical Medicine and Surgery.* 2 vols. Philadelphia: Lea, 1841.

Chitnis, Anand. C. *The Scottish Enlightenment: A Social History.* London: Croom Helm, 1976.

Christie, J. R. R. "Ether and the Science of Chemistry 1740–1790." In *Conceptions of Ether.* Edited by G. N. Cantor and M. J. S. Hodge. Cambridge: Cambridge University Press, 1981, pp. 85–110.

———. "The Origins and Development of the Scottish Scientific Community." *History of Science* 12 (1974): 122–41.

———. "The Rise and Fall of Scottish Science." In *The Emergence of Science in Western Europe.* Edited by M. P. Crosland. London: Macmillan, 1975, pp. 111–126.

Clegg, James. "Diary." Reprinted in part in *The Country Divine.* Edited by Michael Brander. Edinburgh: The Saint Andrew Press, 1981, pp. 47–61.

Clerke, Agnès. Mary. "Gregory, James (1638–1675)." In *Dictionary of National Biography*, vol. 23. Edited by Leslie Stephen and Sidney Lee. London: Smith, Elder & Co., 1890, pp. 98–99.

Cobbs v. Grant 502 P.2d 1 (Cal. 1972).

Commission for Visiting the Universities and Colleges in Scotland. *Evidence, Oral and Documentary, Taken and Received by The Commissioners Appointed by His Majesty George IV, July 23d, 1826; and Re-appointed by His Majesty, William IV, October 12th, 1830; for Visiting the Universities of Scotland, Volume I. University of Edinburgh.* London: Printed by W. Clowes and Sones, Stamford Street, for His Majesty's Stationery Office, 1837.

Cooke, Robert E., Andre E. Hellegers, Robert G. Hoyt, and Herbert W. Richardson, eds. *The Terrible Choice: The Abortion Dilemma, Based on the Proceedings of the International Conference on Abortion Sponsored by the Harvard Divinity School and the Joseph P. Kennedy Jr. Foundation.* New York: Bantom Books, 1967.

Coughtrey, Millen, M. B., C. M., with Hons., Edin. "The Graduation Address, on the Occasion of the Conferring, for the first time in New Zealand, of the Degrees of LL.D. and M.B. of the New Zealand University, Dunedin, New Zealand, August 19, 1887." Dunedin: Printed by G. R. Smith, *Otago Daily Times* Office, 1887.

———. "The Introductory Address in the Faculty of Medicine of Otago University, Delivered at Dunedin, May 31, 1875." Dunedin: MacKay, Risk, Munro, & Co. 1875.

Coxe, John Redman. An Inquiry into the Claims of Doctor William Harvey to the Discovery of the Circulation of the Blood: with a More Equitable Retrospect of That Event; to Which Is Added an Introductory Lecture, Delivered on the Third of November,

1829, in Vindication of Hippocrates from Sundry Charges of Ignorance Preferred Against Him by the Late Professor Rush. Philadelphia: C. Sherman & Co., 1834.

———. *The Writings of Hippocrates and Galen. Epitomised from the Original Latin.* Philadelphia: Lindsay and Blakiston, 1846.

Crowther, M. Anne, "Forensic Medicine and Medical Ethics in Nineteenth-Century Britain." In Baker, Robert, ed. *The Codification of Medical Morality: Historical and Philosophical Studies of the Formalization of Western Medical Morality in the Eighteenth and Nineteenth Centuries. Volume Two: Anglo-American Medical Ethics and Medical Jurisprudence in the Nineteenth Century.* Dordrecht, The Netherlands: Kluwer Academic Publishers, pp. 173–90.

Cushing, Harvey. *The Life of Sir William Osler.* London: Oxford University Press, 1940.

Daiches, David, Peter Jones, and Jean Jones, eds. *A Hotbed of Genius: The Scottish Enlightenment, 1730–1790.* Edinburgh: Edinburgh University Press, 1986.

Dalzel, Andrew. *History of the University of Edinburgh from Its Foundation.* 2 vols. Edinburgh: Edmonston and Douglas, 1862.

Davie, George. E. *The Democratic Intellect: Scotland and Her Universities in the Nineteenth Century.* Edinburgh: Edinburgh University Press, 1961.

———. *The Scottish Enlightenment.* London: Historical Association, 1981.

Davis, N. S. *History of the American Medical Association from its Organization up to January 1855.* Edited by S. W. Butler, MD. Philadelphia: Lippincott, Grambo, & Co., 1855.

D'Elia, Donald J. "Benjamin Rush: Philosopher of the American Revolution." *Transactions of the American Philosophical Society* 64 (new series), Part 5 (1974): 1–113.

Donnachie, Ian, and George Hewitt. *A Companion to Scottish History from the Reformation to the Present.* London: B. T. Batsford Ltd., 1989.

Douglas, Sholto [pseud.]. "Some Account of a Secret Society in New York entitled the "Kappa Lambda" in A Letter to Alexander H. Stevens MD LLD by a Retired Physician." 1859. Available in the library of the College of Physicians of Philadelphia.

Dow, Derek, ed. *The Influence of Scottish Medicine: An Historical Assessment of Its International Impact.* Carnforth, Lancs, Great Britain: The Parthenon Publishing Co., 1988.

Dukeminier, Jesse, and David Sanders. "Organ Transplantation: A Proposal for Routine Salvaging of Cadaver Organs." *New England Journal of Medicine* 279 (1968): 413–19.

Duncan, A. S., G. R. Dunstan, and R. B. Welbourn, eds. *Dictionary of Medical Ethics.* London: Darton, Longman & Todd, 1977.

Edelstein, Ludwig. "The Hippocratic Oath: Text, Translation and Interpretation." In *Ancient Medicine: Selected Papers of Ludwig Edelstein.* Edited by Owsei Temkin, and C. Lilian Temkin. Baltimore: The Johns Hopkins Press, 1967, pp. 3–64.

Edinburgh, University of. *Record University of Edinburgh Laureations and Degrees 1585 to 1809.* Unpublished. Available from the University Library Special Collections.

———. *Record University of Edinburgh Laureations and Degrees 1810 to 1896.* Unpublished. Available from the University Library Special Collections.

———. *University of Edinburgh: Record of Degrees in Medicine, 1897–1953.* Unpublished. Available from the University Library Special Collections.

———. *University of Edinburgh: Record of Degrees in Medicine 1954–; Degrees in Dental Surgery, 1954–; Degrees in Veterinary Medicine and Surgery, 1957–1964; Degrees in Medical Sciences, 1966–.* Unpublished. Available in the Registry Office, University of Edinburgh.

Edwards, Maldyn. *John Wesley and the Eighteenth Century*. London: George Allen & Unwin Ltd., 1933.

Eli, R. George. *Social Holiness: John Wesley's Thinking on Christian Community and its Relationship to the Social Order*. New York: Peter Lang, 1993.

Ellis, Joseph J. *Founding Brothers: The Revolutionary Generation*. New York: Alfred A. Knopf, 2000.

Emanuel, Ezekiel J. *The Ends of Human Life: Medical Ethics in a Liberal Polity*. Cambridge, Ma.: Harvard University Press, 1991.

Engelhardt, H. Tristram. *The Foundations of Bioethics*. Second Edition. New York: Oxford University Press, 1996.

Erlam, H. D. "Alexander Monro, Primus." *University of Edinburgh Journal* (1954): 77–105.

Espinasse, Francis. "Ferguson, Adam." In *Dictionary of National Biography*, vol. 18. Edited by Leslie Stephen. London: Smith, Elder & Co., 1889, pp. 336–340.

"Extracts from the Medical Ethics of Dr. Percival." Philadelphia, 1823.

Faculty of Medicine Minutes, Vol. 1, 28 April 1891 to 29 April 1902. Dunedin, New Zealand: University of Otago Faculty of Medicine, n.d.

Faculty of Medicine Minutes, Vol. 6, 3 June 1947 to 12 December 1952. Dunedin, New Zealand: University of Otago Faculty of Medicine, n.d.

Fagley, Richard M. *The Population Explosion and Christian Responsibility*. New York: Oxford University Press, 1960.

Farlow, John W. "Fleet, John." In *Dictionary of American Medical Biography*. Edited by Howard A. Kelly and Walter L. Burrage. New York: D. Appleton & Co., 1928, pp. 413–14.

Feldman, David M. *Birth Control in Jewish Law*. New York: New York University Press, 1968.

Finney, Charles G. *Revivals of Religion*. 1835. Chicago: The Moody Bible Institute, 1962.

Finney, Patrick, and Patrick O'Brien. *Moral Problems in Hospital Practice: A Practical Handbook*. St. Louis: B. Herder Book Co., 1956.

Fitts, William T., Jr, and I. S. Ravdin. "What Philadelphia Physicians Tell Patients with Cancer." *Journal of the American Medical Association* 153 (1953): 901–04.

Fleet, John. *A discourse relative to the subject of animation delivered before the Humane Society of the Commonwealth of Massachusetts, at their semiannual meeting June 13th, 1797*. Boston: John & Thomas Fleet, 1797.

———. *Dissertatio inauguralis medica, sistens observationes ad chirurgiae operationes pertinentes, apud interrogationem publicam prolocutas et sustentatas die Julii III, habitam, quam annuente summo numine ex auctoritate Reverendi Josephi Willard, praesidis, &c. Honoratorum et reverendorum curatorum et etiam senatus academici consensu, nec non institutionis medicae decreto*. Boston: Typis Thomae Fleet, 1795.

Fletcher, John C. "Realities of Patient Consent to Medical Research." *Hastings Center Studies* 1, no. 1 (1973): 39–49.

———. "A Study of the Ethics of Medical Research." Th.D. thesis, Union Theological Seminary, 1969.

Fletcher, Joseph. *The Ethics of Genetic Control: Ending Reproductive Roulette*. Garden City, NY: Anchor Books, 1974.

———. *Morals and Medicine*. Princeton, NJ: Princeton University Press, 1954.

———. "Our Shameful Waste of Human Tissue." In *Updating Life and Death*. Edited by Donald R. Cutler. Boston: Beacon Press, 1969, pp. 1–27.

———. *Situation Ethics: The New Morality*. Philadelphia: Westminster Press, 1966.

Flint, Austin (1812–1886). *Medical Ethics and Etiquette: The Code of Ethics Adopted by the American Medical Association,* with Commentaries by Austin Flint. New York: Appleton, 1883.

Ford, John, and J. E. Drew. "Advising Radical Surgery: A Problem of Medical Morality." *Journal of the American Medical Association* 151 (1953): 714.

———. "Human Experimentation in Medicine: Moral Aspects." *Clinical Pharmacology and Therapeutics* 1 (1960): 396–400.

———. "Notes on Moral Theology," *Theological Studies* 6 (1945): 543–44.

Fox, Renée C. *Experiment Perilous: Physicians and Patients Facing the Unknown.* Glencoe, IL: The Free Press, 1959.

_____, and Judith P. Swazey. *The Courage to Fail: A Social View of Organ Transplants and Dialysis.* Chicago: University of Chicago Press, 1974.

Fuller, Louis. *The Crusade Against Slavery: 1830–1860.* New York: Harper & Row, 1960.

Fuller, Robert C. *Alternative Medicine and American Religious Life.* Oxford: Oxford University Press, 1989.

"General Medical Council: Disciplinary Committee." *British Medical Journal Supplement,* no. 3442, March 20 (1971): 79–80.

Gihon, A. L., ed. United States Navy Dept. Bureau of Medicine and Surgery. *Medical Essays; Compiled from Reports to the Bureau of Medicine and Surgery by Medical Officers of the U.S. Navy.* Washington, DC: Government PrintingOffice, 1872.

Gillon, Raanan, ed. *Principles of Health Care Ethics.* New York: Wiley, 1994.

Girdwood, RH. "The Influence of Scotland on North American Medicine." In *The Influence of Scottish Medicine: An Historical Assessment of Its International Impact.* Edited by Derek Dow. Carnforth, Lancs, Great Britain: Parthenon, 1988, pp. 33–42.

Gisborne, Thomas. *An Enquiry into the Duties of Men in the Higher and Middle Classes of Society in Great Britain Resulting from their Respective Stations, Professions and Employments.* London: Printed by J. Davis, for B. and J. White, 1794.

———. *On Slavery and the Slave Trade.* London: J. Stockdale, J. Debrett, and J. Phillips, 1792.

———. *On the Duties of Physicians: Resulting from Their Profession.* Edited by W. A. Greenhill. Oxford: John Henry Parker; London: John Churchill, 1847.

———. *The Principles of Moral Philosophy Investigated, and Briefly Applied to the Constitution of Civil Society: Together with Remarks on the Principle Assumed by Mr. Paley as the Basis of All Moral Conclusions, and on Other Positions of the Same Author.* London: Printed by T. Bensley, for B. White and Son, 1789.

Gold, Hal. *Unit 731 Testimony: Japan's Wartime Human Experimentation Program.* Tokyo: Yenbooks, 1996.

Gomperz, Theodor. *Greek Thinkers: A History of Ancient Philosophy.* 1900–12. London: John Murray, 1929–39.

Good, Frederick L., and Otis F. Kelly. *Marriage, Morals and Medical Ethics.* New York: P. J. Kenedy, 1951.

Goodman, Nathan G. *Benjamin Rush: Physician and Citizen: 1746–1813.* Philadelphia: University of Pennsylvania Press, 1934.

Gorovitz, Samuel, Andrew L. Jameton, Ruth Macklin, John M. O'Connor, Eugene V. Perrin, Beverly Page St. Clair, and Susan Sherwin. *Moral Problems in Medicine.* Englewood Cliffs, NJ: Prentice-Hall, Inc., 1976.

Green, Richard. *The Works of John and Charles Wesley,* 2nd ed. London: Charles H. Kelly, 1896.

Gregory, [James]. *Answer to Dr James Hamilton, Junior.* Edinburgh: no publisher, 1793.

Gregory, James. *Philosophical and Literary Essays*. Vols. Edinburgh: Sold by T. Cadell, London, and W. Creech, Edinburgh, 1792.

Gregory, John. *A Comparative View of the State and Faculties of Man with Those of the Animal World*. London: Printed for J. Dodsley in Pall-Mall, 1765.

———. [1774]. In *Letters on the Improvement of the Mind*. Edited by Mrs. Chapone [Hester Mulso]. *A Father's Legacy to His Daughters* by Dr. Gregory. *A Mother's advice to Her absent Daughters* by Lady Pennington. with Lives of the Author. Edinburgh: Printed for Fairbairn & Anderson; William Whyte & Co.; William Oliphant; James Robertson; and T. Tegg, London, 1821.

———. *John Gregory's Writings on Medical Ethics and Philosophy of Medicine*. Edited by Laurence B. McCullough. Dordrecht: Kluwer, 1998.

———. *Lectures on the Duties and Qualifications of a Physician*. London: W. Strahan and T. Cadell, in the Strand, 1772.

———. *Lectures on the duties and qualifications of a physician*. Revised and corrected by James Gregory. Edinburgh: Printed for William Creech; and T. Cadell & W. Davies, London; Alex Smellie, Printer, 1805.

———. *Lectures on the Duties and Qualifications of a Physician*. Philadelphia: M. Carey & Son, 1817.

[Gregory, John]. *Observations on the Duties and Offices of a Physician; and on the Method of Prosecuting Enquiries in Philosophy*. London: W. Strahan; and T. Cadell, (successor to Mr. Millar) in the Strand, 1770.

Grisez, Germain G. *Abortion: The Myths, The Realities, and the Arguments*. New York: Corpus Books, 1970.

Grosart, A. B. "Beattie, James." In *Dictionary of National Biography*, Vol. 4. Edited by Leslie Stephen. London: Smith, Elder & Co., 1885, pp. 22–25.

Gury, Jean Pierre. *Casus conscientiae in praecipuas guestiones theologiae moralis*, 6th ed. Lyons: Briday, 1881. First published 1866.

———. *Compendium theologiae moralis*, 18th ed. Paris: H. Pelaguad, 1869.

Gustafson, James M. "Context Versus Principles: A Misplaced Debate in Christian Ethics. In *New Theology No. 3*. Edited by Martin E. Marty and Dean G. Peerman. New York: Macmillan, 1966, pp. 69–102.

———. "Mongolism, Parental Desires, and the Right to Life." *Perspectives in Biology and Medicine* 16 (Spring 1973): 529–557.

———. *Treasures in Earthen Vessels: The Church as a Human Community*. New York: Harper, 1961.

Guttentag, Otto E. "The Physician's Point of View." *Science* 117 (1953): 207–214.

Guttmacher, Alan F., ed. *The Case for Legalized Abortion Now*. Berkeley, CA: Diablo Press, 1967.

Haakonssen, Lisbeth. *Medicine and Morals in The Enlightenment: John Gregory, Thomas Percival, and Benjamin Rush*. Amsterdam: Rodopi, 1997.

Hamilton, D. "The Scottish Enlightenment and Clinical Medicine." In *The Influence of Scottish Medicine: An Historical Assessment of Its International Impact*. Edited by Derek Dow. Carnforth, Lancs, Great Britain: The Parthenon Publishing Co., 1988, pp. 105–11.

Harris, Sheldon H. *Factories of Death: Japanese Biological Warfare, 1932–45, and the American Cover-up*. London: Routledge, 1994.

Harvard Medical School. "A Definition of Irreversible Coma. Report of the Ad Hoc Committee of the Harvard Medical School to Examine the Definition of Brain Death." *Journal of the American Medical Association* 205 (1968): 337–340.

Harvey, D. C. *An Introduction to The History of Dalhousie University*. Halifax: McCurdy Printing Co., 1938.

Hathout, Hassan. "Islamic Basis for Biomedical Ethics." In: *Transcultural Dimensions in Medical Ethics*. Edited by Pellegrino, Edmund D., Patricia Mazzarella, and Pietro Corsi. Frederick, MD: University of Publishing Group, Inc., 1992, pp. 57–72.

Hawes, W. *An Examination of The Rev. Mr. John Wesley's Primitive Physic: Shewing That Great Number of the Prescriptions therein contained, are founded on Ignorance of the Medical Art, and of the Power and Operation of medicines; and that it is a Publication calculated to do essential Injury to the Health of those Persons who may place Confidence in it. Interspersed with Medical Remarks and Practical Observation*. London: Printed for the Author; and sold by J. Dodsley, Pall-Mall; T. Cadell, Strand; B. Jonson, St. Paul's Church-yard; and W. Fox, Holborn, 1776.

———. *Memoirs of William Hawes, M.D. of London*. London: W. Phillips, 1802.

Hawke, David Freeman. *Benjamin Rush: Revolutionary Gadfly*. Indianapolis: Bobbs-Merrill, 1971.

"Hays, Isaac." In *Appleton's Cyclopaedia of American Biography*, Vol. 3. Edited by James Grant Wilson and John Fiske. New York: D. Appleton & Co., 1888–1889. Reprint. Detroit: Gale Research, 1968, p. 146.

"Hays, Isaac." In *The National Cyclopaedia of American Biography*, Vol. 11. New York: James T. White & Co., 1901. Reprint. Ann Arbor, MI: University Microfilms, 1967–1971, pp. 256–57.

"Hayward, Lemuel." In *The National Cyclopedia*, Vol. 11. New York: J. T. White, 1930, p. 484.

Healy, Edwin F. *Medical Ethics*. Chicago: Loyola University Press, 1956.

Hercus, Charles, and Gordon Bell. *The Otago Medical School Under the First Three Deans*. Edinburgh: E & S Livingstone Ltd., 1964.

Hill, A. Wesley. *John Wesley Among the Physicians: A Study of Eighteenth-century Medicine*. London: Epworth Press, 1958.

"Hippocratic Oath, The." *British Medical Journal* 309 (October 8, 1994): 952–53.

Holifield, E. Brooks. *Health and Medicine in the Methodist Tradition: Journey Toward Wholeness*. New York: Crossroad, 1986.

Hooker, Brad, and Margaret Olivia Little, eds. *Moral Particularism*. New York: Oxford University Press, 2000.

Hooker, Worthington. *Dissertation on the Respect Due the Medical Profession, and the Reasons that It is not Awarded by the Community*. Norwich, CT: J. G. Cooley, 1844.

———. *A First Book in Physiology. For the Use of Schools. An Introduction to the Larger Work by the Same Author*. New York: Sheldon and Company, [1883].

———. *Homeopathy: An Examination of Its Doctrines and Evidences*. New York: Scribner, 1851.

———. *Human Physiology: Designed for Colleges and the Higher Classes in Schools, and for General Reading*. New York, Farmer, Brace, & Co., 1854.

———. *Lessons from the History of Medical Delusions*. New York: Baker & Scribner, 1850.

———. *Physician and Patient: Or, a Practical View of the Mutual Duties, Relations and Interests of the Medical Profession and the Community*. New York: Baker & Scribner, 1849.

Howard, J. K. "Dr. Thomas Percival and the Beginnings of Industrial Legislation." *Journal of the Society of Occupational Medicine* 25, no. 2 (1975): 58–65.

Hume, David. *An Enquiry Concerning the Principles of Morals*. 1751. Edited by Charles W. Hendel. New York: Liberal Arts Press, 1957.

————. *A Treatise of Human Nature.* 1739–40. Edited by L. A. Selby-Bigge, revised by P. Nidditch, 2nd ed. Oxford: Clarendon, 1978.

Huntley, Frank Livingstone. *Sir Thomas Browne: A Biographical and Critical Study.* Ann Arbor: University of Michigan Press, 1962.

Hutcheson, Francis. *Illustrations on the Moral Sense.* 1728. Cambridge, MA: The Belknap Press of Harvard University Press, 1971.

Institute of Society, Ethics and the Life Sciences. *Directory: 1976.* Hastings-on-Hudson, NY: The Institute of Society, Ethics and the Life Sciences, 1976.

————. *Ethics, Population and the American Tradition.* Vol. III, *A Report to the Commission on Population Growth and the American Future.* Hastings-on-Hudson, NY: The Institute of Society, Ethics and the Life Sciences, 1971f.

————. "Program in the Ethical, Social and Legal Issues of Behavior Control." Unpublished document, Institute Program Series Number Four. Hastings-on-Hudson, NY: The Hastings Center Institute of Society, Ethics and the Life Science, [ca. 1971a].

————. "Program in the Ethical, Social and Legal Issues of Death and Dying." Unpublished document, Institute Program Series Number Two. Hastings-on-Hudson, NY: The Hastings Center Institute of Society, Ethics and the Life Science, [ca. 1971b].

————. "Program in the Ethical, Social and Legal Issues of Genetic Counseling and Genetic Engineering." Unpublished document, Institute Program Series Number Five. Hastings-on-Hudson, NY: The Hastings Center Institute of Society, Ethics and the Life Science, [ca. 1971c].

————. "Program in Ethics and Population Policy." Unpublished document, Institute Program Series Number Three. Hastings-on-Hudson, NY: The Hastings Center Institute of Society, Ethics and the Life Science, [ca. 1971d].

————. "Program in Medical Ethics." Unpublished document, Institute Program Series Number Five. Hastings-on-Hudson, NY: The Hastings Center Institute of Society, Ethics and the Life Science, [ca. 1971e].

————. *Program in Medical Ethics: Columbia University College of Physicians and Surgeons and the Institute of Society, Ethics and the Life Sciences: Final Report.* Hastings-on-Hudson, NY: The Institute of Society, Ethics and the Life Sciences, [ca. 1972].

Institute on Human Values in Medicine. *Proceedings of the First Session: Arden House, Harriman, New York, April 12–14, 1971.* Project director, Lorraine L. Hunt. Philadelphia: Society for Health and Human Values, [1972].

Jackson, Joseph. *Encyclopedia of Philadelphia,* Vol. 1. Harrisburg: The National Historical Association, 1931.

Jakobovits, Immanuel. "Judaism." In *Encyclopedia of Bioethics,* Vol. 2. Edited by Warren T. Reich. New York: The Free Press, 1978, pp. 791–802.

————. *Jewish Medical Ethics: A Comparative and Historical Study of the Jewish Religious Attitude to Medicine and Its Practice.* New York: Bloch, 1959.

Jarboe, Betty M. *John and Charles Wesley: A Bibliography.* Metuchen, NJ: The American Theological Library Association and The Scarecrow Press, Inc., 1987.

Jenkins, Daniel Thomas. *The Doctor's Profession.* London: SCM Press, [1949].

Jennett, B., and F. Plum. "Persistent Vegetative State after Brain Damage." *Lancet* 1 (1972): 734–737.

Johnson, W. H. "Civil Rights of Military Personnel Regarding Medical Care and Experimental Procedures." *Science* 117 (1953): 212–15.

Jones, D. W. Carmalt. *Annals of the University of Otago Medical School 1875–1939.* Wellington, NZ: A. H. and A. W. Reed, 1945.

Jones, R. Kenneth, ed. *Sickness and Sectarianism.* Hampshire, England: Gower, 1985.

Jones, W. H. S. *The Doctor's Oath: An Essay in the History of Medicine*. Cambridge: At The University Press, 1924.

Jonsen, Albert R. *The Birth of Bioethics*. New York: Oxford University Press, 1998.

————, and Andre E. Hellegers. "Conceptual Foundations for an Ethics of Medical Care." In *Ethics of Health Care*. Edited by Laurence R. Tancredi. Washington, DC: National Academy of Sciences, 1974, pp. 3–20.

————, and Stephen Toulmin. *The Abuse of Casuistry: A History of Moral Reasoning*. Berkeley: University of California Press, 1988.

Jouffroy, Théodore. *Introduction to Ethics*. Boston: J. Munroe and Company, 1848.

Kappa Lambda. *Constitution and By-Laws*. Philadelphia: Kappa Lambda, 1825.

————. "Extracts from the Medical Ethics of Dr. Percival" Philadelphia: Kappa Lambda, 1829.

————. "Formula To Be Observed at the Initiation of a Member Elect, Together with the Address To Be Delivered on This Occasion." Unpublished manuscript, [ca. 1824–26].

————. "Initiation Ceremony." Unpublished manuscript dated "11-27-22," that is, Nov. 27, 1822.

Katz, Jay. *Experimentation with Human Beings*. New York: Russell Sage Foundation, 1972.

Kelly, David F. *The Emergence of Roman Catholic Medical Ethics in North America: An Historical–Methodological–Bibliographical Study*. New York: The Edwin Mellen Press, 1979.

Kelly, Gerald. *Medico-Moral Problems*. St. Louis: The Catholic Hospital Association, 1958.

Kelly, Margaret K. "Emerson, Gouberneur." In *Dictionary of American Medical Biography*. Edited by Howard A. Kelly and Walter L. Burrage. New York: D. Appleton & Co., 1928, pp. 379–80.

Kelly, William D. and Stanley R. Friesen. "Do Cancer Patients Want to Be Told?" *Surgery* 27 (June 1950): 822–26.

Kendrick, Francis Patrick. *Theologia Moralis*. Mechlin: H. Dessain, 1860–61.

Kidd, Alexander M. "Limits of the Right of a Person to Consent to Experimentation on Himself." *Science* 117 (1953): 211–12.

King, Lester S. *American Medicine Comes of Age 1840–1920*. Chicago: American Medical Association, 1984.

————. "The 'Old Code' of Medical Ethics and Some Problems It Had to Face." *Journal of the American Medical Association* 248 (1982): 2329–33.

————. *Transformations in American Medicine: From Benjamin Rush to William Osler*. Baltimore: The Johns Hopkins University Press, 1991.

Konings, A. *Theologia moralis novissimi ecclesiae doctoris S. Alphonsi, in compendium redacta, et usui venerabilis cleri americana accomodata*, 4th ed. New York: Benziger Brothers, 1880.

Konold, Donald E. *A History of American Medical Ethics 1847–1912*. Madison: State Historical Society of Wisconsin, 1962.

Kuhn, Thomas S. *The Structure of Scientific Revolutions*. Chicago: University of Chicago Press, 1962.

Lader, Lawrence. *Abortion*. Boston: Beacon Press, 1966.

Ladimer, Irving, and Roger W. Newman. *Clinical Investigation in Medicine: Legal, Ethics and Moral Aspects: An Anthology and Bibliography*. Boston: Boston University Law-Medicine Research Institute, 1963.

Lansing, D. I. "Hays. Isaac." In *Dictionary of American Medical Biography*, Vol. 1. Edited by Martin Kaufman, Stuart Galishoff, and Todd L. Savitt. Westport, CT: Greenwood Press, 1984, p. 333.

Lanza, Conrad H. "Chapman, Nathaniel." In *Dictionary of American Biography*, Vol. 2. Edited by Allen Johnson and Dumas Malone. New York: Charles Scribner's Sons, 1957, pp. 19–20.

Lawrence, Christopher. "Alexander Monro *Primus* and the Edinburgh Manner of Anatomy." *Bulletin of the History of Medicine* 62 (1988a): 193–214.

———. "The Edinburgh School and the End of the 'Old Thing' 1970–1830." *History of Universities* 7 (1988b): 259–86.

———. "Ornate Physicians and Learned Artisans: Edinburgh Medical Men, 1726–1776." In *William Hunter and the Eighteenth-century Medical World.* Edited by W. F. Bynum and Roy Porter. London: Cambridge University Press, 1985, pp. 153–76.

Lehmkuhl, Augustin. *Casus conscientiae ad usum confessariorum compositi et soluti*, 3rd ed. Fribourg: Herder, 1907.

Lenman, Bruce. *Integration, Enlightenment and Industrialisation: Scotland 1746–1832*. London: Edward Arnold, 1981.

Lifton, Robert J. *Nazi Doctors: Medical Killing and the Psychology of Genocide*. New York: Basic Books, 1986.

Liguori, Alfonso Maria de'. *Theologia moralis* (1748–85). Editio nova. Edited by Leonard Gaude. 4 vols. Rome: Vaticana, 1905–12.

Lipsett, Mortimer B, John C. Fletcher, and Marian Secundy. "Research Review at NIH." *Hastings Center Report* 9, (no. 1 (1979): 18–21.

MacArthur, Kathleen Walter. *The Economic Ethics of John Wesley*. New York: Abingdon, 1936.

Maclaurin, Colin. *An account of Sir Isaac Newton's Philosophical Discoveries, in Four Books*. London: A. Millar, and J. Nourse, 1748.

"Majority Papal Commission Report." In Callahan, Daniel, ed. *The Catholic Case for Contraception*. New York: Macmillan, 1969, pp. 149–73.

Marquardt, Manfred. *John Wesley's Social Ethics: Praxis and Principles*. Nashville: Abingdon, 1992.

Mather, Cotton. "The Angel of Bethesda," In *Cotton Mather: First Significant Figure in American Medicine*. By Otho T. Beall and Richard H. Shryock. Baltimore: Johns Hopkins University Press 1954, pp. 127–234.

May, William F. "Code, Covenant, Contract, or Philanthropy?" *Hastings Center Report* 5 (December 1975): 29–38.

McCrae, Thomas. "Hays, Isaac." In *Dictionary of American Biography*, Vol. 4. Edited by Allen Johnson and Dumas Malone. New York: Scribner's, 1957, pp. 462–62.

McCulloch, Thomas. *The Stepsure Letters*. Toronto: McClelland and Street, 1960.

McCulloch, William. *Life of Thomas McCulloch, D.D.* Truro, Nova Scotia: privately published, 1920.

McCullough, Laurence B. *John Gregory and the Invention of Professional Medical Ethics and The Profession of Medicine*. Dordrecht: Kluwer, 1998.

———. "John Gregory's Medical Ethics and Humean Sympathy." In *The Codification of Medical Morality: Historical and Philosophical Studies of the Formalization of Western Medical Morality in the Eighteenth and Nineteenth Centuries*. Vol. 1, *Medical Ethics and Etiquette in the Eighteenth Century*. Edited by Robert Baker, Dorothy Parker, and Roy Porter. Dordrecht: Kluwer, 1993, pp. 145–60.

———. "Virtue, Etiquette, and Anglo-American Medical Ethics in the Eighteenth and Nineteenth Centuries." In *Virtue and Medicine: Exploration in the Character of Medicine*. Edited by Earl E. Shelp. Dordrecht: Reidel, 1985, pp. 88–89.

McFadden, Charles J. *Medical Ethics*, 6th ed. Philadelphia: F. A. Davis, 1967.

McLachlan, Herbert. *Warrington Academy, Its History and Influence.* [Manchester:] Printed for the Chetham Society, 1943.

McVicker, John. *A Domestic Narrative of the Life of Samuel Bard, M.D., LL. D.: Late President of the College of Physicians and Surgeons of the University of the State of New York.* New York: Literary Rooms [Columbia College], 1822.

Medical Association of the District of Columbia. *Regulations and System of Ethics of the Medical Association of Washington.* Washington, DC: Barron, 1833.

Medical Society of the State of New York. *A System of Medical Ethics.* New York: Grattan, 1823.

Medico-Chirurgical Society of Baltimore. *A System of Medical Ethics.* Baltimore: Printed by James Lucas and E. K. Deaver, 1832.

"Minority Papal Commission Report." In *The Catholic Case for Contraception.* Edited by Daniel Callahan. New York: Macmillan, 1969, pp. 174–211.

Monro, Alexander, Primus. "Life of Dr. Are. Monro Sr. in His Own Handwriting." Manuscript in the collection of the Medical Library of the University of Otago, New Zealand. [ca. 1760]

———. "The Professor's Daughter: An Essay on Female Conduct Contained in Letter from a Father to his Daughter, 1739. Transcribed from Original Manuscripts with Introduction and Notes by P. A. G. Monro, M.D." *Proceedings of the Royal College of Physicians of Edinburgh* 26, no. 1, Suppl. 2 (January 1996):

Monro, Alexander Secundus. "An Account of the Life of the Author." In *The Works of Alexander Monro, M.D., Fellow of the Royal Society, Fellow of the Royal College of Physicians, and late Professor of Medicine and anatomy in the University of Edinburgh. Published by his Son, Alexander Monro, M.D., President of the Royal College of Physicians, and Professor of Medicine and of anatomy and Surgery in the University of Edinburgh, to which is Prefixed, the Life of the author.* By Alexander Monro, [Primus]. Edinburgh: Printed for Charles Elliot, Parliament-Square; and George Robinson, No. 25, Paternoster-Row, London, 1781.

Moore, Norman. "Monro, Alexander." In *Dictionary of National Biography,* Vol. 38. Edited by Sidney Lee. London: Smith, Elder & Co., 1894, pp. 179–80.

Moreno, Jonathan D. *Undue Risk: Secret State Experiments on Humans.* New York: W. H. Freeman, 2000.

Mumford, James Gregory. *A Narrative of Medicine in America.* Philadelphia: Lippincott, 1903.

———. "Warren, John Collins." In *Dictionary of American Medical Biography.* Edited by Howard A. Kelly and Walter L. Burrage. New York: D. Appleton & Co., 1928, pp. 1263–64.

Murdock, Kenneth B. "Mather, Cotton." In *Dictionary of American Biography,* Vol. 6. Edited by Dumas Malone. New York: Scribners, 1957, pp. 386–89.

Murray, John. *System of Materia Medica and Pharmacy.* Edited by Nathaniel Chapman. Philadelphia: Thomas Dobson, 1815.

Murray, T. J., and Suellen Murray. "The History of Dalhousie Medical School." *MeDal 1982–83,* n.d., pp. 12–14.

National Commission for the Protection of Human Subjects of Biomedical and Behavioral Research. *The Belmont Report: Ethical Principles and Guidelines for the Protection of Human Subjects of Research.* Washington, DC: U.S. Government Printing Office, 1978.

New Zealand University, Supplementary Calendar, 1877. Christ Church: Printed for the New Zealand University, by W. Reeves, at The Lyttelton Times Office, Glouster

Street, 1877. (Important information also appeared in the calendar for the following years.)

Nicholson, Albert. "Percival, Thomas." In *Dictionary of National Biography*, Vol. 15. Edited by Leslie Stephen and Sidney Lee. London: Smith, Elder & Co., Reprint edition 1937–38, pp. 828–29.

"Nomina Eorum, qui gradum Medicinae Doctoris in Academia Jacobi Sexti Scotorum Regis, quae Edinburgi est, Adepti Sunt. Edinburgi: Exciebant Neill et Soch, 1846" [Edinburgh medical graduates, 1705 to 1845].

Noonan, John T. *Contraception: A History of Its Treatment by the Catholic Theologians and Canonists*. Cambridge, MA: Harvard University Press, 1966.

——. *The Morality of Abortion: Legal and Historical Perspectives*. Cambridge, MA: Harvard University Press, 1970.

Norgate, Gerald Legrys. "Ryan, Michael." In *Dictionary of National Biography*, Vol. 17. Edited by Leslie Stephen and Sidney Lee. London: Oxford University Press, 1937, pp. 525–26.

Novack, Dennis H., Robin Plumer, Raymond L. Smith, Herbert Ochitill, Gary R. Morrow, and John M. Bennett. "Changes in Physicians' Attitudes Toward Telling the Cancer Patient." *Journal of the American Medical Association* 241 (March 2, 1979): 897–900.

Nutton, Vivian. "What's in an Oath?" *Journal of the Royal College of Physicians of London* 29 (Nov/Dec 1995): 518–24.

O'Donnell, Thomas J. *Morals in Medicine*. Westminster, MD: Newman, 1956.

Olson, William C., and A. J. R. Groom. *International Relations Then & Now: Origins and Trends in Interpretation*. London: Routledge, 1991.

Osler, William. *Aequanimitas, with Other Addresses to Medical Students, Nurses and Practitioners of Medicine, by William Osler*. Philadelphia: P. Blakiston's Son & Co., 1905.

——. "After Twenty-five Years." *Montreal Medical Journal* 28 (1899): 823–33. Reprinted in *Aequanimitas, with Other Addresses to Medical Students, Nurses and Practitioners of Medicine, by William Osler*. Philadelphia: P. Blakiston's Son & Co., 1905a, pp. 197–215.

——. "Alfred Stillé." *University of Pennsylvania Medical Bulletin* 15 (1902): 126–32. Reprinted in Osler, William. *An Alabama Student and Other Biographical Essays*. London: Oxford University Press, 1908a, pp. 232–47.

——. "Aristotle, Greek Thinkers by Gomperz, Vol. iv." *Canadian Medical Association Journal* 3 (1913): 416–17.

——. *Bibliotheca Osleriana: A Catalogue of Books Illustrating the History of Medicine and Science*. Collected, Arranged and Annotated by Sir William Osler. Oxford: Clarendon, 1929.

——. "Books and Men." (1901) *In A Way of Life and Selected Writings of Sir William Osler 12 July 1849 to 29 December 1919*. New York: Dover, 1958a, pp. 34–39.

——. "British Medicine in Greater Britain." *British Medical Journal* 2 (1897): 576–81. Reprinted in *Aequanimitas, with Other Addresses to Medical Students, Nurses and Practitioners of Medicine, by William Osler*. Philadelphia: P. Blakiston's Son & Co., 1905b, pp. 168–96.

——. *Creators, Transmuters, and Transmitters. As Illustrated by Shakespeare, Bacon, and Burton*. London: Oxford University Press, 1916. Reprinted in *A Way of Life and Selected Writings of Sir William Osler 12 July 1849 to 29 December 1919*. New York: Dover, 1958b, pp. 1–7.

———. *Elisha Bartlett: A Rhode Island Philosopher.* Providence: Snow & Furnham, 1900. Reprinted in Osler, William. *An Alabama Student and Other Biographical Essays.* London: Oxford University Press, 1908b, pp. 108–58.

———. *The Evolution of Modern Medicine; A Series of Lectures Delivered at Yale University on The Silliman Foundation in April, 1913, by William Osler.* New Haven: Yale University Press, 1921.

———. Greek at Oxford." *The Nation* 91 (1910): 544–45. Reprinted in Cushing, Harvey. 1940a, pp. 938–41.

———. *The Growth of Truth as Illustrated in the Discovery of the Circulation of the Blood.* London: H. Frowde, 1906. Reprinted in *A Way of Life and Selected Writings of Sir William Osler 12 July 1849 to 29 December 1919.* New York: Dover, 1958c, pp. 205–36.

———. "Intensive Work in Science at the Public Schools in Relation to the Medical Curriculum." 1916. Extract reprinted in Cushing, Harvey. *The Life of Sir William Osler.* 1925. London: Oxford University Press, 1940b, p. 1195.

———. *John Keats, The Apothecary Poet.* Baltimore: Friedenwald Co. 1896. Reprinted in Osler, William. *An Alabama Student and Other Biographical Essays.* London: Oxford University Press, 1908c, pp. 37–54.

———. "Locke as a Physician." *Lancet* 2 (1900): 1115–23. Reprinted in Osler, William. *An Alabama Student and Other Biographical Essays.* London: Oxford, 1908d, pp. 68–107.

———. *The Master-Word in Medicine.* Baltimore: J. Murphy Co., 1903. Reprinted in *Aequanimitas, with Other Addresses to Medical Students, Nurses and Practitioners of Medicine, by William Osler.* Philadelphia: P. Blakiston's Son & Co., 1905c, pp. 364–88.

———. *Michael Servetus.* London: Oxford, 1909.

———. "Nerve and 'Nerves." Address at the Leeds Luncheon Club, October 1, 1915. Privately printed, [1915a].

———. "The Old Humanities and the New Science." Presidential address delivered before Classical Association, Oxford, May 16, 1919. *British Medical Journal* 2 (1919): 1–7. Reprinted in Osler, William. *A Way of Life and Selected Writings of Sir William Osler 12 July 1849 to 29 December 1919.* New York: Dover, 1958d, p. 8–33.

———. "Oliver Wendell Holmes." *Johns Hopkins Hospital Bulletin* 5 (1894): 85–88.

———. "On the Educational Value of the Medical Society." *Boston Medical and Surgical Journal* 148 (1903): 275–79. Reprinted in *Aequanimitas, with Other Addresses to Medical Students, Nurses and Practitioners of Medicine, by William Osler.* Philadelphia: P. Blakiston's Son & Co., 1905d, pp. 345–62.

———. "On the Library of a Medical School." *Johns Hopkins Hospital Bulletin* 18 (April 1907): 109–11. Excerpt reprinted in Cushing, Harvey. *The Life of Sir William Osler.* 1925. London: Oxford University Press, 1940c, pp. 761–62.

———. "The Past Century: Its Progress in Great Subjects: Medicine." *The [New York] Sun,* January 27, 1901. Reprinted as "Medicine in the Nineteenth Century" in *Aequanimitas, with Other Addresses to Medical Students, Nurses and Practitioners of Medicine, by William Osler.* Philadelphia: P. Blakiston's Son & Co., 1905e, pp. 229–76.

———. "Physic and Physicians as Depicted in Plato." *Boston Medical and Surgical Journal* 128 (1893): 129–33, 153–56. In *Aequanimitas, with Other addresses to Medical Students, Nurses and Practitioners of Medicine, by William Osler.* Philadephia: P. Blakiston's Son & Co., 1905f, pp. 47–76.

———. *The Principles and Practice of Medicine: Designed for the Use of Practitioners and Students of Medicine.* New York: D. Appleton and Company, 1892.

———. *Science and War* [an address delivered at the University of Leeds Medical School, October 1, 1915]. Oxford: Clarendon Press, 1915b.

———. "Sir Thomas Browne." *British Medical Journal* 2 (1905): 993–98. Reprinted in Osler, William. *An Alabama Student and Other Biographical Essays.* London: Oxford University Press, 1908e, pp. 248–77.

———. "Some Aspects of American Medical Bibliography." *Bulletin of the Association of Medical Librarians* 1 (1902): 19–32. Reprinted in *Aequanimitas, with Other Addresses to Medical Students, Nurses and Practitioners of Medicine, by William Osler.* Philadelphia: P. Blakiston's Son & Co., 1905g, pp. 309–26.

———. "The Study of the Fevers in the South." *Journal of the American Medical Association* 26 (1896): 999–1004.

———. *Teacher and Student.* Baltimore: J. Murphy & Co., 1892. Reprinted in *Aequanimitas, with Other Addresses to Medical Students, Nurses and Practitioners of Medicine, by William Osler.* Philadelphia: P. Blakiston's Son & Co., 1905h, pp. 22–43.

———. *Thomas Linacre.* Cambridge: The University Press, 1908f.

———. "Vienna After Thirty-four Years." *Journal of the American Medical Association* 1 (1908g): 1523–25.

———. "Pascalis-Ouvière, Felix." In *Dictionary of American Biography*, Vol. 7. Edited by Dumas Malone. New York: Charles Scribner's Sons, 1928–1936, pp. 286–87.

"Pascalis-Ouvière, Felix." In *Appleton's Cyclopaedia of American Biography*, Vol. 4. Edited by James Grant Wilson and John Fiske. New York: D. Appleton & Co., 1888–1889. Reprint. Detroit: Gale Research, 1968, p. 667.

Payne, J. F. "Sir John Pringle." In *Dictionary of National Biography*, Vol. 46. Edited by Sidney Lee. London: Smith, Elder & Co., 1896, pp. 386–88.

Pellegrino, Edmund D. "Percival's *Medical Ethics*: The Moral Philosophy of an 18th-Century English Gentleman." *Archives of Internal Medicine* 146 (1986): 2265–69.

———. "Toward an Expanded Medical Ethics: The Hippocratic Ethic Revisited." In *Hippocrates Revisited: A Search for Meaning.* Edited by Roger J. Bulger. New York: Medcom Press, 1973, pp. 133–47.

———. "The Virtuous Physician, the Ethics of Medicine." In *Virtue and Medicine.* Edited by Earl E. Shelp. Dordrecht: Reidel, 1985, pp. 237–55.

———, and David C. Thomasma. *For the Patient's Good: The Restoration of Beneficence in Health Care.* New York: Oxford University Press 1988.

———, and Thomas K. McElhinney. *Teaching Ethics, the Humanities, and Human Values in Medical Schools: A Ten-Year Overview.* Washington, DC: Institute on Human Values in Medicine, Society for Health and Human Values, [1982].

Pennington, T. H., and C. I. Pennington. "The Hippocratic Oath: Is Not Administered in the Strictly Legal Sense." *British Medical Journal* 309 (October 8, 1994): 952.

Percival, Edward. "Memoirs of his Life and Writings." In *The Works, Literary, Moral, and Philosophical, of Thomas Percival; to which are Prefixed, Memoirs of his Life and Writings, and a Selection from his Literary Correspondence. A new edition.* 2 vols. Edited by Edward Percival. Bath: Printed by Richard Cruttwell for J. Johnson, St. Paul's Church-yard, London, 1807, pp. i–cclxii.

———. *Practical Observations on the Treatment, Pathology, and Prevention of Typhous Fever.* Bath: Printed by R. Cruttwell, and sold by Longman, Hurst, Rees, Orme, and Browne, London, 1819.

Percival, Thomas. "Essay on the Small-pox and Measles (1789)." In *Population and Disease in Early Industrial England*. Introduced by B. Benjamin. Hants, England: Gregg International, 1973, pp. 68–84 [photographic reproduction of 1789 edition].

———. *Essays Medical and Experimental. To which are added, select histories of diseases, with remarks; and proposals for establishing More Accurate and Comprehensive Bills of Mortality*. London: Printed for Joseph Jackson . . . , 1773a.

———. *Essays Medical and Experimental*, 2nd ed., revised, and considerably enlarged. To which is added an appendix. London: Printed for J. Johnson, 1772.

———. *Essays Medical, Philosophical, and Experimental*, 4th ed., revised and enlarged. Warrington, London: Printed by W. Eyres for J. Johnson, 1788–89.

———. *Extracts from the Medical Ethics of Dr. Percival*. Philadelphia: [Clark and Raser], 1823.

———. *Experiments and Observations on Water; Particularly on the Hard Pump Water of Manchester*. London: Printed for J. Johnson, 1769.

———. *Experiments on the Peruvian Bark*. London: L. Davis &c. Reymers, 1768a.

———. *A Father's Instructions to His Children Consisting of Tales, Fables, And Reflection Designed to Promote The Love of Virtue, a Taste For Knowledge, And an Early Acquaintance With The Works of Nature*. London: Printed for J. Johnson, 1776a.

———. *Further Observations on the State of Population in Manchester, etc*. Manchester, 1774a.

———. *Medical Ethics*. 1803. NP: DevCom, 1987.

———. *Medical Ethics; or, a Code of Institutes and Precepts, adapted to the Professional Conduct of Physicians and Surgeons; To which is added An Appendix; containing A Discourse on Hospital Duties; [by Rev. Thomas Bassnett Percival, LL.B.] and Notes and Illustrations* Manchester: Printed by S. Russell, for J. Johnson, St. Paul's Church Yard, and R. Bicherstaff, Strand, London, 1803.

———. *Medical Ethics; Or, a Code of Institutes and Precepts, Adapted to the Professional Conduct of Physicians and Surgeons. With additions [by the editor]. illustrative of the past and present state of the profession and its collegiate institutions, in Great Britain*. London: W. Jackson, 1827.

———. *Medical Ethics; or, a Code of Institutes and Precepts, Adapted to the Professional Conduct of Physicians and Surgeons . . .* 3rd ed. Oxford: John Henry Parker. London: John Churchill, Princes Street, Soho, 1849.

———. *Medical Jurisprudence; Or, a Code of Ethics and Institutes, Adapted to the Professions of Physic and Surgery*. [Manchester, 1794].

———. *Moral and Literary Dissertations, on the following subjects: 1. On truth and faithfulness. 2. On habit and association. 3. On inconsistency of expectation in literary pursuits. 4. On a taste for the general beauties or nature. 5. On a taste for the fine arts. 6. On the alliance of natural history, and philosophy, with poetry. To which are added a tribute to the memory of Charles de. Polier, Esq. and an appendix*. Warrington: Printed by W. Eyres, for J. Johnson, London, 1784.

———. *Observations and Experiments on the Poison of Lead*. London: J. Johnson, 1774b.

———. *Observations on the State of Population in Manchester, and Other Adjacent Places*. [Manchester?: s.n., 1773b].

———. *Observations on the State of Population in Manchester and Other Adjacent Places*. [Warrington?: no publisher, 1789].

———. "Observations on the State of Population in Manchester (1789)." In *Population and Disease in Early Industrial England*. [Photographic reproduction of 1789 edition,] with an introduction by B. Benjamin. Hants, England: Gregg International, 1973, pp. 1–67.

———. *On the Disadvantages Which Attend the Inoculation of Children in Early Infancy.* London: J. Johnson & T. Cadell, 1768b.

———. *Percival's Medical Ethics, 1803.* Reprint. Edited by Chauncey D. Leake. Baltimore: Williams and Wilkins, 1927.

———. *Philosophical, medical, and experimental essays . . . To which is added an appendix; containing a letter to the author from Dr. Saunders, on the solution of human calculi.* London: J. Johnson, 1776b.

———. *A Socratic Discourse on Truth and Faithfulness in which the Nature, Extent, and Obligation, together with the Various Branches and Subordinations of these Moral Duties are Explained, Illustrated, and Enforced by Examples: Being the Sequel to A Father's Instructions.* Warrington: printed by W. Ashton, 1781.

———. *Thoughts on Hospitals/ with a letter to the author.* London: Joseph Johnson, 1771.

———. *The Works, Literary, Moral, and Philosophical, of Thomas Percival; to which are Prefixed, Memoirs of his Life and Writings, and a Selection from his Literary Correspondence. A new edition.* 2 vols. Edited by Edward Percival. Bath: Printed by Richard Cruttwell for J. Johnson, St. Paul's Church-yard, London, 1807.

Pickstone, John V. "Thomas Percival and the Production of Medical Ethics." In *The Codification of Medical Morality: Historical and Philosophical Studies of the Formalization of Western Medical Morality in the Eighteenth and Nineteenth Centuries.* Vol. 1, *Medical Ethics and Etiquette in the Eighteenth Century.* Edited by Robert Baker, Dorothy Parker, and Roy Porter. Dordrecht: Kluwer, 1993, pp. 161–178.

Pilcher, Lewis S. *Clinical Studies of the Surgical Diseases of the Female Generative Organs; from Observations Made During Ten Years' Work in the Methodist Episcopal Hospital in Brooklyn.* Philadelphia: Lippincott, 1898.

———. "Codes of Ethics." In *An Ethical Symposium: Being a Series of Papers Concerning Medical Ethics and Etiquette from the Liberal Standpoint.* Edited by Alfred C. Post et al. New York: Putnam, 1883a, pp. 42–55.

———. *Fractures of the Lower Extremity or Base of the Radius.* Philadelphia: Lippincott, 1917.

———. *The Treatment of Wounds; its Principles and Practice, General and Special.* New York: W. Wood & Company, 1883b.

Pilcher, Lewis Stephen. *A List of Books by Some of the Old Masters of Medicine and Surgery: Together with Books on the History of Medicine And on Medical Biography in the Possession of Lewis Stephen Pilcher: with Biographical and Bibliographical Notes and Reproductions of Some Title Pages and Captions.* Brooklyn: no publisher, 1918.

Pope Paul VI. "Encyclical Letter on the Regulation of Births (July 25, 1968)." In *Medical Ethics: Sources of Catholic Teachings.* Edited by Kevin D. O'Rourke and Philip Boyle. St. Louis: The Catholic Health Association of the United States, 1989, pp. 85–91.

Pope Pius IX. "Const. *Apostolicae Sedis*, 12 Oct. 1869." In *Codicis Iuris Canonici Fontes*, Vol. 3. Edited by Peter Gasparri. Rome: Typis Polyglottis Vaticanis, 1923, pp. 24–31.

Pope Pius XII. "The Prolongation of Life: An Address of Pope Pius XII to an International Congress of Anesthesiologists." *The Pope Speaks* 4 (Spring 1958): 393–398.

Porter, Roy. "Thomas Gisborne: Physicians, Christians and Gentlemen." In *Doctors and Ethics: The Earlier Historical Setting of Professional Ethics.* Edited by Andrew Wear, Johanna Geyer-Kordesch, and Roger French. Amsterdam: Rodopi, 1993, pp. 252–73.

Post, Alfred C., et al. *An Ethical Symposium: Being a Series of Papers Concerning Medical Ethics and Etiquette from the Liberal Standpoint.* New York: Putnam, 1883.

Potter, Ralph B. "The Paradoxical Preservation of a Principle." *Villanova Law Review* 13 (Summer 1968): 784–792.

Potter, Van Rensselaer. Biocybernetics and Survival." *Zygon* 5 (1970a): 229–46.

———. *Bioethics: Bridge to the Future.* Englewood Cliffs, NJ: Prentice-Hall, 1971.

———. "Bioethics, the Science of Survival." *Perspectives in Biology and Medicine* 14 (1970b): 127–53.

Ramsay, John. *Scotland and Scotsman in the Eighteenth Century.* 2 vols. Edinburgh: William Blackwood and Sons, 1888.

Ramsey, Paul. "Commentary: Jonsen and Hellegers." In *Ethics of Health Care.* Edited by Laurence R. Tancredi. Washington, DC: National Academy of Sciences, 1974, pp. 21–29.

———. *Deeds and Rules in Christian Ethics.* New York: Charles Scribner's Sons, 1967.

———. *Fabricated Man.* New Haven: Yale University Press, 1970a.

———. "On Updating Death." In *Updating Life and Death.* Edited by Donald R. Cutler. Boston: Beacon Press, 1969, pp. 31–53.

———. *The Patient as Person.* New Haven: Yale University Press, 1970b.

Rawls, John. "Two Concepts of Rules." *The Philosophical Review* 44 (1955): 3–32.

Reich, Warren T., ed. *The Encyclopedia of Bioethics.* New York: The Free Press, 1978.

———. *The Encyclopedia of Bioethics,* revised edition. New York: Simon & Schuster Macmillan, 1995a.

———. "The Word 'Bioethics': Its Birth and the Legacies of Those Who Shaped Its Meaning." *Kennedy Institute of Ethics Journal* 4 (1994): 319–35.

———. "The Word 'Bioethics': The Struggle over Its Earliest Meanings." *Kennedy Institute of Ethics Journal* 5 (1995b): 19–34.

Reid, Alexander Peter. *An Inaugural Dissertation on Strychnia.* Montreal: Printed by J. Lovell, 1858.

Reid, Edith Gittings. *The Great Physician: A Short Life of Sir William Osler.* London: Oxford University Press, 1934.

Reid, Thomas. *An Inquiry into the Human Mind, on the Principles of Common Sense.* Dublin: Printed for Alexander Ewing, 1764.

———. *An Inquiry into the Human Mind, on the Principles of Common Sense*, 5th ed. Edinburgh: Printed for Bell and Bradfute, and William Creech; and for T. Cadell jun. & W. Davies, London, by Ad. Neill & Co., 1801.

———. *An Inquiry into the Human Mind, on the Principles of Common Sense*, Critical Edition. Edited by Derek R. Brookes. University Park, PA: The Pennsylvania State University Press, 1997.

Reiser, Stanley Joel. "Creating a Medical Profession in the United States: The First Code of Ethics of the American Medical Association." In *The Codification of Medical Morality: Historical and Philosophical Studies of the Formalization of Western Medical Morality in the Eighteenth and Nineteenth Centuries.* Vol. 2, *Anglo-American Medical Ethics and Medical Jurisprudence in the Nineteenth Century.* Edited by Robert Baker. Dordrecht: Kluwer, 1995, pp. 89–103.

"Report of the Committee of the Medical Society, of the City and County of New York, Appointed to Investigate the Subject of a Secret Medical Association." 1831. Reprint in Douglas, Sholto [pseud.] *Some Account of a Secret Society in New York entitled the "Kappa Lambda" in a Letter to Alexander H. Stevens MD LLD by a Retired Physician.* 1859. Available in the library of the College of Physicians of Philadelphia.

Richman, Irwin. *The Brightest Ornament: A Biography of Nathaniel Chapman, M.D.* Bellefonte, PA: Pennsylvania Heritage, Inc., 1967.

Roe v. Wade, 410 U.S. 113, 93 S. Ct. 705, 1973.

Rogal, Samuel J. *John and Charles Wesley*. Boston: Twayne Publishers, 1983.

Rosen, Harold. *Abortion in America: Medical, Psychiatric, Legal, Anthropological, and Religious Considerations*. Boston: Beacon Press, 1967.

Rosner, Fred. "The Definition of Death in Jewish Law." *Tradition*, 10, no. 4 (1969): 33–39.

———. *Modern Medicine and Jewish Law*. New York: Yeshiva University Press, 1972.

Rosner, Lisa. *Medical Education in the Age of Improvement: Edinburgh Students and Apprentices 1760–1826*. Edinburgh: University of Edinburgh Press, 1991.

Roth, Russell B. "Medicine's Ethical Responsibilities." *Journal of the American Medical Association* 215 (1971): 1956–1968.

Rothman, David J. *Strangers at the Bedside: A History of How Law and Bioethics Transformed Medical Decision Making*. New York: Basic Books, 1991.

Rothstein, William G. *American Physicians in the Nineteenth Century: From Sects to Science*. Baltimore: The Johns Hopkins University Press, 1972.

Rush, Benjamin. *The Autobiography of Benjamin Rush: His "Travels through Life" Together with his Commonplace Book for 1789–1813*. Princeton, NJ: Published for The American Philosophical Society By Princeton University Press, 1948.

———. *Benjamin Rush's Lectures on the Mind*. Edited, annotated, and introduced by Eric T. Carlson, Jeffrey L. Wollock, and Patricia S. Noel. Philadelphia: American Philosophical Society, 1981.

———. *Essays, Literary, Moral & Philosophical*. Philadelphia: Thomas & Samuel F. Bradford, 1798.

———. "Observations on the Duties of a Physician, and the Methods of Improving Medicine Accommodated to the present state of society and manners in the United States." Delivered at the University of Pennsylvania, February 7, 1789. Philadelphia: Printed and sold by Prichard & Hall, 1789.

———. *The Selected Writings of Benjamin Rush*. New York: Philosophical Library, 1947.

———. *Sermons to the rich and studious, on Temperance and Exercise*. With a dedication to Dr. Cadogan. /By a physician. London: Printed for E. and C. Dilly, 1772.

———. *Six Introductory Lectures to Courses of Lectures upon the Institutes and Practice of Medicine*. Delivered at the University of Pennsylvania. Philadelphia: John Conrad, 1801.

———. *Sixteen Introductory Lectures to Courses of Lectures upon the Institutes and Practice of Medicine: with a syllabus of the latter: to which are added, two lectures upon the pleasures of the senses and of the mind, with an inquiry into their proximate cause: delivered in the University of Pennsylvania*. Philadelphia: Bradford and Innskeep, [Philadelphia]: Fry and Kammerer, 1811.

———. "To John Morgan. Edinburgh, January 20, 1768." In *Letters of Benjamin Rush*, Vol. 1. Edited by L. H. Butterfield. Princeton: The American Philosophical Society and the Princeton University Press, 1951, pp. 49–51.

Ryan, Michael. *A manual of medical jurisprudence and state medicine, compiled from the latest legal and medical works, of Beck, Paris, Christison, Fodere, Orfila, etc. . . . Intended for the use of legislators, barristers, magistrates, coroners, private gentlemen, jurors, and medical practitioners. Containing part I. Medical ethics . . . Part II. Laws relating to the medical profession . . . Part III. Medical jurisprudence and state medicine . . . Part IV. Laws relating to the preservation of public health.* 2nd ed., considerably enlarged and improved. London: Sherwood, Gilbert, and Piper, 1836a.

―――. *A Manual of Medical Jurisprudence, Compiled from the Best Medical and Legal Works Comprising an Account of I. the Ethics of the Medical Profession; Ii. The Charters and Statutes Relating to the Faculty; And, Iii. All Medico-legal Questions, with the Latest Decisions: Being an Analysis of a Course of Lectures on Forensic Medicine, Annually Delivered in London. And Intended as a Compendium for the Use of Barristers, Solicitors, Magistrates, Coroners, and Medical Practitioners.* London: Renshaw and Rush, 1831.

―――. *A Manual of Midwifery, and Diseases of Women and Children. Being a Companion to All Obstetric Works,* 4th ed., re-written. London: [the author], 1841.

―――. *A Manual on Midwifery; or a Summary of the Science and Art of Obstetric Medicine, Including the Anatomy, Physiology, Pathology, and Therapeutics, Peculiar to Females; Treatment of Parturition, Puerperal, and Infantile Diseases; and an Exposition of Obstetrico-legal Medicine.* London: for Longman, 1828a.

―――. *A New Practical Formulary of Hospitals of England . . . France, Germany, Italy, Spain, Portugal, Sweden, Russia, and America; of Mm. Magendie, Lugol, Etc. or a Conspectus of Prescriptions in Medicine, Surgery, and Obstetrics . . . / Translated and considerably augmented.* With M. Magendie's last additions, 2nd ed. London: G. Henderson, 1836b.

―――. *A New Practical Formulary of Hospitals of England, Scotland, Ireland, France, Germany, Italy, Spain, Portugal, Sweden, Russia, and America; of Mm. Magendie, Lugol, Etc. or a Conspectus of Prescriptions in Medicine, Surgery, and Obstetrics. With the Doses of All New and Ordinary Medicines / Translated from the new French ed. of Milne Edwards and P. Vavasseur, and considerably augmented.* London: G. Henderson, 1835.

―――. *The Obstetrician's Vademecum; or Aphorisms on Natural and Difficult Parturition; the Application and Use of Instruments in Preternatural Labours; on Labours Complicated with Hemorrhage, Convulsions, Etc / Considerably Augmented and Arranged According to the Present State of Obstetricy,* 9th ed. London: E. Cox, 1836c.

―――. *The Philosophy of Marriage, in its Social, Moral, and Physical Relations; with an Account of the Diseases of the Genito-urinary Organs . . . with the Physiology of Generation in the Vegetable and Animal Kingdoms; Being Part of a Course of Obstetric Lectures Delivered at the North London School of Medicine,* 4th ed. London: H. Bailliere, 1843.

―――. *Remarks on the Supply of Water to the Metropolis: with an Account of the Natural History of Water in its Simple and Combined States, and of the Chemical Composition and Medical Uses of All the Known Mineral Waters Being a Guide to Foreign and British Watering Places.* London: Printed for Longman and Co., Anderson, and Messrs. Underwood, and Highley, 1828b.

―――. *A Treatise on the Most Celebrated Mineral Waters of Ireland Containing an Account of the Waters of Ballyspellan, Castleconnel, Ballynahinch, Mallow, Lucan, Swadlinbar, Goldenbridge, Kilmainham, &C. &C.: and of the Spa Lately Discovered at Brownstown, near Kilkenny, with Plain Directions During the Use of Mineral Waters and an Account of Some of Those Diseases in Which They Are Most Useful.* Kilkenny: Printed and published by J. Reynolds, for Hodges, M'Arthur, and J. Cumming, Dublin, and Longman, Hurst, Rees, Orme, Brown and Green, London, 1824.

Sabetti, Aloysius. *Compendium theologiae moralis a Joanne Gury, S. J. primo exaratum et deinde ab Antio Ballerini . . . auctum nunc vero ad breviorem formam redactum atque ad usum seminariorum hujas reegionis accomodatum*, 4th ed. New York: F. Pustet, 1889.

Sadler, A. M., B. L. Sadler, and E. Blythe Stason. "The Uniform Anatomical Gift Act." *Journal of the American Medical Association* 206 (Dec. 9, 1968): 2501– 06.

Samp, Robert J., and Anthony R. Curreri. "A Questionnaire Survey on Public Cancer Education Obtained from Cancer Patients and their Families." *Cancer* 10 (1957): 382–84.

Sandys, John Edwin. *A History of Classical Scholarship.* 3 vols. Hafner Publishing Co., 1967 (reprint, first published in 1920s).

Scavini, Pietro. *Theologia moralis universa ad menetem S. Alphonsi M. de Ligorio*, 8th ed. Milan: Ernesto Oliva, 1860.

Scotti, Angelo Antonio. *Catechismo medico ossio suiluppo delle dottrine cotta che conciliano la religione cotta medicina de piu nuovi capi cresciuto nella presente edizione dal ch. suo autore.* Facolta, 1836.

Scrimshaw, Susan C., and Bernard Pasquariella. "Obstacles to Sterilization in One Community." *Family Planning Perspectives* 2 (1970): 40–42.

Shepherd, T. B. *Methodism and the Literature of the Eighteenth Century.* New York: Haskell House, 1966.

Shimkin, Michael B. "The Research Worker's Point of View." *Science* 117 (1953): 205–07.

Shotter, Edward, ed. *Matters of Life and Death, by Francis Camps [and others].* London: Darton, Longman & Todd, 1970.

Smellie, William. *Lives of John Gregory, M.D. Henry Home, Lord Kames. David Hume, Esq., and Adam Smith, L.L.D. to which are Added a dissertation on Public Spirit; and Three Essays.* Edinburgh: Alex. Smellie, Anchor Close etc., 1800.

Smith, Adam. *The Theory of Moral Sentiments.* 1759. Edited by D. D. Raphael and A. L. Macfie. Indianapolis: Liberty Classics, 1976.

———. *The Wealth of Nations.* 1776. Edited by Edwin Cannan. London: Methuen & Co., 1904.

Smith, Wesley D. *The Hippocratic Tradition.* Ithaca: Cornell University Press, 1979.

Sperry, Willard L. *The Ethical Basis of Medical Practice.* New York: Paul B. Hoeber, 1950.

———. "Moral Problems in the Practice of Medicine." *New England Journal of Medicine* 239 (Dec. 23, 1948): 985–90.

Stephen, Leslie. "Gisborne, Thomas." In *Dictionary of National Biography*, Vol. 7. Edited by Leslie Stephen. London: Smith, Elder & Co., 1886, pp. 1280–81.

———. "Hume, David." In *Dictionary of National Biography*, Vol. 53. Edited by Sidney Lee. London: Smith, Elder & Co., 1898, pp. 3–10.

———. "Reid, Thomas." In *Dictionary of National Biography*, Vol. 47. Edited by Sidney Lee. London: Smith, Elder & Co., 1896, pp. 436–439.

Steptoe, Patrick C., and Robert G. Edwards. "Birth After The Reimplantation of a Human Embryo." *Lancet* 2, no. 8085 (1978): 366.

Stewart, Dugald. "Account of the Life and Writings of Thomas Reid, D.D., F.R.S.E." In *The Collected Works of Dugald Stewart, Esq., F.R.S.* 1802. Edited By Sir William Hamilton, Bart. Edinburgh: Thomas Constable and Co., 1858, pp. 243–328.

Stillé, Alfred. *Cholera: Its Origin, History, Causation, Symptoms, Lesions, Prevention, and Treatment.* Philadelphia: Lea Brothers & Co., 1885.

———. *Elements of General Pathology; a Practical Treatise on the Causes, Forms, Symptoms, and Results of Disease.* Philadelphia: Lindsay and Blakiston, 1848.

————. *Epidemic Meningitis; Or, Cerebro-spinal Meningitis*. Philadelphia: Lindsay and Blakiston, 1867.

————. "Memoir of Isaac Hays." *Transactions of the College of Physicians* 3rd Series 5 (1881): 27–60.

————. *Therapeutics and Materia Medica, a Systematic Treatise on the Action and Uses of Medicinal Agents, Including Their Description and History,* 1st ed. Philadelphia: Lea, 1860.

————, and John M. Maisch. *The National Dispensatory, Containing the Natural History, Chemistry, Pharmacy, Actions and Uses of Medicines, Including Those Recognized in the Pharmacopoeias of the United States and Great Britain,* 1st ed. Philadelphia: Lea, 1879.

Styrap, Jukes. "A Code of Medical Ethics." In *The Codification of Medical Morality: Historical and Philosophical Studies of the Formalization of Western Medical Morality in the Eighteenth and Nineteenth Centuries.* Vol. 2, *Anglo-American Medical Ethics and Medical Jurisprudence in the Nineteenth Century.* Edited by Robert Baker. Dordrecht: Kluwer, 1995, pp. 149–71.

Styrap, Jukes de. *A Code of Medical Ethics: with General and Special Rules for the Guidance of the Faculty and the Pubic in the Complex Relations of Professional Life,* 2nd revised and enlarged ed. London: J. & A. Churchill, 1886.

————. *A Code of Medical Ethics: With General and Special Rules for the Guidance of the Faculty and the Pubic in the Complex Relations of Professional Life,* 3rd ed. London: H. K. Lewis, 1890a.

————. *A Code of Medical Ethics: With General and Special Rules for the Guidance of the Faculty and the Pubic in the Complex Relations of Professional Life,* 4th ed. revised and enlarged. London: H. K. Lewis, 1895.

————. *The Medico-chirurgical Tariffs Prepared for the Late Shropshire Ethical Branch of the British Medical Association,* 5th ed. revised and enlarged. London: H. K. Lewis, 1890b.

————. *The Young Practitioner: with Practical Hints and Instructive Suggestions as Subsidiary Aids for His Guidance on Entering into Private Practice.* London: H. K. Lewis, 1890c.

Sudds, R. H. "Rush, Benjamin." In *Dictionary of American Biography*, Vol. 8. Edited by Dumas Malone. New York: Charles Scribner's Sons, 1957, pp. 227–31.

Taylor, Alfred Swaine. *Elements of Medical Jurisprudence.* London: Deacon, 1836.

————. *Elements of Medical Jurisprudence, Interspersed with a Copious Selection of Curious Cases and Analyses of Opinions Delivered at Coroners' Inquests.* London: Deacon, 1843.

————. *A Manual of Medical Jurisprudence.* London: J. Churchill, 1844.

————. *The Principles and Practice of Medical Jurisprudence.* London: J. Churchill & Sons, 1865.

Taylor, Douglass W. *The Monro Collection in the Medical Library of the University of Otago.* Dunedin, New Zealand: University of Otago Press, 1979.

Temkin, Owsei. *Hippocrates in a World of Pagans and Christians.* Baltimore: Johns Hopkins University Press, 1991.

Thacher, James. *American Medical Biography: or Memoirs of Eminent Physicians who have Flourished in America to which is prefixed a Succinct History of Medical Science in the United States from the First Settlement of the Country.* Boston: Richardson & Lord and Cottons & Barnard, 1828.

Thompson, G. E. *History of the University of Otago (1869–1919).* Dunedin, New Zealand: J. Wilkie & Co., Ltd, 1920.

Thoms, Herbert. "Hooker, Worthington." In *Dictionary of American Biography,* Vol. 5. Edited by Dumas Malone. New York: Scribner's, 1957, pp. 201–02.

Tissot, S. A. A. D. *Advice with Respect to HEALTH. Extracted from a late Author.* Bristol: Printed by W. Pine, in Wine-Street, 1769 [bound together with John Wesley's *Primitive Physic*, 1770].

Todd, James S. "Report of the Ad Hoc Committee on The Principles of Medical Ethics [of the American Medical Association]." Unpublished report, [1979].

United States Catholic Conference, Department of Health Affairs. *Ethical and Religious Directives for Catholic Health Facilities.* Washington, DC: United States Catholic Conference, 1971.

U.S. Department of Health, Education, and Welfare. *The Institutional Guide to DHEW Policy on Protection of Human Subjects.* Washington, DC: U.S. Government Printing Office, 1971.

U. S. Government. "Public Law 93-348: Title II—Protection of Human Subjects of Biomedical and Behavioral Research." July 12, 1974.

U.S. Public Health Service. *Final Report of the Tuskegee Syphilis Study Ad Hoc Advisory Panel.* Washington, DC: U.S. Government Printing Office, 1973.

U.S. Senate. Committee on Labor and Public Welfare. Subcommittee on Health. *Quality of Health Care—Human Experimentation, 1973: Hearings Before the Subcommittee on Health of the Committee on Labor and Public Welfare on S. 974, S. 878, S.J. Res. 71: Part 1*, 93rd Cong., 1st sess., February 21 and 22, 1973a.

U.S. Senate. Committee on Labor and Public Welfare. Subcommittee on Health. *Quality of Health Care—Human Experimentation, 1973: Hearings Before the Subcommittee on Health of the Committee on Labor and Public Welfare on S. 974, S. 878, S.J. Res. 71: Part 2*, 93rd Cong., 1st sess., February 23 and March 6, 1973b.

U.S. Senate. Committee on Labor and Public Welfare. Subcommittee on Health. *Quality of Health Care—Human Experimentation, 1973: Hearings Before the Subcommittee on Health of the Committee on Labor and Public Welfare on S. 974, S. 878, S.J. Res. 71: Part 3*, 93rd Cong., 1st sess., March 7 and 8, 1973c.

U.S. Senate. Committee on Labor and Public Welfare. Subcommittee on Health. *Quality of Health Care—Human Experimentation, 1973: Hearings Before the Subcommittee on Health of the Committee on Labor and Public Welfare on S. 974, S. 878, S.J. Res. 71: Part 4*, 93rd Cong., 1st sess., April 30, June 28, 29, and July 10, 1973d.

Vanderpool, Harold Y. "John Wesley's Medicine for the Masses." Unpublished.

———. "The Wesleyan-Methodist Tradition." In *Caring and Curing: Health and Medicine in the Western Religious Traditions.* Edited by Ronald L. Numbers and Darrel W. Amundsen. New York: Macmillan, 1986, pp. 317–53.

Vastyan, A. E. "Medical Ethics Teaching: A Departmental Approach." In *The Teaching of Medical Ethics.* Edited by Robert M., Veatch, Willard Gaylin, and Councilman Morgan. Hastings-on-Hudson, NY: The Hastings Center, 1973, pp. 66–70.

Veatch, Robert M. "The Function of Philosophical Concepts in the Neuro-Medical Sciences" [Pain: A Neuropharmacological–Philosophical Paradox]. In *Philosophical Dimensions of the Neuro-Medical Sciences.* Edited by Stuart Spicker and H. Tristram Engelhardt, Jr. Dordrecht: D. Reidel Publishing Co., 1976a, pp. 252–57.

———. "Internal and External Sources of Morality for Medicine." In *The Health Care Professional as Friend and Healer.* Edited by David Thomasma and Judith Lee Kissell. Washington, DC: Georgetown University Press, 2000, pp. 75–86.

———. "Medical Ethics Teaching: Report of a National School Survey." *Journal of the American Medical Association* 235 (1976b): 1030–1033.

———. "National Survey of the Teaching of Medical Ethics in Medical Schools." In *The Teaching of Medical Ethics*. Edited by Robert M. Veatch, Willard Gaylin, and Councilman Morgan. Hastings-on-Hudson, NY: The Hastings Center, 1973, pp. 97–102.

———. "Teaching Medical Ethics: An Experimental Program." *Journal of Medical Education* 47 (October 1972): 779–785.

———. *A Theory of Medical Ethics*. New York: Basic Books, 1981.

———. *Value-Freedom in Science and Technology*. Missoula, MT: Scholars Press, 1976c.

———, and Carol G. Mason. "Hippocratic vs. Judeo-Christian Medical Ethics: Principles in Conflict." *The Journal of Religious Ethics* 15 (Spring 1987): 86–105.

———, and K. Danner Clouser. "New Mix in the Medical Curriculum." *Prism* (November 1973): 62–66.

Veitch, John. "Memoir of Dugald Stewart." In *Works of Dugald Stewart*, Vol. 10. Edited by Sir William Hamilton. Edinburgh: Thomas Constable and Co., 1858, pp. i–cxv.

Verhey, Allen. "The Doctor's Oath—and a Christian Swearing It." In *Respect and Care in Medical Ethics*. Edited by David Smith. Lanham, MD: University Press of America, 1984.

Viets, Henry R. "Ware, John." In *Dictionary of American Biography*, Vol. 10. Edited by Dumas Malone. New York: Scribners, 1964a, pp. 449–50.

———. "Warren, John." In *Dictionary of American Biography*, Vol. 10. Edited by Dumas Malone. New York: Scribners, 1964b, pp. 479–80.

V[illada], P[aul]. *Casus conscientiae his praesertim temporibusaccomodati, propositi, ac resoluti*. Brussels: Alfred Vromant, 1885–87.

Waite, P. B. *The Lives of Dalhousie University*. Vol. 1, 1818–1925. Montreal: McGill-Queen's University Press, 1994.

Walker, George Leon. *Thomas Hooker: Preacher, Founder, Democrat*. New York: Dodd, Mead, 1891.

Walker, Williston. *A History of the Christian Church*. New York: Charles Scribner's Sons, 1959.

Walsh, James F. *History of the Medical Society of the State of New York*. NP: Medical Society of the State of New York, 1907.

Ware, John. *Address Delivered Before the Massachusetts Peace Society, at Their Ninth Anniversary, Dec. 25, 1824*. Boston: Office of the Christian Register. F.Y. Carlile, printer, 1825.

———. *Contributions to the History, Diagnosis and Treatment of Croup*. Boston: no publisher, 1850a.

———. *Discourses on Medical Education, and on the Medical Profession*. Boston: J. Monroe and Company, 1847.

———. *Hints to Young Men, on the True Relation of the Sexes. Prepared at the Request of a Committee, and Published under Their Direction*. Boston: Tappan, Whittemore & Mason, 1850b.

———. *An Introductory Lecture Delivered Before the Medical Class in Harvard University, on the 16th of Oct. 1833*. Boston: Hilliard, Gray, 1833.

———. *Medical Dissertations on Hemoptysis or the Spitting of Blood, and on Suppuration, Which Obtained The Boylston Premiums for the Years 1818 & 1820*. Boston: Published by Cummings and Hilliard, 1820a.

———. *Memoir of the Life of Henry Ware, Jr. / by His Brother, John Ware*. Boston: J. Munroe; London: John Chapman, 1846.

———. *On Haemoptysis: Its Different Species, and the Method of Treatment Adapted to Each*. No publisher, 1818.

————. *Remarks on the Employment of Females as Practitioners in Midwifery. By a Physician.* Boston: Published by Cummings and Hilliard, 1820b.

Warren, Edward. *The Life of John Collins Warren, M.D., Complied Chiefly from His Autobiography and Journals.* Boston, Ticknor and Fields, 1860.

————. *The Life of John Warren, M.D., Surgeon-General During the War of the Revolution; First Professor of Anatomy and Surgery in Harvard College; President of the Massachusetts Medical Society, etc.* Boston: Noyes, Holmes and Company, 1874.

Warren, J. Collins. "Warren, John." In *Dictionary of American Medical Biography.* Edited by Howard A. Kelly and Walter L. Burrage. New York: D. Appleton & Co., 1928, pp. 1260–63.

"Warren, John." In *The National Cyclopedia.* Vol. 10, New York: James T. White, 1900, p. 288.

Warren, John, Lemuel Hayward, and John Fleet. "Boston Medical Police." In *The Codification of Medical Morality: Historical and Philosophical Studies of the Formalization of Western Medical Morality in the Eighteenth and Nineteenth Centuries.* Vol. 2, *Anglo-American Medical Ethics and Medical Jurisprudence in the Nineteenth Century.* Edited by Robert Baker. Dordrecht: Kluwer, 1995, pp. 41–46.

Waterson, Davina. "Coxe, John Redman." In *A Cyclopedia of American Medical Biography: Comprising the Lives of Eminent Deceased Physicians and Surgeons From 1610 to 1910*, Vol. 1. Edited by Howard A. Kelly. Philadelphia: W.B. Saunders Company, 1912, p. 204.

Webb, William Wilfrid. "Taylor, Alfred Swaine (1806–1880)." In *Dictionary of National Biography*, Vol. 29. Edited by Leslie Stephen and Sidney Lee. London: Oxford University Press, 1921–22, pp. 402–03.

Welsome, Eileen. *The Plutonium Files: America's Secret Medical Experiments in the Cold War.* New York: The Dial Press, 1999.

Wesley, John. *A Christian Library.* 50 vols. Bristol: F. Farley, 1749–55.

————. *The Desideratum: or, Electricity Made Plain and Useful. By a Lover of Mankind, and Common Sense.* Bristol, England: W. Pine, in Wine-Street, 1771.

————. *Primitive Physick: or, An Easy and Natural Method of Curing Most Diseases*, 1st ed. London: Thomas Trye, 1747.

————. *Primitive Physick: or, An Easy and Natural Method of Curing Most Diseases*, 21st ed. London: J Paramore, 1785.

————. *The Works of John Wesley.* London: Oxford University Press, 1975.

————. *The Works of the Rev. John Wesley, MA.* 14 vols. Edited by Thomas Jackson. Grand Rapids, MI: Zondervan Publishing House, 1958 (reprint of the 1872 edition).

————. *The Works of the Rev. John Wesley, MA.* 32 vols. Bristol: William Pine, 1771–74.

————. *Wesley's Primitive Physick 1791.* Abingdon Press, 1999.

Wharton, Francis, and Moreton Stillé. *Treatise on Medical Jurisprudence . . . the Medical part revised and corrected, with numerous additions, by Alfred Stillé*, 2nd and revised ed. Philadelphia: Kay, 1860.

Whibley, Charles. *Essays in Biography.* New York: E. P. Dutton & Co., 1913, pp. 288–89.

Whitelaw, Marjory. *Thomas McCulloch: His Life and Times.* Halifax: Nova Scotia Museum, 1985.

Wilder, Franklin. *The Remarkable World of John Wesley, Pioneer in Mental Health.* Hicksville, NY: Exposition Press, 1978.

Wilkins, Henry. *The Family Advisor or A Plain and modern Practice of Physic; Calculated For the Use of Families who have not the Advantages of a Physician, and Ac-*

commodated to the Diseases of America. The Second Edition, corrected. To which is annexed Mr. Wesley's Primitive Physic, revised. Philadelphia: Printed by Henry Dickins, No. 44 North Second St. Near Arch St., 1795.

Williams, Thomas Franklin. "Cabot, Peabody, and the Care of the Patient." *Bulletin of the History of Medicine* 24 (1950):462–81. Reprinted in *Legacies in Ethics and Medicine.* Edited by Chester R. Burns. New York: Science History Publication, 1977, pp. 307–26.

Wilson, Carroll L. Letter to Dr. Robert R. Stone dated 5 Nov. 1947. Photocopy reprinted in Advisory Committee on Human Radiation Experiments. *Final Report. Supplemental Volume I Ancillary Materials.* Washington, DC: U.S. Government Printing Office, 1995, pp. 93–94.

Wise, Thomas Alexander. *Commentary on the Hindu System of Medicine.* Calcutta: Thacker and Co., 1845.

Wolstenholme, G. E. W, and Maeve O'Connor, eds. *Ethics in Medical Progress: With Special Reference to Transplantation.* Boston: Little, Brown and Company, 1966.

Wood, Paul B. *The Aberdeen Enlightenment: The Arts Curriculum in the Eighteenth Century.* np: Aberdeen University Press, 1993.

Wright St. Clair, R.E. "The Edinburgh Influence on New Zealand Medicine." *Proceedings of the XXIII International Congress of the History of Medicine* 2 (1974): 750.

Index

Osler, William, 134, 135, 259
Percival, Thomas, 69
Rush, Benjamin, 91, 93
significance in nineteenth and twentieth
centuries, 27, 31–35, 72–74, 144, 158–
161, 224, 244, 245
Sperry, Willard, 179, 180
Hippocratic principle, 68
Hippocratism, 15, 68, 158
History of medicine, xii, xvi, xvii, 72, 77,
103, 104, 134, 135, 196, 230, 257
HIV, 76, 204, 205
Hobbes, Thomas, 66, 90, 104, 119, 173
Hodge, Hugh L., 110, 113, 250
Holme, Edward, 63
Holmes, Oliver Wendell, 132, 133, 258
Home, John, 226
Homeopathy, 123, 254
Homicide, 243
Homosexuality, 150
Honesty, 15, 94, 121, 124, 136–139, 219,
261
lying, 15, 67, 68, 137–139, 211, 215
Hooker, Thomas, 123
Hooker, Worthington, 122–125, 137, 143,
211, 259
on homeopathy, 254
*Lessons from the History of Medical
Delusions*, 125
Hope, Thomas Charles, 30
Horace, 67, 132
Horner, William, 113, 250
Hospice, 200
House, Jeffrey, xvii
Human subjects research. *See* Research with
human subjects
Hume, David, 4–6
Complete Works, 164
consequentialism of, 18, 65, 68, 209
Cullen, William, 15, 18, 230
Gregory, James, 19, 231
Gregory, John, 10–13, 226
History of England, 61, 241
Hooker, Worthington, 124
Monro, Alexander, Primus, 24, 25
Osler, William, 130, 257
Percival, Thomas, 59, 61, 64, 65, 68
Reid, Thomas, 226
reason and the passions, 14
religion, 24, 61, 64
Rush, Benjamin, 87, 88, 90, 248
sensory physiology, 101
skepticism, 10, 11, 226
sympathy, 100
Treatise on Human Nature, 10

virtues, 14
Wesley, John, 52
Hutcheson, Francis, 4–6, 10, 57, 90
Cabot, Richard, 137
Hooker, Worthington, 124
Monro, Alexander, Primus, 233
moral sense, 13
Osler, William, 130, 257
Percival, Thomas, 61, 64, 65, 67
Pictou Academy, Nova Scotia, 164
Rush, Benjamin, 90, 248
Seddon, John, 57
System of Moral Philosophy, 64
Taylor, John, 57
Hutton, Captain, 157, 162
Hutton, James, 4
Hydration, 215
Hydrophobia (rabies), 98

Ideal types, x, xii, 7, 23
Imagination, 4, 14, 64, 127, 226–228
In vitro fertilization, 201, 216
Incest, 150
Individual vs. Social, 210
Individualism, 14, 207, 210
Industrial Revolution, 5
Infanticide, 74
Informed consent, 69, 171, 192, 201, 211,
215–217. *See also* Consent
Institute on Human Values in Medicine,
197, 267
Institute of Medical Ethics (Great Britain),
199, 200
Institute of Society, Ethics and the Life
Sciences. *See* Hastings Center
Interests of the patient, 201, 210, 244
Intuitionism, 139
Ireland, 40, 76, 245
Islam, 261, 265
Italy, 245
Ives, Ansel, 112
Ivy, Andrew, 174

Jacobite rebellion, 163
Jacobs, H. B., 257, 258
Jakobovits, Immanuel, 147, 174
James I, 33
James, Henry, 132
Jameson, George, 8
Japanese physicians, 170
Jay, John, 83
Jefferson, Thomas, 88, 99
Jenkins, Daniel, 174, 177–179
Jenkins, Jas. A., 159, 160
Jennett, Bryan, 201